Social Participation in Occupational Contexts

In Schools, Clinics, and Communities

Social Participation in Occupational Contexts
In Schools, Clinics, and Communities

Marilyn B. Cole, MS, OTR/L, FAOTA

Professor Emerita of Occupational Therapy

Quinnipiac University

Hamden, Connecticut

Mary V. Donohue, PhD, OTL, FAOTA

Retired Clinical Professor, Department of Occupational Therapy

New York University

New York, New York

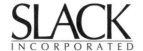

www.slackbooks.com

ISBN: 978-1-55642-900-2

Social Participation in Occupational Contexts: In Schools, Clinics, and Communities includes ancillary materials specifically available for faculty use. Included are PowerPoint slides. Please visit www.efacultylounge.com to obtain access.

SLACK Incorporated uses a review process to evaluate submitted material. Prior to publication, educators or clinicians provide important feedback on the content that we publish. We welcome feedback on this work.

Published by: SLACK Incorporated
                 6900 Grove Road
                 Thorofare, NJ 08086 USA
                 Telephone: 856-848-1000
                 Fax: 856-848-6091
                 www.slackbooks.com

Contact SLACK Incorporated for more information about other books in this field or about the availability of our books from distributors outside the United States.

Library of Congress Cataloging-in-Publication Data

Cole, Marilyn B., & Donohue, Mary V.
  Social participation in occupational contexts : in schools, clinics, and communities / Marilyn B. Cole and Mary V. Donohue.
     p. ; cm.
  Includes bibliographical references and index.
  ISBN 978-1-55642-900-2 (alk. paper)
  1. Interpersonal relations. 2. Psychology, Industrial. 3. Organizational behavior. I. Donohue, Mary V. II. Title.
  [DNLM: 1. Social Behavior. 2. Human Development. 3. Interpersonal Relations. 4. Occupational Therapy. 5. Personal Satisfaction. HM 1106 C689s 2010]
  HM1106.C645 2010
  302.3'5--dc22
                            2010009250

Printed in the United States of America.

Last digit is print number: 10 9 8 7 6 5 4 3 2 1

Dedication

This book is dedicated to my husband Marty, and to our family and friends who have contributed greatly to my appreciation of the multiple facets of social participation and occupation in life.

Marilyn B. (Marli) Cole

To Malcolm Milligan, this book is dedicated for dialogue, encouragement, and sustaining energy in the writing and living of social participation.

Mary V. Donohue

Contents

About the Authors

Marilyn B. Cole, MS, OTR/L, FAOTA, retired from Quinnipiac University in Hamden, Conn., after 25 years of full-time teaching and became a Professor Emerita of Occupational Therapy in the fall of 2007. Her first book, *Group Dynamics in Occupational Therapy,* published by SLACK (1993, 1998), is now in its third edition (2005). In 2008, Professor Cole co-authored a second textbook, *Applied Theories in Occupational Therapy,* with colleague Roseanna Tufano, and has recently contributed a chapter titled "Retirement, Volunteering, and End of Life Issues" to Meriano and Latella's *Occupational Therapy Interventions,* (2008, SLACK); a chapter titled "Theories of Aging" to Coppola, Elliott, and Toto's *Strategies to Advance Gerontology Excellence* (2008); a chapter on "Client Centered Groups" for Creek and Lougher's *Occupational Therapy and Mental Health, 4th Ed.* (2008); and a chapter titled "Occupational Therapy Theory Development and Organization" for Sladyk, Jacobs, and MacRae's *Occupational Therapy Essentials for Clinical Competence* (2010, SLACK). Current activities include working on a survey research study on retirement and volunteering with colleague Karen Macdonald, pursuit of fiction writing, and joining co-author Mary Donohue in promoting issues of social participation and occupation at professional conferences. At home in Connecticut or Freeport, Bahamas, Professor Cole and her husband, Martin Schiraldi, enjoy traveling, cruising, skiing, sailing, and scuba diving.

Mary V. Donohue, PhD, OTL, FAOTA, a retired clinical professor from New York University and currently Clinical Professor at Stony Brook University, Department of Occupational Therapy, specializes in psychosocial mental health. She worked for 13 years at Hillside Psychiatric Hospital, leading activity therapy rehabilitation groups. She is co-editor of the journal, *Occupational Therapy in Mental Health,* assisting guest editors in publishing books, and has recently contributed a chapter, "Evaluation of Social Participation," to Sladyk, Jacobs, and MacRae's text *Occupational Therapy Essentials for Clinical Competence* (2010, SLACK). Dr. Donohue has developed the Social Profile assessment tool, and her research articles using the Profile can be found on the Web. She is Metro NYD Research Co-Chair and NYSOTA Research Representative, providing grants for occupational therapy research projects, consulting with research applicants, and presenting Research Forums with grant awardees. She serves on the MNYD Mental Health Task Force, helping to plan events for OT's Walk with NAMI. She also serves on the State Board for Occupational Therapy of the New York State Board of Education for adjudicating licensure issues. Dr. Donohue has served as Commodore of New York Sailing Club, an educational, safety-oriented, and social club, pairing skippers and crew.

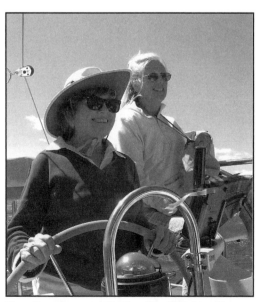

Mary Donohue and Marilyn (Marli) Cole sailing on the Long Island Sound.

Foreword

Social Participation in Occupational Contexts is a book for occupational therapists who are interested in expanding the scope of their practice on a sound theoretical basis. This new text gives an overview of a range of explanatory theories relevant to social participation, as well as predictive theories to support occupational therapy interventions in this area.

In the late 1950s, occupational therapists began to build an explicit theory base for their practice by selecting and adapting the most relevant theories from medicine, psychiatry and psychology. From the 1960s onward, there was a drive to develop occupational therapy theories based on a thorough understanding of occupation. For example, Mary Reilly, at the University of Southern California, developed the paradigm of occupational behaviour, which has been described as "one of the most significant influences on the evolution of the OT profession" (Van Deusen, 1988, p. 146). During the 1970s and 1980s, as more occupational therapy theories were developed, they were incorporated into a variety of models for practice, applicable in different fields. Mosey's adaptive skills, including five levels of social interaction skill, represents one of several theories supporting group interventions (Mosey, 1986). Models for practice offer explanations of occupational dysfunction and set out the process of intervention with a range of client groups.

With its revitalised commitment to enabling occupation, occupational therapy expanded into new areas of practice throughout the latter part of the 20th century. Then, in 1998, Ann Wilcock published *An Occupational Perspective of Health.* This book, which presented an occupational theory of human nature, introduced the possibility of a role for occupational therapy in the field of public health. Wilcock (1998) drew on theories from an array of disciplines to support her contention that occupational therapy is compatible with current public health objectives and therefore has the potential to be a health promoting profession. She set occupational therapists the challenge of finding ways to realise that potential in action.

In 2004, a group of South African occupational therapists took up the challenge and published a collection of essays describing health promoting projects undertaken with groups whose occupations were limited by poverty, disability, or serious illness (Watson & Swartz, 2004). While some authors used theories from the field of public health to support their work (for example, Lorenzo, 2004), others began to develop their own theories of a population approach to transformation through occupation (for example, Duncan, 2004). The following year saw the publication of another occupational therapy book about social and population approaches to promoting health: *Occupational Therapy Without Borders* (Kronenberg, Algado, & Pollard, 2005). Many of the contributors to this text also explored relevant theories for explaining and guiding practice, such as community development (Thibeault, 2005), or developed their own theories, such as social occupational therapy (Barros, Ghirardi, & Lopes, 2005). However, others attempted to apply theories or models designed for individual interventions to new ways of working (for example, Abelenda, Kielhofner, Suarez-Balcazar, & Kielhofner, 2005), with limited success.

For the occupational therapy profession to establish its role and value in working with communities, it is necessary to move away from using the biomedical theories and procedural models that dominated practice in the second half of the 20th century. Occupational therapists need to find or develop appropriate theories and apply them in a more thoughtful way. Community-based interventions require the practitioner to think broadly and flexibly, using a range of thinking strategies. Occupational therapy practice in community settings should be supported by a sound understanding of theory that guides, but does not constrain, the practitioner's clinical reasoning.

Marli Cole and Mary Donohue have written a book that contributes significantly to the project set out by Ann Wilcock (1998). They have selected one of the key concepts underpinning community practice— social participation—and brought together relevant theories from within and outside occupational therapy to explain and explore its meaning and importance. The wealth of theory presented in this book covers individual, group, and community situations and interventions. It is presented clearly and concisely, with examples of how ideas can be used in practice. One of the strengths of the text is that it moves between explaining the normal development of social participation and exploring what can go wrong.

Most importantly, the book provides the reader with various scenarios for analysis and the text is interspersed with questions to stimulate thinking. This is not another recipe book on how to do occupational therapy. It is an invitation to practitioners to think creatively and flexibly about how they can contextualise their practice so that people are enabled to engage in a range of appropriate occupations to support social participation.

References

Abelenda, J., Kielhofner, G., Suarez-Balcazar, Y., & Kielhofner, K. (2005). The Model of Human Occupation as a conceptual tool for understanding and addressing occupational apartheid. In F. Kronenberg, S. S. Algado, N. Pollard (Eds.), *Occupational therapy without borders: Learning from the spirit of survivors* (pp. 183-196). Edinburgh, UK: Elsevier Churchill Livingstone.

Barros, D. D., Ghirardi, M. I. G., & Lopes, R. E. (2005). Social occupational therapy: a socio-historical perspective. In F. Kronenberg, S. S. Algado, N. Pollard (Eds.), *Occupational therapy without borders: learning from the spirit of survivors* (pp. 140-151). Edinburgh, UK: Elsevier Churchill Livingstone.

Duncan, M. (2004). Promoting mental health through occupation. In R. Watson, L. Swartz (Eds.), *Transformation through occupation* (pp. 198-218). London, UK: Whurr.

Kronenberg, F., Algado, S. S., & Pollard, N. (2005). *Occupational therapy without borders: learning from the spirit of survivors.* Edinburgh, UK: Elsevier Churchill Livingstone.

Lorenzo, T. (2004). Equalizing opportunities for occupational engagement: Disabled women's stories. In R. Watson, L. Swartz (Eds.), *Transformation through occupation* (pp. 85-102). London, UK: Whurr.

Mosey, A. C. (1986). *Psychosocial components of occupational therapy.* New York, NY: Raven Press.

Thibeault, R. (2005). Connecting health and social justice: A Lebanese experience. In F. Kronenberg, S. S. Algado, N. Pollard (Eds.), *Occupational therapy without borders: Learning from the spirit of survivors.* (pp. 232-244). Edinburgh, UK: Elsevier Churchill Livingstone.

Van Deusen, J. (1988). Mary Reilly. In B. R. J. Miller, K. W. Sieg, F. M. Ludwig, S. D. Shortridge, J. Van Deusen (Eds.), *Six perspectives for the practice of occupational therapy* (pp. 143-167). Rockville, MD: Aspen.

Watson R., & Swartz L. (2004). *Transformation through occupation.* London, UK: Whurr.

Wilcock, A. A. (1998). *An occupational perspective of health.* Thorofare, NJ: SLACK Incorporated.

Jennifer Creek, MSc, DipCOT, FETC
Freelance Occupational Therapist
North Yorkshire, UK

Introduction

In its own inimitable way,
Occupational therapy has moved from
Immersion in clinics and hospitals,
Largely expanding into schools,
And penetrating on into the community.

This book traces developmental social growth
Across the lifespan,
Then looks at evidence-based practice
With chapters on research
And assessment tools of social participation.

How do we build and restore social participation?
That's presented across the lifespan, too,
With thought provoking, dramatic interactions
Apropos of social participation connectedness,
Desiring to be acted out or read aloud in class,
Inspired by the topics herein,
Bringing the text alive.

-mvd, 2010

Social Participation From an Occupational Perspective

chapter 1

Social Participation in Everyday Life

Marilyn B. Cole, MS, OTR/L, FAOTA

From the moment a child enters the world, cultural and social norms begin to unfold. After childbirth, a mother may be surrounded by relatives and friends as well as by doctors, nurses, and other medical workers. She interacts with each in culturally specific ways. The family becomes the first of many social groups to which each person belongs. As children grow and develop, they learn how to participate socially through imitation and direction from parents and others around them, together with their own reactions and emotions. The child's need for nurture, safety, love, and acceptance may all be met through social interaction. Later, children will learn more reciprocal social roles, seeking satisfaction of their own needs while also meeting the needs of others. Such is the nature of social learning (Bandura, 1977).

Adults rarely go through a day without encountering other people. Social participation may occur between two individuals or many. For example, a college student interacts daily with roommates, classmates, dining hall staff, faculty members, advisors, librarians, and others. Past social groups also continue as parents and friends from home visit, call, or e-mail. Working adults interact with coworkers, supervisors, and clients. Additionally, everyone engages in social transactions with store clerks, bankers, hair stylists or barbers, and other service providers throughout the course of any given day. Considering the central role of social interactions in everyone's life, it is surprising that professionals often do not recognize the importance of social participation as an occupation, parallel with work, leisure, and activities of daily living (American Occupational Therapy Association [AOTA], 2008; World Health Organization [WHO], 2001).

This chapter will review some basic concepts of social participation in everyday life: social groups and occupation, social skills, culture and social roles, conflict resolution, group leadership, teams and teamwork, and facilitators and barriers to social participation. Each topic will highlight some ways that these concepts relate to occupations in therapy and education, and will include some learning activities to reinforce application. Finally, a script from groups in everyday life is presented for role playing and analysis at the end of this, and every, chapter. Each script contains problems that interfere with social participation and group goal achievement. The scripts form a basis for role playing, problem identification, and discussion of potential social participation interventions. As such, they illustrate the scope of social participation issues from the client's perspective and serve as an introduction to the complex nature of social groups for both clients and therapists.

Social Groups and Occupation

This book will explore social participation at many levels. The highest level represents a "top-down" approach to problems with participation in life, obligating therapists and educators to first address the primary social roles people consider necessary for their well-being and life satisfaction. Social participation becomes the motivation for clients and

Cole, M.B., & Donohue, M.V. *Social Participation in Occupational Contexts: In Schools, Clinics, and Communities* (pp. 3-28).

students to engage in therapeutic or educational activities. Children want to learn to read, to practice their handwriting, and to listen as well as speak out in the classroom in order to earn the respect and admiration of peers and parents. People with disabilities want to wash and dress themselves in order to appear presentable when interacting with intimate partners or groups of friends; they are motivated to regain physical skills and endurance in order to continue performing valued work roles.

This chapter begins with the groups most familiar to everyone, linking everyday activities with participation in life experiences (WHO, 2001). Social participation as an occupation is defined by the AOTA practice framework as "activities associated with organized patterns of behavior that are characteristic and expected of an individual or an individual interacting with others within a given social system" (adapted from Mosey, 1996, p. 340; AOTA, 2008, p. 633). Three specific types of social participation fall into this category of the framework: community, family, and peer/friend. The categories of social participation tend to overlap with the other areas of occupational performance in real life as the activities associated with family, friends, and community are often shared or performed by the group as a whole. For example, members of family groups often cook and eat together, share household chores (instrumental activities of daily living), take turns in caregiving roles (activities of daily living), and celebrate holidays together. Even those occupations performed individually, such as dressing and grooming, have a social component, such as dress codes at work. Clients need to think about what the social activities of the day will be in order to dress appropriately and to comply with the social norms of their specific group culture.

Among the social participation activities at the community level are work, school, and neighborhood organizations. Educational groups for children involve not only classroom learning, but also working with partners, participating in group projects, playing team sports, and joining after-school activities such as writing for a school newspaper or performing in a school play or concert. Examples of work groups include construction teams, medical teams, marketing or sales divisions, research and development teams, or customer service departments. Community group participation has many forms—religious groups (Bible study), voluntary community service groups (Lyons Club, American Association of University Women [AAUW]), and special interest groups (book discussions, political debates) are some examples.

Peer or friendship groups may occur in individual homes or at the community level. Play groups for children may be formal (dance classes) or informal (neighborhood kids shooting hoops). Adult leisure groups may also be formal (couples bridge night) or informal (parents chatting at the school bus stop). Many social structures within neighborhoods and communities support group leisure activities, such as golf courses, fitness/health clubs, pools or beaches, libraries, and senior centers. Social participation also includes "engaging in desired sexual activity" (AOTA, 2008, p. 663). The nature of these activities is highly individualized and is often guided by the values and beliefs of one's culture.

Implied within the social participation activities listed is the concept of social roles. Some roles are more highly defined than others. Within families, roles such as breadwinner, home manager, financial manager, and caregiver of children or older adults might be shared between mother, father, older children, or grandparents. Work and leadership roles within the community are often associated with specific occupations. Most elementary school children could describe what activities are associated with the roles of a dentist, family doctor, teacher, priest or rabbi, policeman, or mayor. Other leadership roles are less well known and may vary according to location or demographic area.

Occupations cannot easily be separated from their social contexts, and the meaning of a specific activity for the client is highly influenced by the social role within which it is performed. A mother wishes to re-enter her kitchen after an episode of illness so that she can cook for her family, pack her children's school lunches, and fulfill what she perceives to be the role of a good mother, however she might perceive that role. Occupational therapists need to work closely with clients to define the specific social roles associated with the occupational performance activities chosen as priorities for intervention. Social roles are highly defined by one's culture, as will be described in the next section (Table 1-1).

What Are Social Skills?

Participating with others requires the use of social interaction skills. Social interaction is exceedingly complex, and books and workshops on social skills training for every population abound. The same skills needed for one-on-one interaction also apply in groups. Successful interaction begins with some basic skills, such as self-awareness, listening and empathizing with others, effective communication, and understanding the nuances of social situations. More specific information about the basic skills of social participation will be covered in Chapter 3.

Table 1-1

PERSONALIZING SOCIAL GROUP PARTICIPATION

Directions: To personalize the meaning of social groups for you, briefly answer the following:

1. List 10 people whom you consider a part of your immediate family.

2. List the people with whom you interact the most at work or school. What different groups at work or school do you belong to?

3. List the people you consider friends and peers. What groups are associated with your leisure time? What activities do you do together (sports, eating, parties, just hanging out)?

4. What religious, political, and community groups do you most relate to? Name three activities or meetings you have attended in the past month.

Self-Awareness

Self-awareness develops from birth, in large part through social interactions. Daddy smiles, and the child smiles back. Eye contact becomes a norm when communicating with others, even before words are exchanged. Children see themselves reflected in the eyes of their parents, siblings, peers, teachers, and strangers, and incorporate these impressions into their own self-image. The reactions of others to their behavior and the natural consequences of their actions in social situations further contribute to their self-image and sense of self-efficacy. This learning influences their future behavior in social situations. *What kinds of messages might a physically disabled child receive from others? How might a client with an acquired brain injury re-enter his or her social groups?* These self-awareness issues fall within the scope of our work as occupational therapists. Intervention strategies for these and other client factors will be discussed later.

Listening and Empathizing

Listening and empathizing with others is necessary in order to truly connect with someone else. Children must learn to listen and obey their parents, teachers, and caregivers. They also listen in order to follow instructions and to learn. Children learn early that they need to empathize with their friends in order to keep the friendship. Empathy is the skill of understanding someone else's feelings and point of view. It involves careful observation of nonverbal cues such as facial expression, body language, gestures, and tone of voice, as well as understanding the meaning of someone's words. These are the same skills that occupational therapy students learn in the "therapeutic use of self" and in forming therapeutic relationships. Empathy may

be expressed by asking clarifying questions and by accurately identifying the feelings of the other person, whether or not we agree with his or her point of view. Empathy often occurs naturally among friends who share similar views. However, the skill of empathy may be even more useful when interacting with those with whom we disagree, such as in resolving conflicts, debating political issues, or solving group problems. The script at the end of this chapter (and other chapters) provides some good examples of the need for empathetic responses.

Nuances of Social Situations

Understanding the nuances of social situations incorporates self-awareness, listening, and empathy. People seeking to participate with others first need a clear understanding of their own position and potential roles within a group. This requires both self-awareness and a realistic perception of the roles of other members of the group, their expectations of participants, and their positions of authority or power relative to one another. For example, at a job interview, the applicant who has taken some time to research and understand the company's organizational structure, the people holding positions of power, and the expectations of the position offered has an advantage over other applicants. During the interview, careful observation and asking the right questions may be more important than one's qualifications.

Clients who seek to re-enter their communities after illness or injury need help in reassessing their own position relative to their previous social groups. *How has absence affected their role within the group? How has their own ability to perform a former role been changed by their illness experience?* A high school student with a sports injury may not be able to participate with his or her team as before.

Table 1-2

EXPANDING YOUR FEELING VOCABULARY

Write five alternative words that describe the emotion listed at the top of each column.

ANGRY	AFRAID	SAD	ASHAMED

After a heart attack, a worker may be viewed differently by coworkers, supervisors, and clients. A child diagnosed with attention deficit disorder (ADD) may need help to understand the social expectations of a classroom, and teachers and other students may need help in understanding what adaptations the child with ADD needs in order to participate and learn in that environment.

Effective Communication

Effective communication is the social skill most often associated with social participation, yet awareness of self and others must pave the way. When a person understands what appropriate social participation means, using language and nonverbal behaviors to communicate with others flows more easily. The most important skills within this area are starting conversations, asking appropriate questions, expressing emotions in ways that are acceptable to the group, and taking on various roles to help the group meet its goals. For example, participation in a community fundraising effort may require seeking ideas from members, making phone calls, taking meeting notes, selling items in a food booth, or organizing an event. All of these roles require effective communication.

Verbal communication is particularly important when clients need to manage their emotions because their nonverbal expression often creates interpersonal conflicts. For example, a teen who keeps anger bottled up inside may be acting out by drinking alcohol, driving too fast, or staying out late. A worker frustrated with his job may communicate this by coming to work late and performing poorly on the job. Verbal expression can help clients to use emotional energy in more positive ways, such as

suggesting constructive changes in one's social roles or contexts. Therapists and teachers can help others to expand their emotional vocabulary through modeling and empathy. Use the learning activity above in Table 1-2 for practice.

Culture and Social Roles

Social interactions occur both within and between cultures. The social norms within each culture may differ greatly. *How do people greet one another?* In some families, relatives hug and kiss each time they meet, while others shake hands or just smile and say hello. In the Japanese culture, a bow replaces the hug or handshake, and making eye contact may be a sign of disrespect, depending on the role and position of each participant. A recent television advertisement depicts the fiancé of a Chinese girl greeting his future Chinese in-laws for the first time. He rushes up to hug his future father-in-law, sees the alarm in the man's face, then wisely backs away and gives a polite bow. In the television version everyone laughs, but in real life such clashes of culture often cause misunderstanding, confusion, and hostility.

Social Norms

Culture shapes the social norms of any group and defines what forms of interaction are acceptable and which are not. According to Bonder, Martin, and Miracle, "Defining culture is notoriously difficult" (2002, p. 3). A simple definition of culture is "learned patterns of behavior shared by a social group" (Brown, 1998, p. 10). Culture tends to be invisible to those within the group and only becomes an issue when people fail to recognize cultural differences, as in the TV ad example. Social roles are also defined differently within each culture. *What is the appropriate role for a mother or father within the family? What expressions of emotion are acceptable for the child in the classroom or on the playground? How do teens behave on dates? What activities can married people do for fun? What are appropriate interactions at work, with one's boss and coworkers, or with students or clients? How should people treat an elderly or disabled person?* In these examples, culture goes beyond a shared language or ethnicity and opens up a plethora of potential social dilemmas. For this reason, occupational therapists and other health professionals need to develop a keen sensitivity to cultural differences, not only when interacting with clients of diverse cultures, but also in assisting clients with developing appropriate social participation behaviors within today's multicultural environment.

Social and Cultural Contexts

Social and cultural contexts for occupations of everyday life have been defined by the AOTA's (2008) framework domains as separate but interrelated environmental factors that highly influence a person's occupational performance. Cultural context and environment are defined as "customs, beliefs, activity patterns, behavior standards, and expectations accepted by the society of which the client is a member. Includes ethnicity and values as well as political aspects, such as laws that affect access to resources and affirm personal rights. Also includes opportunities for education, employment, and economic support" (2008, p. 645). According to this definition, while culture shapes the relationships, interactions, and social behaviors for social participation, social context involves the actual presence of one or more people (groups/systems) who expect certain types of social behaviors from the individual. Social context "is constructed by presence, relationships, and expectations of persons, organizations, populations.

- Availability and expectations of significant individuals, such as spouse, friends, and caregivers
- Relationships with individuals, groups, or organizations
- Relationships with systems (eg, political, legal, economic, institutional) that are influential in establishing norms, role expectations, and social routines" (AOTA, 2008, p. 645)

As an example, Wilma, age 66, who has undergone a hip replacement, may not resume cooking and housecleaning activities even after she has regained her strength and flexibility because her husband considers these duties a part of caregiving. Thus, his expectations may unintentionally create a barrier to her full functional recovery. The health care system may represent a different expectation, one in which Wilma will participate in physical and occupational therapy in order to regain her previous level of occupational functioning after 4 weeks of rehabilitation. Two different cultures (family versus institutional) may thus be in conflict with regard to what occupations Wilma should perform.

Social Roles

Roles may be defined as "sets of behaviors expected by society, shaped by culture, and may be further conceptualized and defined by the (person)" (AOTA, 2008, p. 674). Social roles provide a structure for both interactions with others and for the performance of occupations. For example, family caregivers, college students, hospital volunteers, construction workers, chairpersons of committees, or presidents of corporations represent social roles that imply different sets of tasks, social behaviors, and expectations. More about roles will be discussed in later chapters.

Group Leadership in Everyday Life

Who leads family groups, work groups, informal peer groups, and community groups? Many of these individuals may not think of themselves as leaders, such as a parent being leader of the family, or a teen informally leading the activities of a group of peers. Others may take on defined leadership roles, such as a supervisor at work, chairman of a committee, mayor of a town, or president of a community organization. Leadership may not reside in the hands of just one individual, but may be shared or delegated to other members of the group—for example, the board of directors of a company, a charitable organization, or a condominium association. Leadership in business, the topic of much study, is usually thought of as the person who (1) calls the meeting to order, (2) announces the agenda, (3) guides discussion, (4) asks members for input, (5) summarizes interaction, (6) articulates the conclusion, and (7) serves as spokesperson for the group (Gouran, 2003). While these actions describe a formal leadership role, Gouran believes that leadership involves a broader range of attributes best evidenced during the process of group decision making and problem solving, which he calls "the art of counteractive influence" (p. 172). Northouse (2001) offers a broader definition of leadership, a process whereby an individual influences a group of individuals to achieve a common goal. The precise role of a leader, while

Table 1-3		
COLE'S SEVEN STEPS OF GROUP LEADERSHIP		
1.	*Introduction*	Explain the group's purpose. Make sure each member feels included.
2.	*Activity*	Provide clear instructions for the group task. Provide materials and time limits for completion.
3.	*Sharing*	Each member presents his or her own work to others. Members offer feedback to each other.
4.	*Processing*	Members express their feelings about the task and the group experience.
5.	*Generalizing*	Members discuss the meaning of the task and summarize what they learned.
6.	*Application*	Members explore some of the ways that what they learned can be applied to their everyday lives.
7.	*Summary*	Leader and members summarize the group to reinforce learning.

often fitting these definitions, varies according to leader traits, leadership style, and social situation.

Therapeutic Leadership

Leadership of occupational therapy groups, as outlined by Cole (2005), includes seven steps: introduction, activity, sharing, processing, generalizing, application, and summary. Leaders facilitating small groups use these steps to ensure that each member participates, understands the group's purpose, articulates the lessons to be learned, explores possible applications to his or her own life, and practices social skills through interacting with other members in the process. Rarely do leaders in everyday social groups take the time to structure groups in this way or to facilitate social learning. However, when things go wrong and groups do not run smoothly or produce the intended positive outcomes, reviewing these steps may be a helpful way to analyze the leadership and to determine what might have been done differently. Table 1-3 outlines the intent of each of Cole's seven steps of therapy group leadership.

Another guideline, originally outlined by Mosey (1986) and updated by Donohue (2009), suggests that leadership changes according to the level of group interaction. Mosey, and later Donohue, defined five levels of group interaction: (1) *parallel* (side-by-side activity with little interaction), (2) *associative* (minimal interaction centered on similar but individual tasks), (3) *basic cooperative* (individuals interact as they work together toward a common group task or goal), (4) *supportive*

cooperative (members support one another socially and emotionally while participating together in a group activity of their own choosing), and (5) *mature* (social support and productive activity contribute equally to group goal achievement). Most everyday group activities fall into one of these categories, and each requires different social interaction skills. In a parallel group, such as a first-grade classroom, the teacher provides structure, direction, and support to all members—a strong, directive leadership role. With each increase in the level of interaction, more of the leadership roles are shared by members. Finally, in a mature group, leadership is shared equally among members, and they work as a team to produce a defined and often complex end result. More on this theory will be discussed in later chapters.

Family Group Leadership

Even among couples, each partner acts as a co-leader, defining their activities and how they spend their time together. Teens beginning to date and to think about becoming a "couple" experience this type of shared leadership, taking each other's wants, needs, and preferences into account as they plan their life together. By high school, teens, already in the process of separating from parents, often break away from peer groups in order to socialize as a couple with other couples. As young adults, each partner of a couple takes on gender roles, and their culture as well as their natural abilities may influence each to lead in different life areas. For example, the man may make financial decisions, while the

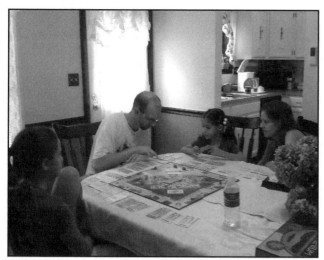

Figure 1-1. Family board games teach children some basic social skills.

woman plans social events for both of them. *In your relationship, who takes the lead? How are decisions made regarding where to go and what to do on dates, who pays for dinner, how much time is spent together or apart? When couples get married or live together, who decides about living arrangements, household responsibilities, or how money will be spent?*

Leading a household becomes even more complicated when couples become parents. The new type of leadership requires adding a common goal of caring and providing for a child, a difficult balancing act when each partner must also continue other life roles, such as worker, friend, home maintainer, and community group participant. Good parenting requires couples to take on leadership roles within the family, set up daily activity schedules, and provide appropriate physical and social environments for the safety and welfare of their children. This leadership ideally extends the love and acceptance couples give each other to providing social and emotional support to their children as well.

Family leadership also involves setting and maintaining moral and ethical standards for all family members. Some couples do this through religious participation or upholding the rituals and traditions of their culture. Teaching children acceptable social behaviors begins as soon as children begin to express their wants and preferences while interacting with others. In doing so, parents often lead best by example, showing children how to share and take turns (Figure 1-1), listen to and consider needs of others, accept different opinions and viewpoints, resolve conflicts with fairness, admit and correct mistakes, and appropriately apologize to others. Parents can also lead by providing enriching experiences for their children, such as opportunities to

learn skills (dance, gymnastics), participate in team sports, or experience other cultures through travel or community service.

Household rules are another way to convey acceptable social norms within the family. Some of these might include listening and showing respect for one another, following parental guidelines, doing chores or meeting obligations, and obeying rules of safety. When children break rules, consequences need to be imposed consistently, not so much as punishment, but as an opportunity for children to learn from their mistakes without compromising their safety and well-being. *What happens when parents do not use consistent discipline to teach their children acceptable social behaviors and the boundaries of safety? What examples can you think of when children (or parents) have lacked self-discipline or demonstrated inappropriate social behaviors?*

Like any other group, a family needs to cooperate for the benefit of all its members. Children should be expected to contribute, to take on household responsibilities as they are able, and to participate in decisions that affect all family members. Children need structure, and whether it's cleaning up their room, washing the dishes, or walking the dog, making a contribution conveys a sense of acceptance and belonging. When everyone helps with chores, there may even be time left over for doing something fun together, such as playing board games, taking a walk, or watching a movie. Family leadership involves setting up the rules and a schedule of activities that balances work and play so that everyone's needs are met, including those of the parents. To fully understand what family leadership means, parents may find it useful to think of their family as a social system with common goals and shared responsibility. Using this analogy, leading a family has many similarities with leading a therapeutic group—including all of the members, understanding the goals, following activity procedures, discussing issues and sharing emotions, supporting one another, and learning from both mistakes and successes, the important lessons of life.

What happens when families fail to lead? How do children get along with others at school? How do they learn the necessary social skills to get along in life?

Leadership at Work

New employees usually begin as followers or trainees, but as workers become experienced, they tend to be promoted to supervisory positions. In the workplace, specific leadership responsibilities may be formally defined according to the organizational plan for the company or corporation. Studies of organizational behavior have identified

---

Table 1-4

TASK ROLES THAT HELP THE GROUP TO GET ITS WORK DONE

1. *Initiator contributor*—Suggests new ideas, innovative solutions to problems, unique procedures, and new ways to organize.

2. *Information seeker*—Asks for clarification of suggestions, focusing on facts.

3. *Opinion seeker*—Seeks clarification of values and attitudes presented.

4. *Information giver*—Offers facts or generalizations spontaneously.

5. *Opinion giver*—States beliefs or opinions.

6. *Elaborator*—Spells out suggestions and gives examples.

7. *Coordinator*—Clarifies relationships among various ideas.

8. *Orienter*—Defines position of group with respect to its goals.

9. *Evaluator critic*—Subjects accomplishments of group to some standard of group functioning.

10. *Energizer*—Prods the group into action or decision.

11. *Procedural technician*—Expedites group's movement by doing things for the group such as distributing materials, arranging seating.

12. *Recorder*—Writes down suggestions and group decisions, acts as the group memory.

Adapted from Benne, K., & Sheats, P. (1948). Functional roles of group members. *Journal of Social Issues, 4*, 41-49.

---

four approaches to defining a leader: (1) the person named by the group as the leader, (2) the person who group members perceive to be performing leader-like behaviors, (3) the person who has the greatest influence on the group's final decision, and (4) the actual performance of leadership behaviors (Shimanoff & Jenkins, 2003). These authors conclude that leadership is best understood as the behaviors that help a group to achieve its goals. Leadership behaviors include the following:

× Appropriate procedural suggestions

× Sound opinions

× Relevant information

× Frequent participation

× Active listening

× Supporting group members

× Asking for opinions of other group members

When focusing on leadership behaviors, leadership can be performed by multiple group members, or it can be the responsibility of the group as a whole (Shimanoff & Jenkins, 2003).

In an older but classic study of group roles conducted by Benne and Sheats (1948, 1978), task roles and group maintenance roles defined the leadership contributions of multiple group members. Group roles are behavior patterns within the group that tend to remain stable regardless of who is in them. Therefore, each member can take on a variety of roles within the group, and members can change their roles as often as they wish. The maturity of an individual member may be viewed as the ability to take on a variety of group roles, and the maturity of a group may be measured by the shared leadership roles of multiple members (Donohue, 1999, 2009). The group task and maintenance roles first defined by Benne and Sheats are listed in Tables 1-4 and 1-5.

Ideally, leaders facilitate or delegate many task roles to members, who carry out these roles as needed when solving problems or making decisions within a mature-level group. The social expectations of a mature-level group (Donohue, 1999, 2009; Mosey, 1986) are outlined in Table 1-6.

Table 1-5

GROUP BUILDING AND MAINTENANCE ROLES THAT KEEP THE GROUP FUNCTIONING TOGETHER

1. *Encourager*—Praises, agrees with and accepts the contributions of others.
2. *Harmonizer*—Mediates the differences between other members.
3. *Compromiser*—Modifies his or her own position in the interest of group harmony.
4. *Gatekeeper and expediter*—Keeps communication channels open by regulating its flow and facilitating participation of others.
5. *Standard setter*—Expresses ideal standards for the group to aspire to.
6. *Group observer and commentator*—Comments on/interprets the process of the group.
7. *Follower*—Passively accepts ideas of others and goes along with the movement of the group.

Adapted from Benne, K., & Sheats, P. (1948). Functional roles of group members. *Journal of Social Issues, 4,* 41-49.

Table 1-6

SOCIAL EXPECTATIONS OF A MATURE GROUP

COOPERATION IN GROUPS

- Members can demonstrate the ability to interact with diverse ages, skills, viewpoints.

GROUP NORMS

- Members can balance energy between needs of task and interactive behaviors.

GROUP ROLES

- Members can balance task, maintenance, mentoring, and mutual group leadership roles.

COMMUNICATION

- Members can verbally identify roles needed and assumed by members.

ACTIVITY BEHAVIORS

- Members make the end products of high quality, while the process of doing the activity is equally as important.

POWER/LEADERSHIP OF GROUP

- Members can take turns sharing expertise in roles needed to achieve goals.

MOTIVATION FOR THE ACTIVITY AND ATTRACTION TO THE GROUP

- Members like to assume a variety of roles, while enjoying efficacy and efficiency as a group.

Adapted from Donohue, M. V. (2009). *The social profile manual.* Retrieved from www.Social-Profile.com

Conflict Resolution and Mature Interaction Skills

Some of the expectations of mature interaction involve skills in confronting others, resolving conflicts, and dealing with emotional discord (sometimes called immediacy). These abilities require a strong sense of self and others and a keen awareness of the social and cultural factors that influence social participation.

Confrontation Skill

A confrontation between two or more people usually means trouble. Many people think of confrontation as something to avoid, but it is actually a constructive process when performed correctly. For example, Dale tells his wife, Sarah, that he wants to spend more time with his family, but he comes home late each night and continues working on his laptop during the weekends. *How should Sarah approach him about his unavailability to enjoy his time off with her and their two young children?* She could get angry and make accusations, but that would only raise the level of hostility. Instead, using the skill of confrontation, she simply points out the discrepancy between what he says and what he does. If she does this without anger or frustration, she can then ask Dale to explain these two seemingly opposite messages without putting him on the defensive. She might say over a late dinner, "Dale, I thought you said you wanted to spend more time with me and the kids. Yet, you got home late every night this week, and the kids were already sleeping. When were you thinking we would spend more time together as a family?"

In relationships, people may at first have difficulty in getting past how the specific words and actions of a significant other make them feel. This happens particularly when the participants have avoided approaching the subject of conflict until they have almost reached the end of their emotional rope. Feelings do build up and need to find expression, but expressing strong emotion during a confrontation only creates barriers to its resolution. Part of the skill of confrontation is timing. Avoiding a difficult issue increases the stress level of one or both partners in a relationship over time, and the bottled-up feelings have a tendency to explode at the least opportune times. Ideally, the first signs of strain in a relationship should signal the need to look for discrepancies before emotions reach the boiling point. For practice, try role playing the situations described in Table 1-7.

Leaders in groups also use the skill of confrontation to address issues between members of the group. For example, a committee might be torn between several different ways to raise funds for an organization, resulting in heated arguments and breakdowns in communication. When dealing with a difficult decision, a leader might use confrontation as a way of clarifying multiple viewpoints about a problem by encouraging the group to reflect upon its own mode of interaction. He or she may stop the discussion and ask the group members to clarify how their current process, with members becoming entrenched in a specific project and refusing to consider other ideas, will help the group reach its goal of raising money for the organization. This question encourages the group members to resolve their differences and refocus on the overall group goal.

Confrontation in groups may be used in the context of member roles defined earlier, such as compromiser, harmonizer, orienter, evaluator critic, or standard setter. These roles, by definition, help group members to define discrepancies in their words and behaviors that help move the group forward toward group cohesiveness and goal achievement.

Emotional Conflicts

The ability to empathize, or to imagine what it would feel like to be in another person's shoes, helps mature individuals to identify the possible causes of stress in relationships. However, no one can read minds, and it is a mistake to assume the reasons for the words and social behaviors of another. Mature social participants learn to trust their own instincts and to ask significant others directly to discuss their thoughts and feelings about their mutual relationship. Therapists call this the skill of immediacy, directly addressing issues of trust, shame, anger, or any other feelings that may affect communication or self-disclosure in the therapeutic relationship. In everyday life, many relationships end when such issues go unresolved. For example, preoccupation with one's work or life issues may be mistaken for unfriendliness, and busy neighbors may misjudge one another without ever talking to each other. Family members may argue about some trivial issue and stop speaking to each other for years.

Emotional discord between people, groups, cultures, or organizations can signal the need for change through its negative, painful, or stressful impact on social participation. Northouse and Northouse (1995) define conflict as "a felt struggle between two or more interdependent individuals over perceived incompatible differences in beliefs, values, or goals, or differences in desire for control, status, and affection." They identifies two kinds of conflict: (1) content (thoughts, goals, beliefs) and

Table 1-7

CONFRONTATION SKILL PRACTICE

Directions: Point out a contradiction in the person's message, body language, or behavior. As a mature friend, helper, or counselor, ask the other person to resolve the discrepancy, using exact words. When appropriate, also express some empathy in your response.

1. *High school freshman, 14, feeling she is being treated unfairly by her teacher:* "I've had a learning disability since I was young, but this year for the first time, I haven't told anyone. It feels so great to be treated like a normal kid. Last week, I flunked my algebra test. All those word problems! I couldn't read them fast enough, and I didn't finish so I guessed. Now, the teacher thinks I'm just stupid."

2. *Woman, 59, recovering from the loss of husband:* "I get so depressed on weekends in this house. No one ever comes to visit. Anyway, I have to get the house cleaned before I could have company over."

3. *Man, 38, diabetic:* "I'd give anything to be normal, just to be well again. My willpower gave out yesterday— I had two pieces of pie and a chocolate bar for dessert."

4. *High school senior, 17:* "I really deserved that scholarship. I have the highest class standing out of all of the college prep students. They gave it to Ellen. She's pretty smart. I'm not angry about that."

5. *Man, 22, enters the room, face flushed, breathing hard:* "Nothing happened. Why are you picking on me?"

6. *Woman, 35:* "I trust my husband implicitly, but just let his brother come and ask him for money again, and who knows what he'll give away next time."

7. *Man, 44:* "My wife is nothing but a bitch... nag, nag, nag! I told her to shut up and leave me alone. I love her, but she doesn't seem to care much about me."

8. *Girl, 15:* "Why should I care anyhow? Nobody else does."

9. *Man, 33, involved in vocational rehab evaluation:* "No, I don't have my project done. I just want to get my own apartment and get out of here. I'm not even interested in this dumb evaluation."

10. *Boy, 17:* "How can you expect me to go back and finish school? My parents threw me out of the house because I broke up their living room, and now I don't even know where my next meal's coming from."

11. *Man, 28, Black, sloppily dressed and smelling of alcohol:* "Nobody hires minorities around here. They take one look at me, and suddenly the door closes. So, I just go to the bar."

---

(2) relational (feelings, control, esteem, or closeness of affiliation) (p. 218). These two types of conflict may occur together. While people may openly discuss conflicting content issues, they often ignore the relational undercurrents of the conflict. When people or groups fail to resolve conflicts of content, the interference of relational factors should be explored. Emotions more than beliefs can create barriers to communication, an essential ingredient in resolving conflicts. Consider the following progression that often follows an argument between individuals. Hostility, once begun, follows a predictable sequence:

× Both parties develop the belief that they are right and the other is wrong

× Communication breaks down

× Opponents stop listening to each other

× Correction of misconceptions is prematurely prevented

× Perceptions of one another are distorted

× Words and actions are skewed by preconceived distortions

× Conciliatory actions may be perceived as deceitful tricks

× Distrust pervades, and connections are often broken

This sequence, when allowed to continue to its conclusion, makes reconciliation among the parties extremely difficult. By applying the skill of immediacy, participants, therapists, or adult helpers can prevent the initial breakdown of communication resulting from emotional discord. Whether you're a family member, friend, or therapist, being able to name and discuss the emotions that create barriers can

---

Table 1-8

IMMEDIACY SKILL PRACTICE

Directions: As a mature friend, family member, or therapist, how would you identify and resolve the emotional barriers to communication in your relationship with the individuals in these scenarios? Use exact words in creating your responses, and continue the role play as needed.

1. *Adolescent girl with eating disorder:* "Why can't you stop asking me about what I eat? It's none of your business anyway."

2. *Woman, 53, overweight with chronic arthritis:* "Sure my doctor told me I have to find ways to exercise, but I don't need to go to the gym with you to do it."

3. *Man, 21, with spinal cord injury:* "I know you're my therapist, but after I'm done with therapy, would you go out with me?"

4. *Man, 45, recovering from bypass surgery:* "I know you mean well, but I don't need you to play cards with me out of pity. When I go back to work, I won't have any leisure time anyway."

5. *Boy, 16, with unexplained hostility in school:* "So, here we are again. My parents can make me stay after school, but they can't make me talk."

6. *Man, 35, having trouble with supervisor at work:* "I need some advice. What's the best way for me to tell my boss he's an idiot?"

---

open up communication and re-establish trust. This skill requires both individuals to risk self-disclosure and should be approached with the recognition that feelings are not right or wrong. Cultural issues such as saving face or maintaining mutual respect also factor into the verbal exchange. Usually, the more mature individual takes the initiative in discussing emotional barriers in relationships.

For therapists and others, immediacy provides a strategy for early intervention to prevent this destructive process:

- Use immediacy *before* communication breaks down
- Therapist models *continued communication*
- Feelings are dealt with directly
- Alternative perceptions are suggested and encouraged
- Therapist models *appropriate reality testing*
- Therapist's role is to "harness conflict and use in the service of client growth" (Yalom, 2005, p. 350)
- Use empathy to soften the intervention.

For example, an adolescent hospitalized for a drug overdose tells you, his peer counselor, "If I talk about my problems, you'll just go and tell my parents. It's them who sent me here, because they just want to get rid of me. How could you help me anyway?" Using immediacy, you might respond,

"You feel abandoned because your parents brought you here for treatment. It sounds like you think if you confide in me, I'll abandon you just like they did. How do you see that?" For practice in the early identification of emotional barriers in relationships, try role playing the scenarios in Table 1-8.

Conflict-Resolution Theories

Many theories of conflict resolution have been developed over the past several decades. While a thorough review of these theories is beyond the scope of this chapter, those offering helpful structures for application in everyday social situations will be discussed. Game theory, the oldest theory, suggests that people use conflict-resolution strategies based on self-interest to increase chances of winning and minimize risk of losing (Deutsch, 1973; Rapoport, 1960). Later, Filley (1975) expanded this model for use in business situations, with three possible resolution alternatives: (1) win-lose (person with most power wins), (2) lose-lose (unintentional outcome of avoidance, in which neither side achieves its goal), or (3) win-win (requires cooperative effort and creative problem solving to achieve goals on both sides). Some of the social conditions that heighten the risk of conflicts in the workplace (Filey, 1975) are as follows:

- Respective roles are ambiguous
- There is competition for limited resources

× Barriers to communication

× Forced dependence on others

× High differentiation in organizational levels/job specialties

× Joint decision making or consensus is necessary

× Inflexible rules, procedures, and policies

× Existence of unresolved prior conflicts

These factors can guide leaders and organizations to take steps to prevent conflicts or at least reduce their frequency and severity. Filley's theory goes on to define the conflict process, which includes identifying the antecedent conditions (listed above) involved in each individual's perceptions of the conflict; emotional issues such as threat, hostility, fear, or mistrust; manifest actions such as overt aggression or active problem solving; resolution or suppression of the conflict; and the aftermath or living with the consequences (Filley, 1975).

Different styles of conflict resolution were defined by Kilman and Thomas (1975) as avoidance, competition, accommodation, compromise, and collaboration. They determined that the resolution style changes to fit different situations. While there isn't just one best way to resolve conflicts, the steps usually follow this general sequence:

1. Mutually define problem

2. Identify potential solutions

3. Assess the advantages and disadvantages of each solution

4. Select the best solution

5. Discuss or evaluate how the solution affects the original problem

This process becomes cyclical as the original problem is reconsidered or redefined, and additional actions are suggested and tried.

Conflicts in schools can be classified into four categories (Johnson & Johnson, 1995):

1. *Controversy:* Occurs when two or more ideas, theories, opinions, or conclusions are incompatible. Debating the pros and cons of different theories or ideas can facilitate learning and high-quality decision making.

2. *Conceptual conflict:* Occurs when new ideas, theories, or arguments are perceived to be incompatible with one's original position on the issue.

3. *Conflicts of interest:* An interpersonal conflict arises when one person's attempts to reach a goal prevents, blocks, or interferes with another person's goal attainment. For example, when two students need to use a computer at the same time.

4. *Developmental conflict:* Incompatible activities of adulthood and childhood are based on opposing sides. For example, a teen wants to become more independent, while the parent wants to keep control for safety reasons.

Current theories view conflicts as not only unavoidable, but valued opportunities to make constructive change. Teaching constructive conflict resolution to groups of students in schools has several advantages, including the following:

× Better preparing students to deal with stress and cope with unforeseen adversities

× Encouraging complex reasoning, creative problem solving, and higher-level decision making

× Greater sense of commitment, joint identity, and cohesiveness among group members

× Fostering care, respect, and trust for others on both sides

× Heightened awareness of problems that need to be solved

× Increased incentive to change

Using this theory, Johnson and Johnson (1995) suggest that schools embrace positive conflict management in classrooms and related educational groups by (1) creating a cooperative context in which students recognize that long-term relationships have a greater importance than the result of any short-term conflict, (2) using academic controversy in cooperative student groups to teach specific social and cognitive skills such as making persuasive arguments, researching relevant topics, applying complex logical thinking, and viewing issues from a variety of perspectives.

Third, Johnson and Johnson (1995) suggest that high school students be taught the skills of peacemaking. These skills include negotiation, mediation, and arbitration. Negotiation begins with problem-solving strategies similar to the sequences mentioned earlier: defining both sides of an issue, identifying feelings, explaining interests as well as positions, taking an opposing perspective, and finding areas of agreement. Creative solutions involve some gains and some concessions on both sides. Students mediating controversies for each other involves reducing hostility, ensuring commitment to the mediation process, facilitating negotiations between involved individuals, and reaching an agreement. When mediation fails, adults must take over and model arbitration of student conflicts. Arbitration involves listening carefully to both sides, deciding who is right and who is wrong. This option is a last resort because students who do not participate in the resolution process lose the opportunity to learn from it.

In summary, social skills, including communication, empathy, emotional expression, and the ability to compromise, play a central role in conflict resolution. Students, families, workers, and community groups may all benefit from knowledge and use of positive conflict resolution skills as not only helpful in resolving differences, but also in facilitating needed changes and higher-level goal achievement for individuals, groups, and society.

Teams and Teamwork

The word *team* brings to mind sports teams such as football, baseball, or soccer. Most people have participated on at least one sports team during their school years. Parents believe that getting their kids involved in sports will teach them some important life lessons, such as teamwork, perseverance, sportsmanship, the value of hard work, and the ability to deal with adversity (Pauch, 2008). Pauch writes,

> This kind of indirect learning is what some of us like to call a "head fake." There are two kinds of head fakes. The first is literal. On a football field, a player will move his head one way so you'll think he's going in that direction. Then he goes the opposite way. It's like a magician using misdirection. Coach Graham used to tell us to watch the player's waist. Where his belly button goes, his body goes (also)… The second kind of head fake is the *really* important one—the one that teaches people things they don't realize they're learning until well into the process…your hidden objective is to get them to learn something you want them to learn. (p. 39)

Successful teamwork requires clear communication skills, trust in one's teammates, and a willingness to cooperate, using each member's strengths in reaching a common goal (Bordessa, 2006). Some people suggest that learning "team skills" on youth teams is not guaranteed, especially when coaches focus solely on winning, learning the basics of the game, or developing specific physical skills and conditioning. Not much research exists on team building for kids. Maybe that's why there are so many corporate team-building programs for adults (2006).

Teams in Education

Teams also commonly occur in classroom settings when groups of students work together on projects or assignments. As a suggestion for teachers with large classes, group projects give students opportunities for active participation and feedback to promote learning. Svinicki (2009) outlines four team models in education, adapted from Mouton and Blake (1984):

1. *Team effectiveness design*—For learning facts and principles
2. *Clarifying attitudes design*—For making good judgments
3. *Performance judging design*—To practice skill or application of knowledge
4. *Team member teaching design*—Each member prepares part of the content

Student teams could use some of the conflict-resolution strategies, taking different positions on issues or applying problem-solving strategies to social or ethical situations. In college-level classes, problem-based learning (PBL) takes this team method to its extreme, allowing small groups of students to teach each other course content through theory, knowledge application, and complex problem solving. Educators facilitate these groups by presenting consecutive parts of carefully laid out case studies and delegating most or all of the leadership roles to group members. More about PBL groups may be found in Chapter 5.

Groups in education have the additional advantage of providing multiple opportunities for students to learn, practice, and model for each other many of the social skills and competencies necessary for successful social participation in everyday life.

In recent years, college and university educators have studied how teams of students can benefit from projects that integrate coursework with community leadership and service learning. For example, Rutgers University students worked in teams with a local charity, Elijah's Promise, which provides nutritious meals, social services, culinary job training, and business training to low-income people in central New Jersey. Student teams collaborated to create a cookbook for this charity as a fundraising and community outreach project, also including personal stories and anecdotes, comments, and reactions to the meals gathered from interviews with diverse clients. These student teams demonstrated the connections between service learning, integrating community, teamwork, and leadership communication (Kuo, 2009).

Work Teams in Business and Community Settings

Currently, the meaning of teams and teamwork extends beyond sports and refers to groups of workers and community volunteers as well. In a corporate setting, a team usually refers to members of a group with different responsibilities and skills working together to achieve a common objective (Spilker, 1998). Occupational therapists might work

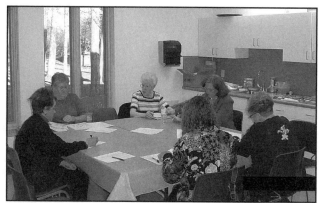

Figure 1-2. A serious discussion in this AAUW Finance Committee requires trust and joint decisions among members.

as a member of a health care team, or teachers may serve together as members of a school faculty. Workers become team members in several ways: (1) appointment by one's supervisor, (2) recruitment by the team leader, (3) appointment by a senior manager, or (4) volunteering (Spilker, 1998). In business settings, there is a prevailing belief that groups make sounder decisions than individuals. However, this only happens when people with the appropriate knowledge, skills, and experiences become team members, and they are given an interaction structure and timeline that allow them to apply their unique contributions to the team problem-solving process, decision, or outcome (Hirokawa, DeGooyer, & Valde, 2003; Spilker, 1998).

Both work and volunteer teams share similar features for which the goal includes solving problems and making decisions for the company or organization. For example, the AAUW raises and manages large amounts of money with which to give scholarships for higher education to deserving women in their communities. The finance committee advises and manages AAUW's investments to maximize the amount of money available for each year's scholarship awards (Figure 1-2).

Teamwork implies that all of the members work together to accomplish a common goal. A team of workers at a restaurant plays separate roles in providing the best possible dining experience, working toward the common goal of a satisfied customer.

Features of Work Teams

A basic way to understand teams and their organization was outlined by Holpp (1999), introduced as the five "Ps": *purpose, place, power, plan,* and *people. Purpose* defines the need to bring people together, to collaborate, to develop direction and commitment, and to work interdependently. At Microsoft Corporation, a research and development team

consisting of workers with various expertise might collaborate to develop a new and better version of the Windows operating systems for personal computers. *How would you describe the purpose of such teamwork?*

Place addresses how a team model fits into the overall organizational structure of a business or community agency. *In the Ford Motor Corporation, how might a sales team fit into the overall structure, and what might be its purpose or goal? How might a fundraising team fit into the structure of a charitable organization, such as the American Cancer Society? Power* refers to who takes the leadership and responsibility for the team's work. Leadership depends on the corporate work group or community culture. In traditional corporations, teams have an appointed leader (director, manager, supervisor) with defined responsibilities, and this person holds the sole responsibility for the performance and outcome of his or her team. For example, in the medical model, the doctor often determines the goals and norms of communication for a medical team, and he or she may delegate different responsibilities to the other team members. In community-based health care agencies, power and responsibility might be more equally shared among team members. Different types of power structures and organizations for medical teams are described in a separate section below.

The team *plan* involves the structure, such as when, where, and how often the team meets, and what types of communication occur between meetings. Some teams may use virtual meetings such as real-time internet conferencing or planned conference calls over the telephone. When the team's purpose involves clients, customers, or other recipients of service, how the team members interact with these entities may also be defined within the team plan. *People* are the last, but not least, important aspect of the work team. As described earlier, members may be recruited or appointed to work on teams, or they may volunteer.

How these five factors define a team depends upon the culture, setting, purpose, and intent of the organizers. For example, work teams at construction sites may include a variety of skilled workers, such as plumbers, carpenters, and assistants working together to repair a roof air conditioner (as shown in Figure 1-3). Health care teams are another example, and their differences are described in the next section.

Corporate culture in the United States today embraces the belief that teams make better decisions than individuals, and that team efforts, when given free reign, produce more creative designs, more effective solutions to problems, and more proactive and comprehensive strategic plans. Another purpose of teams in the workplace is to combine members' visions or perspectives in order to determine a more accurate whole (Cohn, 2008). For example, in public schools, an interdisciplinary team of professionals and family members brings together divergent viewpoints of a child with special needs in order to create an individualized educational plan. According to the McGill Action Plan (MAP) (Swinth, 2008), such educational teams meet together in a 2-hour team session to answer the following seven questions:

1. What is the student's history?

2. What are your dreams for the student?

3. What are your fears?

4. Who is the student (give one-word statements)?

5. What are the student's strengths, gifts, and abilities?

6. What are the student's needs (goals and outcomes)?

7. What would an ideal day at school be like, and how can the team make it happen?

After the meeting, a report is written to which all team members contribute. The Individualized Educational Plan (IEP) spells out in detail how members of the team will work on the goals and objectives on a daily basis and how the outcomes will be measured. Social participation includes ongoing communication between team members throughout the implementation process and collaborative problem solving along the way. See the end of Chapter 12 for a script of an IEP team meeting.

Teams in Health Care

In a study of health care teams inspired by a growing consumer-identified need for more continuous and reliable health care (Institute of Medicine, 2003), Hirokawa and colleagues (2003) identified five characteristics of effective health care teams: (1) external support, (2) member attributes, (3) relationships, (4) organization, and (5) process. External support for the team concept includes rewards and incentives for successful team participation, and accepting team decisions or outcomes. Some team members in the study felt that hospital administrators implicitly undermined the team's value by failing to recognize team efforts or by overriding their recommendations. Beyond knowledge and skill, motivation and commitment ranked high among team member attributes. Relationships greatly influence medical team success or failure—35% of cases in the study alluded to the positive effects of group cohesiveness and mutual respect.

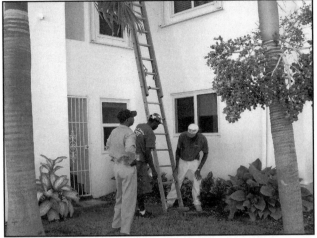

Figure 1-3. Construction work team with ladder: Safety issues require coordination of movement as well as good communication during work tasks.

However, good organization (clearly defined roles, responsibilities, as well as good leadership) ranked highest (47%) in team success, while members blamed a lack of organization for 58% of team failures. The process involved hard work, effective communication, and helping each other out in order to achieve a positive client outcome. Thirty-two percent of medical team members reported effective group process as a factor in success, while 54% blamed failures on faulty group process. These findings suggest that successful social participation on a medical team is highly associated with good communication among members and the presence of group cohesiveness (Hirokawa et al., 2003).

In terms of the structure of health care teams, three types have been identified: (1) multidisciplinary, (2) interdisciplinary, and (3) transdisciplinary (Cohn, 2008; Moyers, 2005). In each type, members share the same goals, but their methods of communication and interaction are different.

The *multidisciplinary* team members work side by side, each having a defined role. The health care team may communicate in writing through the medical chart, while meeting with clients and family members separately. The *interdisciplinary* health care team shares the goals and responsibilities for each client. While evaluations may be separate, the client and family meet with the whole team together to form an integrated intervention plan. In both multidisciplinary and interdisciplinary teams, doctors, nurses, social workers, occupational therapists, and others remain within the boundaries of their own discipline. This sets the first two types apart from the third, the *transdisciplinary* team, which calls for members to cross professional boundaries in order

Table 1-9

KNOWLEDGE, SKILLS, AND ATTITUDES FOR EFFECTIVE TEAMWORK

KNOWLEDGE	SKILLS	ATTITUDES
• Knowledge of other team member's roles	• Collaborate—Work with others to achieve goals	• Respect for others—Appreciate different points of view
• Knowledge of group dynamics	• Cooperate and compromise	• Show team spirit
• Good self-awareness—Knows own role and respects its boundaries	• Communication skills—Express thoughts, emotions, and beliefs appropriately	• Work for the group effort
• Understand the culture of the team	• Empathize with others	• Self-confidence
• Ability to communicate through common language—Avoid professional jargon	• Assertiveness—Speak up but without devaluing others	• Keep an open mind
• Holistic thinking	• Handle conflict	• Trust others
• Use feedback and/or supervision constructively	• Problem-solving skill	• Commitment—Willing to assume responsibility

Adapted from Latella, D. (2002). Teams and teamwork. In K. Sladyk (Ed.), *The successful occupational therapy fieldwork student*. Thorofare, NJ: SLACK Incorporated.

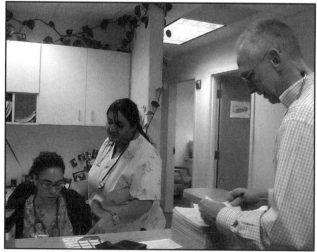

Figure 1-4. Professional collaboration among an office medical team provides the best care for patients.

to work effectively together to meet goals, solve problems, and resolve emerging conflicts. In the transdisciplinary approach, the team works across boundaries in all aspects of health care, evaluation, planning, implementation, and determining outcomes. In the interest of efficiency, one member of the team may be designated to communicate the shared perspective and/or plan with the client. A unique feature of the transdisciplinary team approach is the creation of a common language and shared meaning and values (Figure 1-4).

In order for an individual to participate effectively with a team, Latella (2002) suggests some specific knowledge, skills, and attitudes be in place, as described in Table 1-9. These areas can be selectively applied to any type of team participation and to many naturally occurring groups as well.

Moyers (2005) discusses the competency for occupational therapists in working with interdisciplinary teams, which includes cooperating, collaborating, communicating, and integrating care to ensure continuity and reliability. She suggests as a continuing competency that occupational therapists "develop and sustain team relationships to meet identified client outcomes" (p. 19). This competency includes networking skills to learn about and use local and nonlocal community resources, clearly defining occupational problems with regard to client social participation, and evaluating the effectiveness of the team effort in facilitating client social participation.

The Stanford School of Medicine Web site reports that while sports teams, orchestras, pilots, astronauts, and the military routinely practice team skills, breakdowns in communication are common on health care teams. This Web site suggests good teamwork can best be learned and practiced through challenging situation simulations (Stanford University Center for Immersive and Simulation Based Learning [SISL], 2009).

Facilitators and Barriers to Social Participation

Facilitators are factors that make social participation easier. These factors may be categorized as social support and encouragement, the availability of role models for social learning, rewards and reinforcements for participating, personal motivation and sense of self-efficacy, and the presence of social and cultural contextual factors that support social roles.

As an example, for people with disabilities, caregiver encouragement and skilled cueing can greatly enhance social participation. Judy, a polio survivor, depends on her caregiver to help her dress, gather her materials, and travel to her memoir writing group at a local community center (Figure 1-5).

Some of the barriers of social participation include the following categories: physical constraints such as a lack of mobility, unavailability of transportation, or accessibility issues for people with physical disabilities; lack of social skills and competencies; offensive or problematic behavior of others within the group; poor sense of self-efficacy; and social and cultural contexts that discourage participation.

People with health conditions often wish to continue to participate in former social roles. As part of a team approach, occupational therapists, social workers, psychologists, and other health professionals can help them do so by evaluating the expectations of significant others and the social norms, role expectations, and social routines of the groups in which clients wish to participate. In evaluating social contexts, both the client's perspective and that of others needs to be defined. When comparing these views, barriers are identified, and problem-solving strategies can then be collaboratively developed. Occupational therapists attend not only to clients' occupational performance but also the contexts within which they participate. For example, teaching dressing skills to a child with a physical disability will not work if caregivers do not reinforce these skills. Adapting a work station for a worker with spinal cord injury will only succeed if the corporate culture allows and encourages such adaptations. Social contexts can both facilitate occupational performance and create barriers to it.

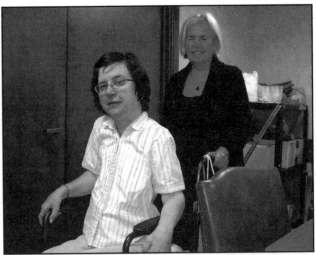

Figure 1-5. Judy, a polio survivor, participates regularly in a memoir writing group thanks to the assistance and encouragement of her caregiver.

Within social or work groups in the community, the social behaviors of some individuals have been found to discourage other members from participating. Sometimes, individual team members use the group to serve their own individual needs. These roles tend to interfere with group functioning. Benne and Sheats (1948, 1978) suggest that a high incidence of individual behaviors is symptomatic of various group malfunctions such as inadequate group skills of members (including the leader), low level of group maturity, discipline and morale, or an inappropriately chosen and inadequately defined group task. Eight individual roles defined by these authors are described in Table 1-10.

The case example below describes the point of view of a person with mature social skills who is highly motivated to continue living her life to the fullest despite physical and emotional setbacks. She describes the barriers to social participation she has encountered along the way.

Case Example: Michele

Michele, an occupational therapist of 30 years, found herself widowed at age 48. She had been disabled since age 13 by transverse myelitis. She continued working as an occupational therapist even after numerous medical issues required her to give up walking on cane or crutches and use a power wheelchair. She had to retire on disability 8 years ago due to shoulder injuries at age 55. In spite of having to downsize from her home to a condo due to cost, the condo is completely wheelchair accessible and has enabled Michele to remain socially

Table 1-10

INDIVIDUAL ROLES THAT CREATE BARRIERS TO SOCIAL GROUP PARTICIPATION

1. *Aggressor*—Deflates the status of others; expresses disapproval of the values, acts, or feelings of others; attacks the group or group task, etc.

2. *Blocker*—Tends to be negativistic or stubbornly resistant, opposing beyond reason or maintaining issues the group has rejected.

3. *Recognition seeker*—Calls attention to self through boasting, acting in unusual ways, or struggling to remain in the limelight.

4. *Self-confessor*—Uses group as an audience for expressing non–group-oriented feelings, insights, or ideologies.

5. *Playboy*—Displays lack of involvement through joking, cynicism, or nonchalance.

6. *Dominator*—Monopolizes group through manipulation, flattery, giving directions authoritatively, or interrupting the contributions of others.

7. *Help seeker*—Looks for sympathy from the group through unreasonable insecurity, personal confusion, or self-depreciation.

8. *Special interest pleader*—Cloaks his or her own biases in the stereotypes of social causes, such as the laborer, the housewife, the homeless, or the small businessman.

Adapted from Benne, K., & Sheats, P. (1948). Functional roles of group members. *Journal of Social Issues, 4,* 41-49.

active and completely independent, participating in volunteer and occupational therapy-related small projects. She travels to social meetings and community events by driving an adapted van. She writes:

> I marvel at how easy my life has become since I have been living here. Because of the sidewalks with curb cuts and the ground level, fully-accessible condo, I don't usually feel "disabled" until I enter a world where I can't use my wheelchair, like my daughter's home, or an inaccessible public area. When I come out of the local movie theater, I have to pay attention to which door to exit, because there is a beam on one side, which blocks my access to the one little curb cut. If I'm not careful, I could go off the curb. I am fortunate that I can still walk on crutches, so I can negotiate some of these barriers. Other disabled people are not so fortunate. Next year, I will be celebrating 50 years living with a disability! When I come out of Home Depot, the entire parking area is accessible because the walk is sloped so ABLE-BODIED people can wheel out loads of lumber. It really is easy to include disabled people in society by thinking ahead, just as those who designed Home Depot stores for their contractor customers' needs. Once people with disabilities have made the effort to modify their homes so they can get out into the world, the world needs to also make itself accessible to them. Public bathrooms designed for the disabled, I now have to share with obese individuals and mothers with little children. By making things convenient for the disabled, we make them convenient for all people. They also seem to be a convenient place to install diaper change tables. We are talking about an ever-increasing population of elderly and disabled people. Why are we not building for this? (M. Mulhall, personal communication, 2009)

Discussion

1. What barriers to social participation did Michele encounter during her adulthood, and how did she overcome them?

2. What social roles are referred to for Michele in this case description?

3. Choose three social roles, and explain how you might enable Michele to continue them if you were her therapist.

4. What mental attitudes did Michele convey in her writing that helped her to make adaptations and to continue her social participation despite disability?

5. If Michele were to plan a road trip to an unknown location, what preparation would she need to do before packing her van and departing?

6. What lessons can be learned from this case that could be used to help other people with disability to continue their social participation?

Summary

This chapter has introduced the concept of social participation as encountered by most adults in their everyday lives: their social interactions one-on-one or in groups at home, school, work, and the community. Hopefully, these topics convey the high levels of social skills, competencies, roles, and relationships that are expected of mature adults in contemporary society. By including the skills of empathetic social interactions, conflict resolution, effective leadership, and team membership in schools, communities, and work settings, students and professionals can appreciate the pivotal nature of social participation as both a motivator and a context for the performance of occupations in achieving the highest potential for individuals and societies.

A Note About Script Analysis

Learning activities have been strategically placed throughout this chapter in order to illustrate step-by-step learning of important basic social skills and competencies. The skills that have been included represent mature social interaction ability: listening, expression of empathy, resolution of conflict through confrontation and immediacy, and a variety of leadership roles and abilities. This sets the standard for high-level participation in mature social groups, which ideally should balance mutual team communication and cooperation with group goal attainment.

Many groups in everyday life, however, do not measure up to ideal expectations. One such group is the Condominium Board Meeting script, which follows. Many other governing bodies, such as town councils and groups of elected officials of public and private community organizations, are charged with the leadership, maintenance, public communication, and financial management that is necessary in order to meet stated goals. Whether goals are met depends largely upon the ability of leaders and members to demonstrate and apply mature social skills. Through the analysis of this and other scripts, students should be able to identify which characters possess and use high-level skills and which do not. If time allows, the missing skills might be added through creative role playing to produce a different outcome.

All of the scripts should be read by groups, with perhaps an audience of the rest of the class, in order to get a sense of how social interactions work in everyday situations. If preferred, the script readings can be videotaped and used for presentation by different groups of students. Each person can then describe the point of view of the character he or she played and the emotions or feelings conveyed by their communications with other characters. Discussion questions at the end of each script serve as a basis for further learning and analysis, either in the classroom, as an assignment, or through journal writing.

Script for Analysis: Condominium Board Meeting

Directions

Student groups take on roles in the script to read, and/or groups can make a video of their role play. Principles from the chapter should be kept in mind during this role play.

Seating Chart

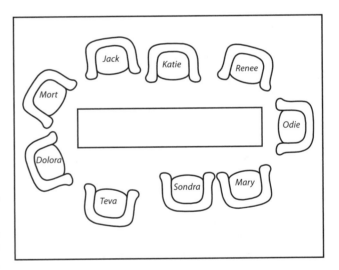

On the table are a portable tape recorder, sheets of paper with the agenda, and glasses of water/soda. Almost everyone has a note pad and pen with them for taking notes.

Characters and Background

Board meetings for this small vacation condo complex in the South Pacific island of "Bliss" are held once a year. Half of the owners live and work on the island, while the other half live and work elsewhere and come periodically for holidays or rent out their condos. This year, the island was hit by a typhoon that blew off part of the roof and flooded the lower units. Luckily, there was no structural damage to the concrete buildings, and most of the windows remained intact. However, the Association received a large sum of money for repairs from the insurance company. Two specific owners, Dolora and Odie, have taken control of these funds and have done extensive work on their own units while preventing other owners from making needed repairs. Additionally, the manager has been "borrowing" some of the money from owners who paid their fees in cash. These are just a few of the problems facing this board of directors at this year's meeting.

Jack: (age 50) British. One of the developers and owner of the loft on the third floor having a spectacular view of the ocean. He is the President of Futura Corporation, which also owns the airport, the seaport, three golf courses, and 10 hotels on the island. He does not live in the loft, but his company uses it for consultants and special guests. He knows everyone on the Island and has an immense dislike for Mort and Dolora. He is here at Joe's request to take the insurance money out of Mort's hands before he spends it all.

Mort: (age 70) A former cruise ship captain, now a permanent resident of the island of Bliss. He's used to getting his own way. He thinks the world of himself and likes to control others by threatening or terrorizing them. He has been known to drink heavily and may have done so prior to the meeting.

Dolora: (age 45) An ex-model, Mort's second wife. Has bleached blond wavy hair, was once very attractive but is now obese. She's terrified of Mort and does whatever he asks.

Dolora and Mort own two of the 15 condos. Dolora had been President and Manager combined for more than 20 years, until 3 years ago when Sondra was elected and took over. Dolora has never forgiven Sondra for taking this position away from her.

Teva: (age 30) A bookkeeper who is good friends with Dolora and with the manager, Victor, and believes that neither can do any wrong.

Sondra: (age 33) An attractive businesswoman who works on the island, but is originally from Los Angeles, California. She has an aggressive side, but also a great sense of humor. Three years ago, she was elected President and Manager, but quit after 1.5 years of being constantly harassed by Mort, who watched and questioned her every move. Dolora filled the rest of her term by default.

Odie: (age 60) Bought her place from Dolora and Mort, but spends very little time there. Odie, not being there, relies on Dolora to tell her what's going on. She often participates in political games invented by Mort and Dolora. Odie is friendly, but very superficial to everyone else.

Mary: (age 80) Walks with a cane because of severe arthritis. She was Jack's predecessor's secretary for more than 50 years, and he gave her the ground floor condo as payment for many loyal years of service.

Renee: (age 23) A dark-haired, slim, and very fit tennis instructor, Tunesian, speaks with an accent. She bought her place 1 year ago from Odie, and Odie took back the mortgage. Renee doesn't make a lot of money and struggles to pay her bills on time. She pays everything in cash, as do many people on the island.

Katie: (age 40) Owns two condos in this complex and serves as Vice President. She rents both condos, and, until recently, Victor has been collecting the rent for Katie.

Absent owners: Joe, an owner who inherited his condo from his father, is married, owns his own business, and lives in Atlanta. Victor, an owner, has managed the condo with the help of Dolora for the past 2 years, ever since Sondra quit. Victor and his wife do whatever Mort and Dolora tell them to do.

Action Begins Here

Dolora: This meeting is called to order.

Mort: We'll need everyone's proxies. (Dolora—for Victor, Odie—for her husband, Jack—for Joe, pass proxies to Mort)

Odie: Where's your proxy, Jack?

Jack: What do you mean? I represent the loft.

Odie: But your company owns the loft. Where is his proxy?

Jack: (incredulous) Yes, my company owns it and I am the President of the company.

Odie: The title isn't in your name. You need a proxy.

Jack: This is preposterous! Don't you know who I am?

Odie: Are you saying everyone else needs a proxy but you don't?

Jack: Who's got some paper? (writes out a proxy, signs it, and passes it to Odie) Does this make you happy?

Odie: It should be on your letterhead, but I guess it's okay. (throws it in center of table, Sondra passes it to Mort)

Jack: What's next?

Dolora: I'll read the minutes of last year's meeting. (begins reading)

Jack: Why don't we all have copies?

Dolora: I thought I'd just read them.

Jack: When were the minutes written? We should have had copies sent to us weeks ago.

Dolora: Well, I'm sorry! You weren't even here last year. Why do you care?

Mort: *(to Dolora)* Just make some copies now. *(she does, and passes them around)*

Jack: Who's supposed to take the minutes today? Don't we have a secretary?

Renee: I'm the secretary. I'm taking notes.

Jack: These are your minutes, then?

Renee: No. Joe was chairman last year. He tape recorded the meeting and summarized it.

Jack: But he's the treasurer, not the secretary. Doesn't anyone do anything right around here?

Renee: I was new last year. No one told me to do it. Joe had the tapes.

Dolora: Look, we can't change that now. Can't we just get on with approving the minutes?

Sondra: Yes, let's. We have a lot of work ahead of us.

Dolora: *(begins reading again)* "The meeting was called to order on March…"

Jack: We have them in front of us. Must you read them aloud?

Sondra: Yes. It's in the bylaws. They must be read aloud. *(checks if tape recorder is on)*

(skip ahead here to finishing the minutes) The meeting was adjourned at 6:30 pm.

Jack: What did we do about the wall and gate? Is it finished?

Sondra: Yes. It cost $19,000. It says right there. *(points to paper)*

Jack: And what about the parking lot?

Dolora: That's old business. We aren't there yet. First, we have to approve the minutes.

Katie: I move that the minutes be approved.

Odie: I second.

Sondra: All in favor. *(chorus of "aye")*

Dolora: Approved. Now we'll move on the treasurer's report. Since Joe's not here, Teva, our accountant, will present the financial statements.

Teva: *(passes out copies of accounting for each member's fee payments, all pause to read)*

Katie: I have a dispute with my statement. I don't owe any fees.

Renee: So do I. I paid all my fees on time. Why do I have all these late fees?

Dolora: Hold on, will you? Let Teva finish her presentation. Then, we'll discuss any issues. *(Renee and Katie roll their eyes at each other, then nod at Dolora; they continue whispered conversation.)*

Teva: *(passes out more papers)* Here is where we stand as of today. (Presents income, expenses, and balances for checking accounts.)

Jack: What about the typhoon insurance settlement? I see $100,000. That's just the first payment. Where's the rest?

Dolora: I have all that on a separate sheet. Let's finish the general account first.

Jack: But here is a check written against it on Teva's sheet. Why doesn't she have all the information together?

Dolora: *(miffed)* It's a separate account.

Jack: Look, you can't have some of the money here *(points to paper)* and the rest somewhere else. And why aren't we getting copies of these accounts ahead of time? For my company's board meetings, we send out financial reports, minutes, and an agenda 30 days ahead of time. People need time to go over all this beforehand.

Teva: I only got the latest information a few days ago. As it was, I had to chase down your manager, Victor, to get the bank statements.

Renee: Where are the bank statements now?

Teva: *(lifts up a basket of file folders and papers)* This is my portable office. *(laughter) (she finishes her report, then gets up to leave)*

Katie: Teva, could you stay a bit longer? I'd like you here for this.

Teva: Okay. *(she sits)*

Renee: I have a question. What is going on with this statement? I paid my fees to Victor in cash. Here are my receipts.

Teva: Victor deposited a check on March 8 for over $8,000. That should have covered your fees and most of Katie's.

Katie: That's not the point. Victor is the manager of our condo. He gets all of our fees twice a year, and part of his job is to deposit them on time. He didn't do that for Renee, and he certainly didn't with my fees.

Mort: But Victor manages your rentals. That's between you and him.

Katie: Not when he's collecting rents that should have been applied to my condo fees. According to this statement, I owed fees from before January as an outstanding balance. Here *(points to statement)*, he wrote a check just prior to last year's meeting, and the next day it bounced.

Renee: And mine go back to last January also. Why aren't we getting notification of these outstanding balances before today?

Sondra: I'll tell you why—because Dolora and Mort don't want you to know. They know you can't vote today if you owe money. They want to take away your votes.

Dolora: How dare you accuse us! We sent out notices, didn't we Teva?

Teva: They're supposed to be sent by the manager. I gave Victor the notices last January and last June. You should have received them months ago.

Renee and Katie: *(glancing at each other)* We didn't.

Jack: I have a dispute also. I have an outstanding balance, and I know I paid these fees.

Mary: Your assistant paid them through me. I've been the secretary for years. There was never a missed fee.

Sondra: You see, Jack? They don't want you to vote either.

Mort: You better stop those accusations, or I'll sue you for slander.

Jack: *(to Mort)* Just hold on. I think we have a bigger problem here. Where is Victor?

Dolora: I have his proxy here. He couldn't come.

Jack: Why not?

Katie: Yes, why isn't he here? I saw him 5 minutes before the meeting, driving out of the parking lot.

Dolora: He dropped off his proxy and a letter to be read at the meeting.

Sondra: I hope it's his resignation as manager.

Dolora: No, it isn't.

Katie: But look what he's done with my money and Renee's. I don't think we can trust him to manage the funds of the Association.

Renee: I agree. He used our money as his own personal bank account.

Sondra: I move that Victor be removed as manager, effective immediately.

Odie: I second. I also think he should be removed from the signature of the Association bank account.

Jack: Absolutely. I second the motion as amended.

Sondra: All in favor? *(chorus of "aye")*

Katie: So what does this mean for Renee and me? Can we vote? *(side conversations arise)*

Sondra: Can we all agree that Katie's and Renee's fees can be considered paid? Victor didn't steal from them. He stole from the Association. It's now the Association's responsibility to collect the money from Victor. Any objections? *(silence)*

Renee: I'm writing that down.

Teva: Do you need me for anything else? *(stands up and gathers her belongings)*

Jack: Yes. I think you should mail the statements to all the owners yourself. Dolora, don't you agree, under the circumstances?

Dolora: *(with a scowl)* Alright. *(Dolora escorts Teva out, then returns)*

Sondra: Let's move on. We need to elect a chairperson for the rest of the meeting.

Katie: I nominate Jack.

Mary: I second.

Dolora: Wait a minute. I'm the President, and I have an agenda all ready. Jack is new to this.

Sondra: *(ignoring Dolora)* All in favor raise your hand.

Odie: *(ignoring Sondra)* I nominate Dolora.

Mort: I second.

Sondra: All in favor of Jack? *(Katie, Jack, Mary, Sondra, and Renee raise hands)*

Dolora: Sondra, you aren't the chairman.

Sondra: Katie has two votes, Jack has three, Renee, Mary, and I make three more. Dolora, I think you're outvoted.

Jack: Alright, then. Are we ready to proceed?

Dolora: *(throws copies of the agenda toward Jack)* Go ahead.

Jack: I think we can postpone old business until the end or take care of it by e-mail. Our priority is the typhoon fund. Dolora, you said you had an accounting?

Dolora: Like Teva said, we got $100,000 last November to get us started with roof repairs. Why don't you tell us the rest, Jack? You were at the meeting.

Jack: Yes. You and Mort were willing to sell us short and accept a settlement of $250,000. Joe, Sondra, and I met with Crane Insurance Adjusters in January and agreed on a much higher figure, $500,000. That's enough to get a new roof on both buildings and all new windows besides.

Mort: You conveniently left us out of that meeting, and Dolora is the President.

Sondra: Thank God, Mort wasn't there. The way he insulted and threatened everyone at the last meeting, it's no wonder we weren't getting anywhere.

Jack: Let's put that behind us. With this settlement, we have enough to pay for all of our repairs and improve the property values in the bargain. But we need to be careful how the money gets spent. Mort, Dolora, and Odie, you can't expect to renovate your condos any longer without all of us approving the expense.

Odie: But why not? In the past, when there's been damage to my unit, I just had it fixed, and the condo always paid.

Sondra: That's because your best friend was President. *(smirks at Dolora)* She controlled the money and didn't tell anyone else.

Dolora: I resent your implications.

Sondra: Just calling 'em like I see 'em.

Jack: We agreed during our conference call last month that we all have to approve how the insurance money is spent. How many bids did you get, Odie?

Odie: One. But the work's already done. Here's the invoice. *(hands it to Jack)*

Mort: I have one, too. *(hands that to Jack)* We had to get the work done before more damage occurred as a result.

Jack: $53,000?? *(outraged, looks at Mort)* Did you have the whole place redecorated?

Renee: I think there should be a committee to make decisions on the insurance money. Otherwise, some of us will spend it all, and the rest will be left out in the cold.

Katie: I agree. I haven't had a chance to make any repairs yet. By the time I do, there won't be any money left.

Sondra: Was that a motion, Renee? I second.

Dolora: Who's going to be on the committee? You?

Renee: Actually, I think we all should be. There are only nine owners.

Jack: That sounds like a good idea. All in favor? *("aye" from everyone except Mort and Dolora; Jack stares at them)* All opposed?

Dolora and Mort: Nay!

Jack: I believe the ayes have it. We'll submit our invoices and get everyone's approval by e-mail. Alright? *(nods from all)* What's next?

Mary: We need to elect a new manager. Who's going to be our manager?

Katie: I nominate Sondra. She did a good job before, and she's here most of the time.

Dolora: *(scowls)* How much is she going to charge?

Sondra: I won't do it for less than $1000/month.

Dolora: Victor was getting $350/month. Can we afford $800?

Mort: I won't approve Sondra for manager at any price. Don't you realize all the money she spent last time? Before we know it, we'll be broke.

Jack: What do you mean, Mort? Sondra runs a business. She's perfectly capable.

Mort: She took out perfectly good plants and bought new ones. She fired the landscaper and got expensive new tiles for the pool. It was just dreadful. *(whispered to Jack)* I'll tell you later.

Sondra: Alright, Mort. *(bangs the table)* Now, I don't want to do it at all. Are you satisfied?

Katie: With Victor in charge, we might be broke soon, too. We need someone we all can trust.

Sondra: I think Renee should do it.

Renee: No. Never!

Mary: *(to Renee)* I think you'd be a great choice. You live here and could keep on top of things. You could keep in contact with us all by e-mail.

Sondra: I wish you'd consider it. Why don't you want to?

Renee: I'll tell you why. Because I feel like I'm dealing with a bunch of children! Mort, you're insulting Sondra and threatening her. Odie, you're telling me don't talk to this one or that one. Dolora, as President you sign all the checks, but you're telling us you didn't know Victor was stealing our money? Jack has to prove he's an owner when we all know each other.

(Sondra and Katie exchange knowing looks; others appear shamed into silence)

Katie: *(to Renee)* I think you should give it a try. We'll all support you. Won't we, Dolora? Mort?

Sondra: I know sometimes the owners can be difficult, but I'll try to help you if you run into difficulty.

Jack: We could hire someone on the outside if she doesn't want to.

Odie: No, I think we really need someone who lives here and not an outsider. Dolora, don't you think you could work with Renee?

Dolora: *(attempting kindness)* How would $400/month be if you decide to try it?

Renee: Alright. I'll do it temporarily for a few months. I'll see how it works out and if I made the right decision.

Mary: Thank you, dear. We'll all support you. I know you can do it.

Jack: There's only one more item on the agenda. We need to elect officers for the next year.

Sondra: I nominate Jack for President.

Mary: I second.

Jack: Alright. I'll do it if no one objects.

Mort: *(grunts to Dolora and Odie)* They've got us outvoted.

Dolora: No objection here.

Jack: Katie, will you stay on as Vice President?

Katie: Sure, and I nominate Sondra for Treasurer.

Jack: Any objections? *(none)* Renee, you'll remain our secretary?

Renee: *(nods)* Alright.

Jack: That's it, then. Can we adjourn?

Dolora: I don't see why Katie should be Vice President. Why can't Mort be VP? He lives here, and he can be more involved.

Jack: Katie can be involved by e-mail. Anyway, the voting is over.

Renee: I'd say the meeting is adjourned. All in favor. *(chorus of "aye")*

The End.

Discussion

1. Describe the role of the person you played on the team. How did it feel to play this role?

2. What group or social roles could you identify during this meeting? How did they affect the group's ability to communicate or work on its task?

3. Who was the designated leader? What leadership roles did this person play?

4. What were the goals of this board meeting? Did the board achieve its goals?

5. List three conflicts that occurred during the meeting. How did the conflicts get resolved?

6. If you were leading this meeting, what would you have done differently and why?

7. Choose one character and describe how you would have changed his or her role if you had the opportunity.

8. What facilitators and barriers for social participation can you identify in this script?

9. What ethical issues does this script bring to mind? How were they addressed?

10. Did this group interact at a mature level (see Table 1-10)? Why or why not?

References

American Occupational Therapy Association. (2008). Occupational therapy practice framework: Domain and process (2nd ed.). *American Journal of Occupational Therapy, 62,* 625-683.

Bandura, A. (1977). *Social learning theory.* New York, NY: General Learning Press.

Benne, K., & Sheats, P. (1948). Functional roles of group members. *Journal of Social Issues, 4,* 41-49.

Benne, K., & Sheats, P. (1978). Functional roles of group members. In L. Bradford (Ed.), *Group development* (2nd ed., pp. 52-61). LaJolla, CA: University Associates.

Bonder, B., Martin, L., & Miracle, A. (2002). *Culture in clinical care.* Thorofare, NJ: SLACK Incorporated.

Bordessa, K. (2006). *Team challenges: Group activities to build cooperation, communication, and creativity.* Retrieved February 10, 2009 from greatsolutions.blogspot.com/youth-sports-and-team-building-html

Brown, P. J. (1998). *Understanding and applying medical anthropology.* Mountain View, CA: Mayfield.

Cohn, E. (2008). Team interaction models and team communication. In E. Crepeau, E. Cohn, & B. Schell (Eds.), *Willard & Spackman's occupational therapy.* Philadelphia, PA: Lippincott, Williams & Wilkins.

Cole, M. (2005). *Group dynamics in occupational therapy* (3rd ed.). Thorofare, NJ: SLACK Incorporated.

Deutsch, M. (1973). *The resolution of conflict: Constructive and destructive processes.* New Haven, CT: Yale University Press.

Donohue, M. V. (1999). Theoretical bases of Mosey's group interactions skills. *Occupational Therapy International, 6,* 35-51.

Donohue, M. V. (2009). *The social profile manual.* Retrieved from www.Social-Profile.com

Filley, A. (1975). *Interpersonal conflict resolution.* Glenview, IL: Scott, Foresman & Co.

Gouran, D. (2003). Leadership as the art of counteractive influence in decision-making and problem-solving groups. In R. Hirokawa, R. Cathcart, L. Samovar, & L. Henman (Eds.), *Small group communication: Theory and practice: An anthology* (pp. 172-183). Los Angeles, CA: Roxbury Publishing.

Hirokawa, R., DeGooyer, D., & Valde, K. (2003). Characteristics of effective health care teams. In R. Hirokawa, R. Cathcart, L. Samovar, & L. Henman (Eds.), *Small group communication: Theory and practice* (pp. 148-157). Los Angeles, CA: Roxbury Publishing.

Holpp, L. (1999). *Managing teams.* New York, NY: McGraw Hill.

Institute of Medicine. (2003). *Health professions education: A bridge to quality.* Washington, DC: National Academy Press.

Johnson, D., & Johnson, R. (1995). *Teaching students to be peacemakers* (3rd ed.). Edina, MN: Interaction Book Company.

Kilman, R., & Thomas, K. (1975). Interpersonal conflict handling behavior as reflections of Jungian personality dimensions. *Psychological Reports, 37,* 971-980.

Kuo, H. (2009). *Unconventional service learning: integrating community, teamwork, and leadership communication.* Paper presentation at NCA 94th Annual Convention, San Diego, CA. Retrieved February 10, 2009 from www.allacademic.com/meta/p_mla_apa_research_citation/2/3/6/5/9/p256592_index

Latella, D. (2002). Teams and teamwork. In K. Sladyk (Ed.), *The successful occupational therapy fieldwork student.* Thorofare, NJ: SLACK Incorporated.

Mosey, A. C. (1986). *Psychosocial components of occupational therapy.* New York, NY: Raven Press.

Mosey, A. C. (1996). *Applied scientific inquiry in the health professions; An epistemological orientation* (2nd ed.). Bethesda, MD: American Occupational Therapy Association.

Mouton, J., & Blake, R. (1984). *Synergogy.* Hoboken, NJ: Jossey-Bass, Inc.

Moyers, P. (2005). Working in teams. *Occupational Therapy Practice,* February 7, 19-20.

Northouse, P. G. (2001). Introduction. In P. Northouse (Ed.), *Leadership: theory and practice* (2nd ed., pp. 1-13). Thousand Oaks, CA: Sage.

Northouse, P., & Northouse, L. (1995). *Health communication: Strategies for health professionals* (2nd ed.). Englewood Cliffs, NJ: Prentice Hall.

Pauch, R. (2008). *The last lecture.* New York, NY: Hyperion Books.

Rapoport, A. (1960). *Fights, games, and debates.* Ann Arbor, MI: University of Michigan Press.

Shimanoff, S., & Jenkins, M. (2003). Leadership and gender: Challenging assumptions and recognizing resources. In R. Hirokawa, R. Cathcart, L. Samovar, & L. Henman (Eds.), *Small group communication: Theory and practice.* Los Angeles, CA: Roxbury Publishing.

Spilker, B. (1998). Using teams and committees effectively. *Drug News Perspect, 11,* 389-393.

Stanford University Center for Immersive and Simulation Based Learning (SISL). (2009). *Teamwork.* Retrieved February 10, 2009 from cisl.stanford.edu/what_is/learning_types/teaamwork.html

Svinicki, M. (2009). *Using small groups to promote learning.* Austin, TX: University of Texas Web site.

Swinth, Y. (2008). Occupational therapy evaluation and intervention related to education. In E. Crepeau, E. Cohn, & B. Schell (Eds.), *Willard & Spackman's occupational therapy* (11th ed., pp. 592-614). Philadelphia, PA: Lippincott, Williams & Wilkins.

World Health Organization. (2001). *International classification of functioning, disability, and health.* Geneva, Switzerland.

Yalom, I. (2005). *Theory and practice of group psychotherapy* (5th ed.). New York, NY: Basic Books.

chapter 2

Theoretical Basis of Social Participation
An Overview

Mary V. Donohue, PhD, OTL, FAOTA

This chapter will present the theoretical bases of social participation including an overview; components; and related constructs of *social learning theory*, *social emotional learning*, and *social capital*. Concepts related to these constructs will be defined, including levels of social participation and measurable social factors that have been studied through empirical research.

Concepts, Constructs, and Definitions

Concepts are ideas or thoughts representing abstract cognitive notions, opinions, states of being, perceptions, principles, emotions, or beliefs, as well as representing concrete objects, realities, and people. Constructs are overarching concepts used in theories or naming theories that integrate subsidiary related concepts into an organized system or group of principles (Burns & Grove, 2009). For varying definitions of concepts and constructs, see Portney and Watkins (2009) and Gliner and Morgan (2000). Concepts and constructs both need to be defined in order to indicate what their labels represent.

Social participation is a major construct that may be defined as interpersonal interaction with others in a verbal or nonverbal mode, with or without involvement in an activity. This definition is designed to distinguish social participation from activity participation. Social participation is a

construct presented in the *International Classification of Functioning, Disability and Health (ICF)* (World Health Organization, 2001) as a chapter/division describing an element of daily life essential to recovery. Social participation incorporates several other social constructs including *social learning theory* (Bandura, 1977), *social emotional learning (SEL)* (Cohen, 2004; Zins, Elias, & Maher, 2007), and *social capital* (Dekker & Uslander, 2001; Field, 2003).

These constructs incorporate a number of related social concepts such as *parallel, associative,* and *cooperative* levels of interaction (Mosey, 1968; Parten, 1932); *sociability, social presence,* and *socialization* (Gough, 1957); and *project, egocentric cooperative,* and *mature* levels of interaction (Mosey, 1968). Table 2-1 presents major authors and their related clusters of concepts or constructs relevant to the construct of social participation, which will be defined, illustrated, and expanded on in later chapters.

Social Participation International

In the ICF, Chapters 7 and 9 in the section on Activities and Participation (WHO, 2001) focus on the construct of social participation. As indicated earlier, this book makes a distinction between social participation and activity participation, although much social participation takes place during activities and can be combined as social activity participation (see Appendix for Outline of ICF Chapters referenced here).

Cole, M.B., & Donohue, M.V. *Social Participation in Occupational Contexts: In Schools, Clinics, and Communities* (pp 29-42).
© 2011 SLACK Incorporated

Table 2-1

AUTHORS AND CONSTRUCTS/CONCEPTS INCLUDED IN THE MAJOR CONSTRUCT OF SOCIAL PARTICIPATION

PARTEN, 1932
Parallel
Association
Cooperative

BANDURA, 1977
Social learning theory

ERICKSON, 1950
Trust
Autonomy
Initiative
Industry
Identity
Intimacy
Generativity
Integrity

GOUGH, 1957
Sociability
Social presence
Socialization

DEKKER & USLANDER, 2001;
FIELD, 2003
Social capital

MOSEY, 1968
Parten's three concepts
Egocentric cooperative
Mature level

COHEN, 2004; ZINS & ELIAS, 2007
Social emotional learning (SEL)

The ICF Chapter 7 of the section on Activities and Participation is devoted to interpersonal interactions and relationships, analyzing both general and particular interpersonal relationships. Social participation is considered to be an integral part of overall health and includes characteristics on a continuum of tolerance, respect, appreciation, and warmth. The ICF explains that complex interpersonal interactions include both forming and ending relationships appropriately, regulating social behaviors, participating according to social norms, and even being aware of providing social space to others when we sense their desire and need for some degree of distance. Distinctions are made among how to relate to strangers, authority figures, peers, coinhabitants, and family members. Romantic, spousal, and sexual relationships are described as intimate and in need of maintaining through emotional, physical, and intellectual sustenance (WHO, 2001).

The ICF Chapter 9 of the section on Activities and Participation explores the parameters of social participation that extend into community and civic life, describing both formal and informal associations such as churches, synagogues, temples, Red Cross, Habitat for Humanity, sports leagues, political parties, and professional associations. These social interactions may include volunteer and charitable organizations providing service to the community and assuming responsibility for citizenship. They may also provide opportunity for play, recreation, and leisure through engaging in or observing sports, fitness, art, and nature in clubs, teams, museums, theaters, sight-seeing, and reunions, convened for inspiration and celebration in memorial and ceremonial gatherings (WHO, 2001).

The ICF mentions human rights recognized by the United Nations' Declaration of Human Rights (United Nations General Assembly, 1948) and its Standard Rules for the Equalization of Opportunities for Persons with Disabilities (United Nations General Assembly, 1993) as under the umbrella of social participation. It emphasizes the right to self-determination of people in governing themselves through political bodies, boards, and committees, which are also social assemblies. In relationship to others in society, the ICF Chapter 9 reminds readers of the right to participate in shaping one's own destiny and lifestyle. A large aspect of social participation is engaged in by those wishing to relate to their community through political office; however, the ICF encourages all to participate in the social responsibility of voting, serving on juries, and contributing to the upkeep of society's superstructure, which supports social interaction (WHO, 2001).

Parten and Social Participation Developmental Concepts

In 1932, Mildred Parten wrote about and researched *social participation* as a developmental continuum of social behavior, motivation, and adjustment increasing through the years of growth of preschool children. Her definition of social participation is operational in nature, including the measurable concepts of unoccupied behavior, onlooker behavior, and solitary play as pregroup interactions, and parallel play, associative

Table 2-2

CONTINUUM OF PARTEN'S SOCIAL-RELATED PLAY BEHAVIORS OBSERVED IN PRESCHOOL CHILDREN

PRE-GROUP BEHAVIORS

Unoccupied behavior → → Onlooker behavior → → Solitary play behaviors → →

GROUP BEHAVIORS

Parallel Play Behavior → → Associative play behavior → → Cooperative organized play

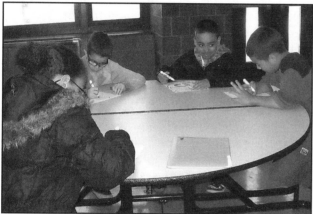

Figure 2-1. Parallel level of participation: children drawing with magic markers.

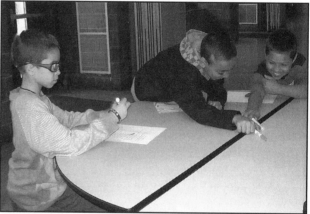

Figure 2-2. Associative level of participation: sharing magic markers.

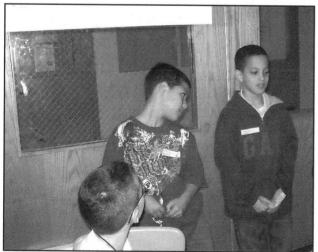

Figure 2-3. Basic cooperative level of participation in role playing scenarios to practice appropriate assertiveness.

play, and cooperative play as organized into groups. She, and others working with her, observed these social-related behaviors during free play periods

of children arriving at preschool early in the day with their parents. The children were coloring; card making; or playing with sandboxes, scooter cars, or dolls. Table 2-2 illustrates a continuum depicting this spectrum of group-related behaviors.

Parten (1932) defined the concept of *parallel* behavior within a group as independent activity among children, using toys like those of others in the group, and playing *beside* others though not *with* them (Figure 2-1). She defined the concept of *associative* behavior as group play in which there is some recognition of others' mutual interests and common activity leading to personal association of children briefly, often paired, without sustained organized interaction (Figure 2-2). Parten defined the concept of *cooperative* behaviors as organized play in which there is agreement on a central activity performed jointly with other children, emergence of separate roles, which supplement existing roles, and recognition of norms of behaviors or goals as characteristic of the group interaction (Parten) (Figure 2-3).

Parten (1932) provides a clear example of the group behaviors comparing the parallel, associative, and cooperative levels of participation at a sandbox. During parallel play at a sandbox, children will typically fill their cups individually, pouring out the contents or making shapes with the sand without looking at what other children are doing, but not hindered by their presence. There is little conversation. When associative play emerges at the sandbox, children begin to borrow one another's cups or plastic shapes, advising and offering sand to other children. They call others to the sandbox and make room for the newcomer. They compare formations of sand shapes. There is much conversation describing this common activity. If someone suggests making a road in the sand, they each make their own road. In cooperative play at the sandbox, a child may suggest that they are all making supper. Children select or are assigned family roles of parents, brothers, and sisters. One child is designated the baby of the family and is told he cannot cook. The children speak about their part in preparing the meal. Children coach each other if the roles are not played correctly. The group may become closed to some newcomers depending on the desires of the group members. One or two children may assert themselves as leaders. The group members are expected to stay with the group until the meal is "finished."

At one point in her discussion, Parten (1932) uses *socialization* as a synonym for social participation. Here, she uses socialization as a global term of interacting with others, which is the sense in which it is often used in educational and clinical work.

In her research, Parten (1932) examined the six social-related behaviors, three pregroup and three group behaviors, with age and experience in preschool. She postulates that as children mature and become acquainted with others in their classes, they gradually add increased levels of participation to their repertoire of social behaviors. In Section III of this book, Social Participation Assessment, the method and results of Parten's research will be presented.

In thinking about concepts such as Parten's *parallel*, *associative*, and *cooperative* social participation concepts, recalling examples from your own life is an excellent way to concretize your understanding and fix this abstract schema in your memory. *Can you recollect examples of instances from your own memories of your preschool childhood days where you participated socially in parallel, associative, and cooperative activities with other young children? What were your favorite social participation activities?*

As you are reading the following section, recall recent examples of *Erikson's social development levels* that you have experienced in your own life, among your family members, friends, teachers, and coaches.

Erikson's Social Developmental Levels

Building on Freud's three earlier sexual developmental levels of oral, anal, and genital stages, Erikson (1950) published his schema for eight social developmental levels in his text, *Childhood and Society*, expanding the developmental age continuum into adolescence and adulthood.

Erikson's (1950) infant stage was focused on the baby's struggle between *trust* and *mistrust* of others in his or her sphere of family and friends. The toddler stage of exploration was identified as locked in a crisis of *autonomy* versus *shame* and doubt in the war between seeing the value of cooperating with others versus having tantrums. Erikson identified his third social developmental level as *initiative* versus *guilt* in expressing preferences for appealing activities and potential roles for the future. Erikson labeled the fourth level of social development as *industry* versus *inferiority* as children begin to enjoy the mastery of hand, body, and cognitive skills in crafts, reading, arithmetic, martial arts, and sports in an effort to experience the satisfaction of competence. In the adolescent period, Erikson emphasizes the tension between one's *identity* in contrast to whom others are and *role confusion*—either experiencing no desirable roles or attraction to many roles accompanied by an unwillingness to make a selection.

Moving into adulthood, Erikson labels the social development level continuum as the dilemma of expanding personhood with experiences of *intimacy* with a partner and family in contrast to isolation or frenetic socializing as a "social butterfly." In adulthood itself, Erikson reflects on the social development period of *generativity* in giving to others and immersion in work roles versus the stagnation and boredom in perspectives asking, "Is that all there is?" and disappointment in the lack of achievement of ambitions.

Finally, in the last stage of life, Erikson points out the desire to find *integrity* in one's use of time and to weave together all of the themes of life in contrast to despair at having wasted one's lifetime of opportunity. These concepts and crises will be expanded upon in specific chapters devoted to the social development of children, adolescents, adults, and seniors, followed by chapters providing interventions designed to enable people to achieve social participation satisfaction during all stages of life's development.

Table 2-3

Have you encountered family members, friends, and professionals (such as teachers, ministers, athletes, nurses, and doctors) who illustrate the *sociability, social presence,* and *socialization* concepts of Gough's social participation factors?

Gough's Concepts of Social Participation

In 1957, Harrison Gough formulated an assessment, the *California Psychological Inventory,* consisting of factors to measure the career characteristics of competence in familiar jobs. These factors included the three concepts of sociability, social presence, and socialization. They are listed here incrementally in terms of level of skill acquisition among social participation behaviors.

Sociability is the capacity to be comfortable with people and to enjoy social encounters (Gough, 1957). Manifestations of sociability include friendliness, agreeableness, and a relaxed affability. It includes liking to hang out in groups with others just to be with people. Sociability is a beginning level social skill and the basis of the other more advanced skills. Examples include people who like to go to cafes and bars to mingle with others and "people watch" or to cluster by the coffee machine in the office.

Social presence is the ability to interact with others in a manner that includes poise, spontaneity, enthusiasm, and self-confidence, including the capacity to enjoy humor and/or flirtatiousness (Gough, 1957). People with social presence are assertive in their presentation, speech, and interactions. As examples, successful salespeople, politicians, and soloists in a band or choir usually manifest high levels of social presence performance.

Socialization, as defined by Gough (1957), is the degree of maturity, integrity, rectitude, prudence, and responsiveness to the obligations of interpersonal life, common needs, and customs of social and work groups. Gough's definition contrasts with the term *socialization* commonly used in clinical settings, which relates to general social competence of children or patients. In clinical or educational settings, the term should be used as it is customary in that particular setting. Gough's concept relates to the extent to which people are embedded in the cultural environmental norms and expectations of behavior of their group's acceptable roles. It relates to the degree to which a professional or group member exemplifies the interpersonal characteristics needed to carry

out his or her job or tasks with devotion to his or her duties. Examples would include teachers and therapists who have become seasoned educators and clinicians exhibiting professional, caring, and respectful attitudes in interpersonal interactions with children, patients, peers, and administrators. Other examples include group officers or members who cooperate with others in the group to achieve their common goals. Little League coaches and scout leaders as volunteers generally exhibit this trait. This concept describes the type of personnel or group members who have grown into their roles and incorporate aspects of social participation in their demeanor, judgments, and interactions around their activities.

Overall, Gough's concepts of social participation of average individuals have assisted educators and therapists in formulating distinctions of social skills required of typical workers in their occupational/vocational and community settings. These concepts facilitate understanding of distinctions among aspects of "normal" social participation in community and work groups and teams (Table 2-3). Research on Gough's concepts will be presented in Section III.

Mosey's Expansion of Parten's Social Participation Developmental Concepts

In 1968, Mosey amplified Parten's continuum of *parallel, associative,* and *cooperative* levels of social participation development to expand the levels of interactive skills into adolescence and adulthood. Mosey perceived the associative level as one emphasizing brief projects, like building blocks or using crayons, and renamed this level of beginning participation the *project* level. She also renamed the childhood years of Parten's cooperative level as *egocentric cooperative,* reflecting the basic cooperation usually manifested by children of 5 to 7 years of age as they experiment with joint goals, norms, and activities of interest to themselves. Mosey moved the *cooperative* concept label upward in years to

Table 2-4

PARTEN AND MOSEY'S GROUP INTERACTION LEVELS

Parallel → →	Project → →	Egocentric Cooperative → →	Cooperative → →	Mature Levels
1½ to 2 yrs	2 to 4 yrs	5 to 7 yrs	9 to 2 yrs	15 to 18 yrs

describe adolescent interactive behavior. Finally, she added the concept of the *mature* group (Lifton, 1966) to describe adult participation in groups as the highest level of social participation development. Mosey's expansion of Parten's spectrum of social participation development in group behavior can be summarized as a continuum of concepts (Table 2-4).

Mosey's age groupings provide ranges of years, which may be disputed by some people; however, the concepts of the social behavioral developmental continuum, in its sequence, reflect observations of growth of group level interaction skills as a gradually acquired spectrum of abilities.

Comparing the five social participation level concepts of the developmental sequence illustrates distinctions among the abilities of each level. At the *parallel* concept level, initially, children are learning to trust others in the group and can tolerate playing in the presence of others. There is some minimal mutual stimulation and awareness of others. Children engage in familiar activities. As the children begin to interact in *associative/project* concept level activities, they briefly choose activities that they and their playmates enjoy together. Children sometimes seek assistance from others and are willing to give concrete assistance to other children. The next level of activity interaction development at the *egocentric* or *basic cooperative* concept stage involves longer involvement with group activity selection, along with understanding of norms and goals of group interaction. Engagement in activities that children select is preferred, and agreement on rules of games is essential (Figure 2-4). There is experimentation with group roles. Respect for others' rights and rules builds basic cooperation (Figures 2-5 and 2-6). As adolescence emerges, teens enjoy homogeneous, compatible companionship as they recognize each others' emotional development and interests. *Supportive cooperative* concept behaviors among teenagers can encourage self-expression of positive and negative feelings. Frequently, activities become secondary to the social participation of hanging out together (Figure 2-7). Adolescents can accurately identify each others' feelings and needs. At the *mature* concept level of participation, adults

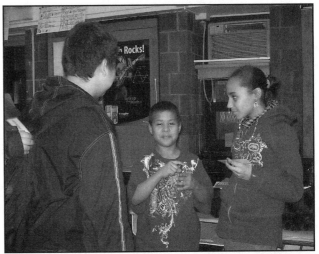

Figure 2-4. Basic cooperative level of participation in role playing scenarios to discuss joint dilemma of choosing a game to play together.

can maintain a balance between activities and social exchange (Figure 2-8 and Table 2-5). They can assess the needs of the group and assume a variety of roles as they are needed for the completion of a task with a near-perfect product and process (Donohue, 1999; Mosey, 1986).

In recommendations that Mosey (1986) provided for encouraging the promotion and practice of the five concepts of social participation development, she indicated how the leader of the group could facilitate a desired level of interaction. Sample selected suggestions from Mosey for the role of the leader and interventions to teach the conceptual social participation skill are described in Table 2-6 (Donohue, 1999).

As can be seen from Table 2-6, the leader's role changes with the expected or desired level of social participation. Philosophically, the good leader enables the group to move on, developing its own collegial mutual leadership, thus avoiding making the group dependent on the leader and thus fostering a higher level of social participation.

Theoretical assumptions are principles or guidelines that link or describe relationships among concepts or constructs. Assumptions regarding social

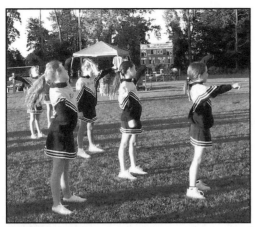
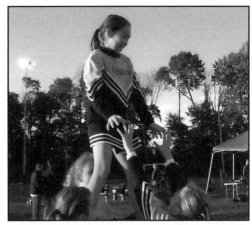

Figure 2-5 and 2-6. Basic cooperative level of participation required for coordinated support in cheerleading interaction.

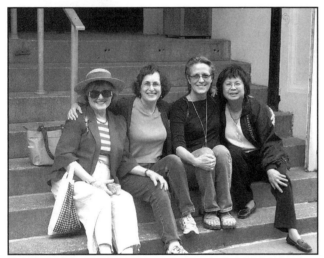

Figure 2-7. Supportive cooperative level of participation in a reunion of former classmates from 35 years ago, from East and West Coasts of the United States.

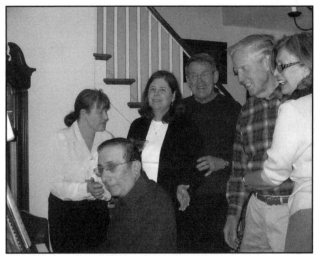

Figure 2-8. Mature level group, playing piano and singing in harmony, combining basic and supportive cooperative participation.

Table 2-5

What memories do you recall from your teen years that are examples of the *supportive cooperative* conceptual level of group camaraderie, sharing feelings, and caring for friends? Do you still sustain some relationships of this type in a group currently? When did you first find yourself a member of a *mature* conceptual type group that could get a task done while encouraging a friendly environment among members? Do any of your work or volunteer groups fit this description?

Table 2-6

FACILITATION OF SOCIAL PARTICIPATION IN GROUPS AT FIVE LEVELS OF GROUP INTERACTION

1. *Parallel level*
   Leader provides toys and material fostering children's play interests.
   Leader provides task assistance and reinforces parallel skills.

2. *Associative/project level*
   Leader helps children select activities they are interested in.
   Leader encourages trial and error and small groupings.

3. *Egocentric/basic cooperative level*
   Leader fosters children's selection of activities and materials.
   Leader serves as a resource person and takes on missing roles.

4. *Supportive cooperative level*
   Leader connects people who are compatible; encourages feelings.
   Leader is a facilitator and nonauthoritative consultant.

5. *Mature level*
   Leader is a peer.
   Leadership role is shared.
   Leader guides discussion on balance of activity and social exchange.

---

participation using this conceptual social developmental framework of five levels of social participation have been observed by numerous group leaders. They include the following:

- When a level of social participation performance has been developed or achieved, it can be used again throughout the lifespan during appropriate activities.

- The type of activity influences the level of social participation performance.

- There is no pure group static at any one level of social skills; rather, groups can perform or interact at a range of contiguous levels during a single activity and across multiple activities (Donohue, 1999).

Mosey did not undertake research regarding her conceptual levels; however, research regarding these assumptions will be presented in Section III (Donohue, 2003, 2005, 2007). *Do these assumptions apply to the groups in your life experience, past or present?* (see Figures 2-3 and 2-4.)

Bandura's Social Learning Theory

In 1977, Bandura published a now famous book, *Social Learning Theory,* that amplified some of his earlier work on social learning and personality development (1973). Bandura is a social science psychologist who carried out research on the role of *social modeling* and *self-efficacy* in motivation, thought, and action in human functioning. He developed these concepts in collaboration with others interested in aspects of the construct of *social learning theory.*

As Bandura is often quoted,

Learning would be exceedingly laborious, not to mention hazardous, if people had to rely solely on the effects of their own actions to inform them what to do. Fortunately, most human behavior is learned observationally through modeling: from observing others one forms an idea of how new behaviors are performed, and on later occasions this coded information serves as a guide for action. (1977, p. 27)

So, Bandura's construct of social learning theory consists of the process of observing and modeling the behaviors, attitudes, and emotional reactions of others. Bandura identified three methods or types of learning by observing others: live models; verbal instructional models; and symbolic media models as represented in books, films, or television.

Social learning theory's modeling process, according to Bandura, requires 4 aspects to be present: (1) paying attention to the model, (2) retention of the modeled information observed, (3) reproduction of the behavior by performing it, and (4) motivation to imitate the modeled behavior. As early as 1977, it can

Table 2-7

BANDURA'S SOCIALLY MODELED SELF-EFFICACY SOURCES WITH GENERAL AND SPECIFIC EXAMPLES

SOURCE	GENERAL EXAMPLES	SPECIFIC EXAMPLES
Performance accomplishments	Participant modeling Performance desensitization Performance exposure Self-instructed performance	Following line dancing or a dance partner Increasing the length of public speaking Joint experiments in a biology lab Holding the railing to skate backwards
Vicarious experience	Live modeling Symbolic modeling	Watching someone's dance steps Reading books, seeing movies
Verbal persuasion	Suggestion Exhortation Self-instruction Interpretive treatments	Counselor's mild recommendations Coach's strong pointers before the game Positive thoughtful self-affirmations Therapist explains rationale for an action
Emotional arousal	Attribution Relaxation Biofeedback . Symbolic desensitization Symbolic exposure	Compliments from friend on a job well done Muscle tensing and release technique Pulse meter on a treadmill Exposure to snake picture/snake skin Support companion for a elevator phobic

be seen that Bandura perceived and incorporated a large cognitive component in his social learning theory. Once this procedure of learning is fully engaged, it can be considered a process of *self-efficacy* in learning. For years, Bandura (1977, 1997; Benight & Bandura, 2004) has focused his theoretical explorations and research writings on self-efficacy, a social cognitive process of bringing about behavioral change as a result of the modeling learning process and positive perspectives through self-affirmation. Bandura (1977) presents four principal sources of information that are a basis of efficacy expectations from various types of modeling (Table 2-7). As you are reading Table 2-7, think of various examples from your life that illustrate Bandura's concepts and methods, in addition to those provided here.

The social aspects of the examples provided indicate the linkage between the concepts of modeling and of self-efficacy in social learning theory. From Bandura's outline of sources and general examples of self-efficacy, an assumption can be formulated that social modeling is an integral part of the self-efficacy processes, illustrating the social cognitive development in social learning (1977).

In the process of explaining social learning theory, Bandura (1973) studied aggression and violence and their sources in the realm of modeling, such as television and cinema. He has lectured on terrorism,

inhumanities, and other ways that people's psychological and social politics are in denial of moral aspects regarding their inhumane actions. Up to this point, the discussion of social participation has focused on the positive aspects of human interaction. Bandura raises and studies the far-reaching consequences of the influences of violence and aggression modeled in public by actors in dramas. His 1997 book on self-efficacy stressed the exercise of control. On the other hand, it has been pointed out that, in most shows and movies, negative behavior is punished and that this modeling does not reinforce aggression and violence. This discrepancy of viewpoints can be discussed in your class.

More recently, Bandura has expanded his construct of social learning theory to incorporate an emphasis on *social cognitive theory* (Benight & Bandura, 2004). In looking at the role of perceived self-efficacy to work with post-traumatic recovery, such as traumatization in military combat or by natural disaster, terrorist attack, sexual and physical assault, and spousal loss, cognitive dimensions are paramount. Bandura perceives that understanding the place of cognitive self-efficacy and social support can assist in the transition to recovery of an individual's beliefs in his or her ability to have some degree of control over the toll of trauma in his or her life.

Another theorist, Vygotsky (1978) has reinforced Bandura's social learning and cognitive theory with his work on the construct of *social developmental theory.* Vygotsky's belief is that social interaction is basic for the development of human cognition; that human functions develop through external, interpsychological observation of others by a child, and then within the child intrapsychologically by intrapersonal integration of potential functions. For example, a child can watch how his or her parents cooperate when solving family problems. Then, the child uses cognition to absorb how to imitate this behavior at his or her level with his or her current abilities of interaction.

The Construct of Social Capital

A brief introduction to the construct of *social capital* will be provided here, with a more in depth discussion to follow in later chapters. Social capital as a construct is historically spread out over time in secondary references dating back to 1916 with the original references lost. Sporadic references merged over the years without continuous follow-up, so the origin is difficult to trace or to ascribe to a single author (Dekker & Uslander, 2001; Field, 2003).

At this point, we can differentiate between two commonplace definitions of the construct of *social capital* as being global or circumscribed in scope. To some, social capital is the everyday social interaction in the daily lives of people with family, friends, neighbors, and workers. To others, social capital, in its global denotation, is the formal networking and outreach to people with potential for shared cultural, religious, political, and economic interests beyond one's daily interaction. It could be interpreted as both.

The construct of *social capital* and *social convoys* will be addressed in Chapter 6. As a parallel to economic capital, social capital may be understood as a resource to be directed toward solving problems of society, such as caregiving of the elderly while remaining at home through community volunteers organized by a church, synagogue, or temple.

Social Emotional Learning

Professionals involved in preschool, school-based, and private practice systems have been acquainted for years with the social participation construct of SEL (Guttman, McCreedy, & Heisler, 2004). It incorporates numerous programs in various educational systems across the country and may be described as processes through which children and adults can develop emotional and social strategies to become aware of and regulate emotions, develop perceptions of others' needs, grow cooperative relationships, problem-solve appropriate decisions, and respond to demanding environments with insight (Cohen, 2006; Cohen & Devine, 2007; Zins, et al., 2007; Zins, Weissberg, Wang, & Walberg, 2004). These skills will be described in Chapter 4.

Meanwhile, various SEL-related programs are introduced on the internet, including the following:

- CASEL—Collaborative for Academic, Social, and Emotional Learning
- National School Climate Center
- CSEFEL—Center on Social and Emotional Foundations for Early Learning
- Caring School Community
- SEL—Illinois Learning Standards for Social/Emotional Learning
- PATHS—Promoting Alternative Thinking Strategies
- The Reggio Emilia Program
- UNICEF
- What Works Clearinghouse

The overall process of education about Social Emotional Learning is of vital understanding to those working with children as therapists, clinicians, and teachers in the general system and in special education systems.

Summary

Social participation theory, with its roots in developmental theory, has grown over the years and is still growing. Both social and theoretical aspects are abstract and need to be anchored in concepts that are agreed upon by professors, researchers, and practitioners. As society follows the trend of socialization of its young by institutions beyond the family, service professionals having a grasp of the foundations of social participation is essential. The subsequent chapters in this text expand on the theories of social participation presented here and build on the basic concepts heuristically, as they lead us to new horizons.

Script: Family Therapy Session

(Adapted from an unpublished novel, *Crystal Clear*, by Marilyn B. Cole)

Seating Chart

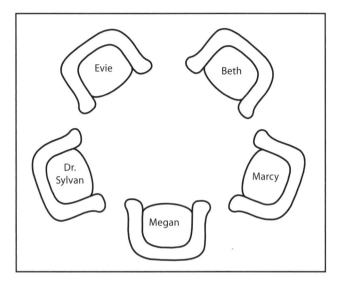

Characters and Background

Evie: (age 24) Evie had an illegitimate daughter (Valerie) at age 15 and was diagnosed with schizophrenia at age 16. Misled by a con-man boyfriend (Mackie), she forged her mother's signature and withdrew a large sum of money from her retirement account. Evie is also a talented artist and has been selling her paintings through an art dealer named Bartel Davidson.

Marcy: (age 28) She is an occupational therapist at Oceanview Day Treatment Center, where Evie was court ordered to be treated for schizophrenia until her trial. Marcy is aware that Evie is imagining an intimate relationship with Bartel that doesn't actually exist.

Megan: (age 30) Evie's older sister, married to a Berkeley professor, has twins age 7, and the adopted Valerie, now 10.

Beth: (age 52) Evie and Megan's mother, Valerie's grandmother.

Dr. Sylvan: (age 45) Female director of Oceanview and a family therapist.

Only Evie and Marcy have arrived. The following conversation occurs in private, while waiting for the others.

Marcy: *(looking concerned)* Evie, is it true what your sister said about Bartel? Are you sleeping with him?

Evie: We're not having sex, if that's what you mean.

Marcy: What exactly is going on between the two of you?

Evie: I asked him to stay over with me. It was only one weekend, and he was great with Valerie. Megan had no right to say any of those things. *(Just thinking about it made Evie feel angry; how could her sister make such a beautiful relationship seem so wrong?)*

Marcy: Bartel isn't there with you all the time, is he?

Evie: No. He had plans this week. But he's coming back.

Marcy: When?

Evie: I don't know. Saturday, maybe. *(Evie smiled thinking of Bartel)*

Marcy: He's kind of old for you. He must be pushing 40.

Evie: Why does that matter? He loves me.

Marcy: Did he say that?

Evie: He didn't have to. I just know.

Marcy: *(alarmed)* Evie, I don't think you understand.

Evie: What? *(An awkward silence)*

Marcy: Look, no matter what your relationship is, or will be, with Bartel, you can't bring it up at the meeting today. If you do, you may as well forget about seeing Valerie.

Evie: Why? What do you mean?

Marcy: Maybe you should try to think of it from Megan's point of view. She's trying to protect Valerie from what she sees as a bad situation. That's her job as a mother.

Evie: You think I'm in a bad situation?

Marcy: No, Evie. I don't think that. But I think the session will go better for you if you can show Megan that you understand her role as a mother to Valerie.

Evie: But I'm her mother. Why can't she live with me now?

Marcy: Evie, please listen. I'm telling you this to help you. If you want to be a part of Valerie's life, you have to set aside any real or imagined relationship with Bartel other than as your art agent. You also have to show Megan that you're willing to share the role of mother. Megan has taken care of Valerie for 9 years. You can't expect her to just hand her over. You have to go into this session with an open mind. Listen to your sister's point of view.

Evie: Okay, I'll try.

Marcy: Good girl, and, remember, don't speak of any special relationship with Bartel. In fact, it would be better if you called him Mr. Davidson.

Evie: *(repeated, as if rehearsing)* Mr. Davidson. If I do that, do you think Megan will let Valerie live with me?

Marcy: Not permanently. But you'll be able to see her more often, maybe on weekends and school vacations. That's the best you can hope for today.

(Dr. Sylvan enters the room with Megan and Beth)

Evie: *(pleading with Marcy)* Are you staying for the meeting?

Marcy: Yes. I volunteered to be cotherapist. One of our students is covering my group.

(Evie stood and greeted her mother and sister; they took their seats)

Dr. Sylvan: Marcy has told me such good things about you, Evie. Why don't you summarize your progress since you left Oceanview?

Evie: So much has happened since then that I hardly know where to begin.

Dr. Sylvan: *(kindly)* Tell us how the trial turned out.

Evie: They found me not guilty, but I'll have to testify against Mackie.

(Dr. Sylvan looks confused)

Beth: Her accomplice. The police are still looking for him, and the bank and insurance company are still debating about how much money I'll recover.

Dr. Sylvan: Some legal issues are still pending, then.

(Evie nods)

Marcy: *(redirected)* Tell Dr. Sylvan about your art career.

Evie: I have my own studio now, and Bar-, I mean, Mr. Davidson has been selling my paintings in his galleries. He's arranging a special showing for my paintings in his New York gallery in January.

Dr. Sylvan: That's wonderful, Evie! *(Dr. Sylvan turns to Beth and Megan)* You must be so proud. We all knew she was talented, but even without the problems Evie has, not many artists achieve so much so quickly. Evie, you are Oceanview's best success story yet.

Evie: *(smiles, welcoming the compliment)* I guess.

Dr. Sylvan: *(looks at each of them expectantly)* What is it that brings us together today?

Marcy: *(to Evie)* Tell us about Valerie.

Evie: Valerie came to stay with me last weekend. She wanted to come back, but my sister doesn't want her to. She knows I'm her mother now, but she's hardly ever seen me. I thought maybe she could stay with me for awhile.

Dr. Sylvan: I don't remember discussing Evie's daughter when she was a patient here.

Megan: Perhaps we didn't discuss Valerie during my sister's family sessions then, but that was almost 2 years ago. Valerie will be 10 in March. Richard and I thought it was time she knew the truth. She knew she was adopted, but only a week ago we told her that Evie is her real mother. We explained that Evie was only 15 when Valerie was born and that she was very sick afterwards, so that's why Mom suggested that Richard and I adopt her.

Marcy: Valerie didn't take the news very well. She responded by running away from home and ended up on Evie's doorstep.

Beth: The child was obviously shocked by the news. Who wouldn't be? Megan and Richard are the only mother and father she's ever known.

Dr. Sylvan: What about the child's biological father? What does he think?

Megan: Evie didn't even know who the father was. No one came forward at the time of her birth. Whoever he was, he didn't want anything to do with Evie once he found out that she was schizophrenic.

Evie: Okay, so that's ancient history. Now, things are different. I have my own place now. I don't see why she can't live with me.

Megan: *(sighs)* So many reasons, Evie.

Evie: Like what?

Megan: First of all, she needs stability. You're asking her to leave her school, all her friends, and the only home and family she's ever known. Just the fact that I have to explain all this tells me you haven't a clue what her needs are.

Evie: But…

Marcy: *(interrupts)* Hold on, Evie. Hear your sister out before you start arguing. Megan, tell us about your other concerns.

Megan: Secondly, my sister has schizophrenia. She may be doing okay right now, but she has a chronic disease. None of us knows when she's going to have another episode, and it's always worse when she's under stress. Her trial ended just 2 weeks ago, and there'll be another one when they find Mackie. What's going to happen then? And that's not even considering the stress involved in taking care of a child.

Marcy: Go on. I want Evie to hear all the reasons.

Megan: Thirdly, she can barely take care of herself, let alone anyone else. Marcy, don't you have to help her every week, doing her shopping, managing her money?

Marcy: Yes, I do help her with those things. As an occupational therapist, I provide the structure she needs so that she can keep on painting. Without producing paintings, Evie couldn't make enough money to pay her expenses.

Megan: *(smirking)* And who pays you to help Evie?

Marcy: Mr. Davidson pays me. He considers it a part of his investment in Evie as an artist. And he's right. With my help, Evie is flourishing as an artist.

Megan: Which brings me to my fourth objection. What about Mr. Davidson? Valerie led me to believe he and Evie had a more intimate relationship.

Evie: *(making eye contact with Marcy)* That's not true.

Megan: Then what was he doing in your home on a Sunday morning, little sister? And why is my daughter calling him Bartel?

Evie: *(without batting an eyelash)* He came to visit, to discuss my new paintings. And I've worked for him for almost 2 years now. Why shouldn't I call him Bartel?

Megan: *(sarcastic)* Why do you think he paid for your defense at the trial? Was that part of your work agreement, too?

Marcy: In fairness to Evie, let me say something. I work for Mr. Davidson, too. And I know that he goes to great lengths to protect all of his clients. He's well aware of Evie's illness, and he's doing his part to keep it under control.

Megan: And buying her a Christmas tree? Cooking dinner? Are those for my sister's protection?

Marcy: *(keeping her voice even)* Sometimes, he goes the extra mile for his clients, but his intentions are always honorable and above board. Are there any other concerns you'd like to discuss?

Megan: That's all I can think of right now.

(There is an awkward silence; Evie shifts nervously in her seat)

Dr. Sylvan: What about you, Mrs. O'Connor? What are your thoughts on where Valerie should stay?

Beth: I do understand Megan's objections, but there must be some way for Evie to spend time with Valerie, especially since she wants to so badly. Did you know the child actually packed a suitcase and got a ride to Evie's studio on her own, without her parents knowing? And you should have seen the fuss she made when Megan wouldn't allow her to go back with Evie after Christmas.

Megan: My mother reminded me on the drive in this morning that Valerie may be young, but she's always had a mind of her own. *(Megan's tone softened)* If I didn't know better, I'd say she took after me.

Evie: *(brightening)* You know, Megan, I said the same thing to Valerie while we were Christmas shopping. She made her list and kept track of the money. I told her she reminded me of you.

Megan: I'm impressed that you noticed, little sis. Maybe there's hope for you yet.

Marcy: *(winked at Evie)* Let me ask you this, Mrs. O'Connor. What might be a possible compromise regarding Valerie?

Beth: *(thought a moment)* What if Valerie could visit Evie on weekends? Often, Evie comes to my house on Saturdays for dinner. Maybe Valerie could come too, and they both could stay the night and spend Sunday with me?

Megan: I'd consider that idea. Then, you could keep them out of trouble.

Marcy: How does that sound to you, Evie?

Evie: *(beaming)* Can we start today?

Megan: I guess tomorrow would be okay.

Marcy: *(looking relieved)* Maybe Evie could do a portrait of Valerie for you and Richard.

Evie: I've already done the sketches for one.

The End.

Discussion

1. How was Evie's life course disrupted by her pregnancy?

2. Which theories discussed in this chapter apply to this scenario and why?

3. What level of social development do you think Evie demonstrates (referring to Erikson, Gough, others)?

4. What mental health services do you observe being used by this family?

5. What manifestations of the application of social capital do this family exhibit?

6. What conflicts can you identify in this scenario and how were they addressed/resolved?

7. How could Evie benefit from exposure to social-emotional learning?

8. What level of group interaction (referring to Parten, Mosey, Donohue) does this session represent and why?

References

Bandura, A. (1973). *Aggression: A social learning analysis.* Englewood Cliffs, NJ: Prentice-Hall.

Bandura, A. (1977). *Social learning theory.* New York, NY: General Learning Press.

Bandura, A. (1997). *Self-efficacy: The exercise of control.* New York, NY: Freeman.

Benight, C. C., & Bandura, A. (2004). Social cognitive theory of posttraumatic recovery: The role of perceived self-efficacy. *Behaviour Research and Therapy, 42,* 1129-1148.

Burns, N., & Grove, S. K. (2009). *The practice of nursing research. Conduct, critique and utilization* (6th ed.). Philadelphia, PA: W. B. Saunders.

Cohen, J. (Ed.). (2004). *Caring classrooms/intelligent schools: The social emotional education of young children.* New York, NY: Columbia University, Teachers College Press.

Cohen, J. (2006). Social, emotional, ethical and academic education. Creating a climate for learning participation in democracy and well-being. *Harvard Education Review, 76,* 201-237.

Cohen, J., & Devine, J. (2007). *Making your school safe: Strategies to protect children and promote learning.* New York, NY: Columbia University, Teachers College Press.

Dekker, P., & Uslander, E. M. (Eds.). (2001). *Social capital and participation in everyday life.* New York, NY: Routledge ECPR.

Donohue, M. V. (1999). Theoretical bases of Mosey's group interactions skills. *Occupational Therapy International, 6,* 35-51.

Donohue, M. V. (2003). Group profile studies with children: Validity measures and item analysis. *Occupational Therapy in Mental Health, 19,* 1-23.

Donohue, M. V. (2005). Social profile: Assessment of validity and reliability in children's groups. *Canadian Journal of Occupational Therapy, 62,* 164-175.

Donohue, M. V. (2007). Social profile: Interrater reliability in psychiatric and community activity groups. *Australian Occupational Therapy Journal, 54,* 49-58.

Erikson, E. H. (1950). *Childhood and society.* New York, NY: W. W. Norton.

Field, J. (2003). *Social capital.* New York, NY: Routledge Taylor & Francis Group.

Gliner, J. A., & Morgan, G. A. (2000). *Research methods in applied settings. An integrated approach to design and analysis.* Mahwah, NJ: Lawrence Erlbaum.

Gough, H. G. (1957). California psychological inventory (CPI). *Administrator's guide.* Palo Alto, CA: Consulting Psychologists Press.

Guttman, S. A., McCreedy, P., & Heisler, P. (2004). The psychosocial deficits of children with regulatory disorders; Identification and treatment. *Occupational Therapy in Mental Health, 20,* 1-32.

Lifton, W. M. (1966). *Working with groups: Group process and individual growth.* New York, NY: John Wiley.

Mosey, A. C. (1968). Recapitulation of ontogenesis: A theory for practice of occupational therapy. *American Journal of Occupational Therapy, 22,* 426-438.

Mosey, A. C. (1986). *Psychosocial components of occupational therapy.* New York, NY: Raven Press.

Parten, M. B. (1932). Social participation among pre-school children. *Journal of Abnormal and Social Psychology, 27,* 243-269.

Portney, L. G., & Watkins, M. P. (2009). *Foundations of clinical research. Applications to practice* (3rd ed.). Upper Saddle River, NJ: Pearson Prentice Hall.

United Nations General Assembly. (December 10, 1948). *Universal Declaration of Human Rights,* Resolution 217 A (III).

United Nations General Assembly. (December, 1993). *Standard rules for the equalization of opportunities for persons with disabilities.* 85th Plenary Meeting, A/Res/48/96.

Vygotsky, L. S. (1978). *Mind in society.* Cambridge, MA: Harvard University Press.

World Health Organization. (2001). *International classification of functioning, disability, and health (ICF).* Geneva, Switzerland: Author.

Zins, J. E., Elias, M. J., & Maher, C. A. (Eds.). (2007). *Bullying, victimization, and peer harassment. A handbook of prevention and intervention.* Binghamton, NY: Haworth Press.

Zins, J. E., Weissberg, R. P., Wang, M. C., & Walberg, H. J. (Eds.). (2004). *Building academic success on social and emotional learning: What does the research say?* New York, NY: Columbia University, Teachers College Press.

Additional Resources

Center for Social Emotional Education. (2008). Retrieved from www.schoolclimate.org

Collaborative for Academic, Social and Emotional Learning. (2010). Retrieved from www.schoolclimate.org

Illinois State Board of Education. (2008). *Illinois learning standards. Social/emotional learning.* Retrieved from www.isbe.net/ils/social_emotional/standards.htm

Reggio Emilia Program. (n.d.). Retrieved from www.reggioemiliaapproach.net

chapter 3

Social Participation Basics

Marilyn B. Cole, MS, OTR/L, FAOTA

This how-to chapter reviews some basic communication skills for dyadic and group interaction, including verbal and nonverbal communication, asking questions, connecting with others, giving and receiving support, assertiveness, emotional expression, and dealing with problems and conflicts. All of these skills apply in the roles people choose or find themselves playing in their everyday lives. This review forms the basis for analyzing social situations and identifying social behaviors that either facilitate or create barriers to participation.

Social groups in real life are seldom perfect. While everyone wishes to have perfect parents and families, ideal educational experiences, and welcoming and supporting communities within which to work and play, people (with or without a disability) often face problems that interfere with social participation. Each chapter in this book ends with a script of an everyday social group situation, which will illustrate some of the problems encountered and will serve as a basis for analysis and discussion. The social skill areas presented here offer some specific guidelines for application in everyday life as well as in professional practice.

Nonverbal Behaviors

Communication, learned from infancy, begins without the use of language. Facial expression, gestures and body language, and cries of hurt or joy form the most basic level of nonverbal communication. As people develop, they incorporate these nonverbal behaviors into their social interactions, and they convey the emotional tone and meaning of their words. Parents read the meaning of their children's nonverbal behaviors in order to meet basic needs; children, likewise, learn to read their parents' facial expression and tone of voice in order to gauge the feelings behind them: "Mommy's really mad at me" or "Daddy's in a bad mood."

For adults, reading nonverbal expressions becomes second nature and is often taken for granted. In many situations, while social norms dictate how and when people can express their emotions in words, nonverbal behaviors remain the best way to recognize how people truly feel. For practice, try the exercise in Table 3-1. Later in the chapter, nonverbal expression will be used in the reflection of empathy.

What attributes of nonverbal communication were used to convey emotion in the above exercise? Facial expression and body movements or gestures may be the most obvious, but, in real life, nonverbal expression includes not only emotion but other aspects of social interaction such as intentions, expectations, judgments, and openness to others. This process is exceedingly complex. Table 3-2 lists some of the ways people communicate nonverbally. Practice your skills of nonverbal observation by filling in column 3 with some possible social interpretations for the examples given in column 2. The first example in each category is interpreted as a guideline.

There are many possible ways to interpret each of the above examples, depending on the interaction

Cole, M.B., & Donohue, M.V. *Social Participation in Occupational Contexts: In Schools, Clinics, and Communities* (pp 43-66).
© 2011 SLACK Incorporated

Table 3-1

RECOGNIZING AND NAMING EMOTIONS

Directions: Consider the following emotions: *pleased, bored, shocked, horrified, elated, miserable, passionate, relieved, embarrassed, ashamed, proud,* and *confident* (add others as needed). Think about a time when you have felt each of these emotions, and write a brief description of the situation. All emotions have different levels of intensity. Write three additional words that describe different levels of each emotion's intensity. These words will be used later when practicing the expression of empathy.

Group activity: Write the above words on index cards. Each member draws a card and takes a turn conveying the emotion on the card nonverbally. The group guesses the emotion, with or without a list of words from which to choose.

of the individual, the activity and its goal, and the social and cultural contexts of the specific situation. This interaction has been described in Baum and Christiansen's (2005) person-environment-occupation-performance model, affirming the influence of social as well as other contexts for an individual's ability to perform occupations. For individuals, the ability to accurately interpret the nonverbal behaviors of others forms a foundation for effective interaction with each other, either in dyads or groups, during the everyday experiences of social participation.

Attending

Attending describes how therapists demonstrate physical and emotional presence with a client (Egan, 2001). When establishing rapport, an effective therapist conveys unconditional positive regard as well as a readiness to listen to a client. Attending, as a skill, transcends any spoken words and nonverbally communicates how interested and emotionally available we are for another person. In everyday relationships, attending nonverbally through direct eye contact, a welcoming facial expression, and an open body position facing the person with whom we are speaking communicates an attitude of caring and acceptance.

Picking up on nonverbal social cues that communicate the opposite of attending is an equally important skill, as this signals us that someone's attention is focused elsewhere and he or she would not wish to be approached or engaged in conversation. Children notoriously ignore their parents' need to focus on a difficult task such as balancing the checkbook or listening to what someone is saying on the other end of the telephone, demanding their attention to ask a question or solve an immediate problem. A socially

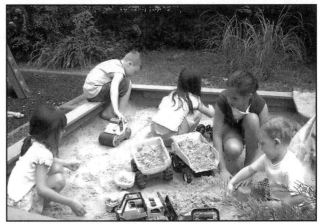

Figure 3-1. Parallel and beginning associative level group.

alert wife will carefully choose the right time to approach her husband about an important purchase or a new vacation plan, making sure she has his full attention. Employees do likewise when approaching their bosses about a problem situation at work. Such timing involves not only interpretation of nonverbal behaviors, but also social judgment. For example, when participating in a parallel group, members may have trouble deciding when to approach the leader with individual problems.

In Figure 3-1, children of different ages appear to be playing side by side in parallel fashion. However, upon closer inspection, Hannah, the child on the left, has a fist full of sand and, a few seconds later, will throw it at Evan, the boy at the rear of the sandbox, an inappropriate attempt to get his attention. A supervising adult might take this opportunity to suggest to Hannah some more appropriate ways to get attention from her peers—a valuable associative level social skill.

Table 3-2

MODES OF NONVERBAL COMMUNICATION

MODE OF EXPRESSION	EXAMPLES	SOCIAL INTERPRETATION
Facial expressions	Smiling	*Happy to see me. In a good mood.*
	Frowning	
	Smirking	
	Stone-faced	
	Other?	
Eye contact	Looking down	*Does not want to talk right now.*
	Eye to eye	
	Rolling eyes up	
	Looking into space	
	Eyes closed	
	Other?	
Sounds	Laughing	*Making fun of me. Not taking me seriously.*
	Crying	
	Screaming	
	Moaning	
	Other?	
Body position	Sitting up straight	*Alert and paying attention. Interested.*
	Sitting slouched	
	Turned away	
	Arms crossed	
	Fists clenched	
	Other?	
Body movement	Hands gesturing	*Excited about the topic. Seeking attention.*
	Hands clapping	
	Hugging someone	
	Patting on the back	
	Tapping feet	
	Other?	
Autonomic responses	Rapid breathing	*Anxious about something. Angry.*
	Blushing	
	Trembling/shaking	
	Sweating	
	Coughing	
	Other?	
Acting out responses	Walking away	*Not interested. Unable to deal with the situation.*
	Slamming the door	
	Pushing/shoving	
	Throwing/breaking something	
	Other?	

Table 3-3

SAMPLE EXPECTATIONS FOR PARALLEL LEVEL SOCIAL PARTICIPATION

COOPERATION IN GROUPS—MOST OF THE TIME, MEMBERS CAN:

- Participate without interfering with others.

GROUP NORMS—MOST OF THE TIME, MEMBERS CAN:

- Occupy themselves within their own space and their own materials.

GROUP ROLES—MEMBERS CAN:

- Engage in solitary activity with others in the room.

COMMUNICATION—MEMBERS DEMONSTRATE:

- Minimal verbal exchange.

ACTIVITY BEHAVIORS—MEMBERS CAN:

- Engage in activity in the presence of others without distraction.

POWER/LEADERSHIP OF GROUP—MEMBERS:

- Look to the leader to select activities to meet safety, love, and esteem needs.

MOTIVATION FOR ACTIVITY AND ATTRACTION TO THE GROUP—MEMBERS:

- Prefer focus on activities rather than peers.

Adapted from Donohue, M. V. (1999). Theoretical bases of Mosey's group interactions skills. *Occupational Therapy International, 6,* 35-51; Donohue, M. V. (2008). *Social profile goals.* Unpublished manuscript.

Nonverbal Learning in Parallel Groups

Because parallel groups involve mainly pre-group behaviors with minimal verbal interaction, communication occurs mainly in nonverbal form. For example, children may begin to notice the nonverbal behaviors of others while participating in a parallel play group. Each 3 year old may be happily focused on a different play task side by side with the others. But, consider what happens when Becky knocks over Johnny's block tower, then laughs when it falls. Johnny responds with a loud cry and throws a block at Becky. *What feeling was Johnny expressing nonverbally? What was Becky's intention—was it a mistake or deliberate? What rules of positive social behavior might be learned from this interaction? How should an adult supervisor handle this situation to facilitate positive social learning for both participants?*

An additional norm for the adult, whether parent, teacher, or therapist, when supervising groups of children (as well as adults with cognitive and emotional dysfunctions) would be to instill an expectation of respect for authority. At the parallel level of group interaction, the leader chooses age-appropriate activities for the group and sets the boundaries and ground rules. Breaches of the rules require leader intervention in order to preserve a safe and supportive social context for the group as a whole. *Left unsupervised, how might the interaction between Becky and Johnny in the above example result in negative social learning?* Within a simple encounter such as this during parallel play, children begin to observe the many nonverbal social nuances that will later influence their interpretations and behaviors in other social situations.

Some adult examples of parallel groups are attending a play or concert, taking notes during a lecture, following a leader's movements in an aerobics class, or praying together in a place of worship. Often, the activity itself, rather than the skill or maturity of the adult participants, determines the level of interaction. *What basic social skills are necessary to participate successfully in these groups?* Some expected behaviors for parallel groups are listed in Table 3-3. Member social behaviors common to most adult parallel groups include waiting turns, respecting space and belongings of others, respecting leader authority and group norms, and having the ability to engage in specified tasks without distracting or being distracted by other members.

In a parallel group, peers mainly interact with leaders, and this provides a good opportunity for learning when and how to ask the leader for help by recognizing nonverbal behaviors that indicate a readiness for solving individual problems.

Script for Nonverbal Communication

The Well Exercise

(A beginning exercise for actors—source unknown)

Directions: Working in pairs, students role play two different scenarios using the same words. The different meanings are conveyed only nonverbally, through facial expression, gestures and movements, and voice tone. While two people role play, the rest of the class fills out the observation worksheet below.

First role play: A and B are good friends who have had a falling out. A is angry at B, B is indifferent and aloof.

Second role play: A meets B in a singles bar. A wants to "hook up" with B. A is flirtatious and seductive toward B. B is not interested and is annoyed by A's advances.

Role Play #1	*Role Play #2*
A. *Well?*	A. *What do you want me to say?*
B. *Well, I'm here.*	B. *Nothing.*
A. *So I see...*	A. *Nothing?*
B. *Yes.*	B. *You don't trust me.*
A. *Well?*	A. *It's not that...*
B. *Is that all you can say?*	B. *Then what?*
A. *Never mind...*	A. *What's the matter?*
B. *Stop it.*	B. *I don't know.*
A. *What?*	A. *You don't know?*
B. *That!*	B. *No.*
A. *I can't...*	A. *Tell me!*
B. *Try.*	B. *I can't.*
A. *Is that better?*	A. *Then go.*
B. *This is hopeless.*	B. *I will.*

Nonverbal Behavior Observation Sheet

Listen to a short conversation, and write down your nonverbal observations for each participant.

Body language—emotions conveyed?
- Gestures, mannerisms
- Posture, head position
- Movements
- Other?

Eyes—emotions conveyed?
- Contact
- Movements
- Looking where
- Other?

Facial expression—emotions conveyed?
- Eyes and eyebrows
- Nose
- Mouth
- Other?

Tone of voice—emotions conveyed?
- Pitch
- Speed
- Attitude
- Other?

Autonomic—emotions conveyed?
- Breathing
- Blushing
- Perspiration
- Trembling
- Other?

Verbal Communication

By age 2, children can usually communicate in single words and short phrases and no longer need to rely on nonverbal methods such as crying or acting out to get their needs met. As speech continues to develop, children expand their verbal interactions beyond basic needs, increasingly using words and sentences as a way to learn, exchange information, and form relationships with others. However, verbal expression in no way negates the importance of nonverbal communication. Throughout life, nonverbal expression of all types continues to elucidate and enrich our words, infusing them with emotional tone and meaning. In order to better understand the

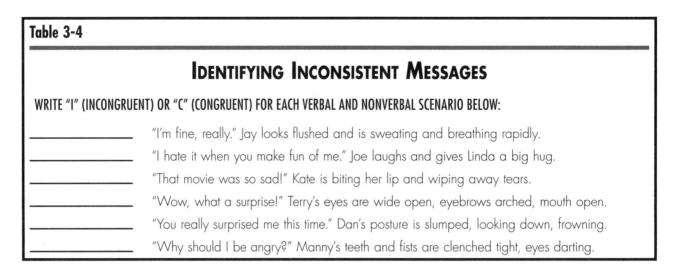

Table 3-4

IDENTIFYING INCONSISTENT MESSAGES

WRITE "I" (INCONGRUENT) OR "C" (CONGRUENT) FOR EACH VERBAL AND NONVERBAL SCENARIO BELOW:

_____   "I'm fine, really." Jay looks flushed and is sweating and breathing rapidly.

_____   "I hate it when you make fun of me." Joe laughs and gives Linda a big hug.

_____   "That movie was so sad!" Kate is biting her lip and wiping away tears.

_____   "Wow, what a surprise!" Terry's eyes are wide open, eyebrows arched, mouth open.

_____   "You really surprised me this time." Dan's posture is slumped, looking down, frowning.

_____   "Why should I be angry?" Manny's teeth and fists are clenched tight, eyes darting.

verbal skills needed for successful social participation, both with individuals and in groups, verbalizations are categorized here according to their purpose, including asking questions, connecting with others, expressing assertiveness, resolving problems and conflicts, and taking on leadership roles.

Listening

After asking a question, it becomes necessary to listen to the response. Careful listening involves the use of both auditory and visual senses. Hearing someone's words does not always lead to understanding the answer to our question. Attending with both eyes and ears to the nonverbal cues, such as tone of voice and facial expression, as well as other aspects described earlier, add significantly to the full meaning of the response. According to Michael P. Nichols, who wrote the book *The Lost Art of Listening*, who we are and what we say triggers other people's response to us (1995). That response and our connection to others remain vital to our psychological well-being.

People who seek to improve their listening skills can borrow some principles from the literature of psychotherapy. As experts in listening to the verbal and nonverbal messages of clients, therapists cite three general purposes for therapeutic listening: (1) to take in information, (2) to bear witness to another's expression and experience, and (3) to recognize the individual as a unique person. Effective listening can have the following outcomes in the therapy process:

* To understand spoken messages

* To strengthen relationships

* To respond to the basic human need of wanting to be understood

* To allow a client to discover himself or herself as understandable and acceptable

* To acknowledge, to take interest, to appreciate others

* To formulate an empathic response

While not everyone aspires to be a therapist, the above goals or outcomes can easily be generalized to everyday conversations with family, friends, or others with whom we seek a trusting or intimate relationship. In order to truly listen and grasp what another person is communicating, an effective listener also considers the context of the conversation and how the messages relate to the respondent's life. A therapist listens for both congruent (matching) and incongruent messages. A genuine response is reflected when both the verbal expressions and nonverbal messages match. For example, a client talks about his loss of functioning following a car accident and shows appropriate sadness in his voice tone and facial expressions. This is an example of a congruent message. Contrast this example with the same client who is discussing loss of functioning and laughs and makes jokes about what an invalid he has become. This represents an incongruent message. Consider the list of verbal comments and their accompanying observable behaviors and characteristics in Table 3-4.

Carl Rogers (1961) emphasized that therapists need to temporarily put aside their own "self" in order to enter the world of the client. Therapeutic listening includes the temporary suspension of one's own personal needs and wants for a designated period of time to fully attend to another. Listening can truly be a gift that we exchange as human beings. It is also natural for people to be "imperfect" in our listening attempts. Here is a list of possible obstacles that could interfere with a therapist's ability to therapeutically listen. *Which of the following might apply also in a person's social relationships?*

- × Prejudgment or assumptions based on the diagnosis, prior experiences, team member's reports, etc

- × Prejudice regarding gender, race, religion, or socioeconomic status

- × Over- or underidentification with the client

- × Rehearsing answers while the client (other person) is presently talking to you

- × Time restraints

- × Preoccupation with personal problems

- × Feelings of boredom, disinterest, depreciation of the client (or other person)

- × Personal illness and physical discomfort

- × Emotional reactions to what the client (or other person) is saying, such as defensiveness or self-righteousness, that are personal rather than professional

- × Fearfulness or anger toward the client (or other person)

Suppose your friend Matt calls you, very upset about a recent argument with his parents. *Which of the above factors might interfere with listening to his story with your full attention?* Now, imagine yourself at work, being called into the boss's office to discuss some problems with your job performance. *Which factors might prevent you from listening to what the boss is saying?*

Active Listening

Active listening has the intent of listening for meaning. Aside from therapy, active listening has been incorporated into many adult interpersonal training programs, such as parent effectiveness, facilitating managers' supervision of employees, social support group leadership, and peer counseling programs. Listening actively implies that the listener engages the speaker through verbal and nonverbal responses that indicate an understanding of the message being conveyed (Robertson, 2005). *How do you know when someone is listening to you? When you are speaking to Sally, is she facing you with an open, relaxed posture? Leaning toward you? Looking at you? Nodding her head with a facial expression that reflects the emotional as well as factual content of your words?* These would represent some nonverbal reactions of a good active listener. While people don't always notice the specific nonverbal responses of a listener, they usually have an immediate unconscious effect upon the speaker. Active listening encourages the speaker to continue making his point or telling her story, facilitates elaboration, and encourages deeper self-disclosure. Passive listening produces the opposite outcome. *For*

example, what might you do if while you are telling Sally a personal story, she turns away from you and stares out the window? How would you feel if Sally's facial expression remained passive and apathetic rather than interested and empathetic? Passive listening usually creates barriers to continued or deepening communication.

Active listening generally facilitates communication through both nonverbal and verbal responses. Two types of verbal responses are *prompts* and *open questions*. Prompts might be simple verbalizations such as "uh huh," "I see," or "go on." These give minimal interruption to the speaker while encouraging continued verbal disclosure. Prompts also reflect the emotional content of messages, such as "oh, dear," "wow!" "how disappointing," or "that's great," said with matching gestures and facial expressions. Additionally, prompts ask for further elaboration, such as "meaning what?" "for instance?" or "give me an example." Open questions asked by the listener, whether starting new aspects ("How did things turn out last time this happened?") or clarifying current topics ("How did this problem begin?") further facilitate continued communication by showing interest and concern for the speaker. These responses might come naturally to experienced listeners and may be taken for granted by people who are speaking. Clearly, active listening can be a useful skill for many different areas of social participation.

When friends respond to each other with active listening, trust develops between them and their relationship deepens and becomes more intimate. When parents actively listen to their children, they facilitate communication while at the same time modeling an effective social skill. This deepens the parent-child relationship, establishes or re-establishes trust that may have been lost, and increases the chances of children reciprocating by actively listening to their parents.

Active listening on the part of group leaders parallels the facilitation of communication for all the members, through the same process of social learning that applies to parents with their children. When therapists model the skill of active listening in a group session, they establish an important therapeutic norm. As group members practice active listening with other members, they begin to facilitate the development of group trust, one of the main characteristics of which therapists have called "group cohesiveness." Cohesiveness is a desirable outcome for many groups in everyday life. For example, social participation is more satisfying and meaningful with groups of friends who truly care about one another. Cohesive work teams cooperate better, make better business decisions, and produce more satisfactory

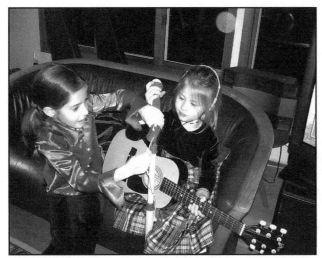

Figure 3-2. Hannah spontaneously helps Noelle to mount her karaoke microphone, a good example of associative level behavior.

outcomes than noncohesive groups (Reich & Wood, 2003). However, the achievement of group cohesiveness also requires additional characteristics and leader facilitation skills, which will be discussed in a later section of this chapter.

Verbal Learning at the Associative Group Level

Children naturally participate in associative peer groups from about age 2, coinciding with the development of beginning verbal communication. These groups can form spontaneously on playgrounds, parks, or neighborhood backyards and are usually at least minimally supervised by parents, caregivers, teachers, or other adults for reasons of safety and boundaries of fair play.

Verbal interactions in this context may be minimal and naturally center upon the toys (a brightly colored ball) or games (jump rope) that children bring with them or equipment that is available (swings, jungle gym). Unlike the parallel group, clusters of two or three children interact together, throwing or kicking a ball to each other or taking turns pushing each other on the swing. Participants express the wish to get the attention of each other ("Now it's my turn.") or might willingly offer to share a treasured toy ("Now it's your turn."). With assistance of a supervising adult, children may ask each other's names and offer to share a slice of stale bread for feeding the pigeons. They may demonstrate techniques for the feeding, breaking bread into small pieces, throwing them all at once or one at a time, seeing what works best, laughing together when the birds steal bread from each other or catch pieces of bread in the air (Figure 3-2).

Table 3-5

SAMPLE EXPECTATIONS FOR SOCIAL PARTICIPATION IN ASSOCIATIVE LEVEL GROUPS

COOPERATION—MEMBERS CAN:

- Begin to share and cooperate briefly when others approach.

GROUP NORMS—MEMBERS CAN:

- Participate in some joint activities.

GROUP ROLES—MEMBERS CAN:

- Participate in activities/games briefly for a few minutes.

COMMUNICATION—MEMBERS CAN:

- Focus on verbal or nonverbal, formal or informal communication around a task.

ACTIVITY BEHAVIORS—MEMBERS:

- Select activities that attract peers.

POWER/LEADERSHIP OF THE GROUP—MEMBERS CAN:

- Respond when the leader reinforces norms and encourages sharing.

MOTIVATION FOR THE ACTIVITY AND ATTRACTION TO THE GROUP—MEMBERS CAN:

- Perceive joint, brief games and tasks as attractive.

Adapted from Donohue, M. V. (2008). *Social profile goals.* Unpublished manuscript.

Verbalization in associative level groups centers around the activity or occupation of the participants. For children, this may take the form of expressions of courtesy, such as saying, "I'm sorry," when a violated social norm has hurt or upset another member. Adult supervisors of children's groups have ample opportunity to facilitate social learning in associative level groups, such as encouraging them to express emotions with words instead of nonverbally, to use courtesy (please and thank you), and to ask rather than demand attention from the leader or peers (Table 3-5).

Examples of adult groups at the associative level may be found in the community, such as making craft items to sell, preparing and serving food at a local charity event, or learning a specific skilled craft, such as woodworking or needlepoint, in adult education. While the activity calls for primarily individual occupational performance, adults verbally ask for or offer help to each other, ask for or offer advice, discuss procedures for completion of the task, and participate in problem solving with an identified leader. Leaders can model active listening to gain a full understanding of social situations when problem solving with individuals or subgroups, a strategy that can facilitate reaching a consensus.

When therapists assist adult clients with community reintegration, the skills and behaviors listed in Table 3-5 can prepare the client for social participation at the associative group level. Clients with acquired cognitive disabilities, such as those caused by stroke or traumatic brain injury, may need to begin with associative level community groups where social participation can be practiced by watching and imitating the leader or other adult members without negative consequences. The feedback provided by other group members can give clients needed self-awareness about how their social interaction skills may have changed and what new learning may be necessary in order to participate successfully in higher level groups.

Connecting With Others

People need increasingly complex social competencies in order to maintain meaningful relationships with others and to effectively participate in cooperative, supportive, and mature groups. From a systems perspective, social participation involves the interaction of personal skills and behaviors, occupational and activity demands, and all of the environmental contexts within which social participation occurs (Baum & Christiansen, 2005). This section focuses on personal skills and competencies that individuals can learn and practice for the purposes of increasing the likelihood of successful social participation, while also considering both the level of intimacy with individuals and the level of group interaction as social contexts that either facilitate or discourage participation. Areas covered are getting to know someone new, awareness of social identity, forming attachments and trust, expressing empathy, and giving and receiving social support.

Getting to Know Someone New

Several studies have been conducted on how long it takes for people to form a "first impression." While the outcomes are varied, with some studies showing it only takes 7 seconds and others showing a more conservative 30 seconds (Laidman, 2009), first impressions are significant to shaping relationships. These impressions can influence relationships in both positive and negative ways, including the possibility that people often make inaccurate judgments of each other (Bernieri, 2005). *How do you want to be remembered by someone who is meeting you for the first time, when all you have is half a minute?*

Appearance and First Impressions

In addition to nonverbal behaviors, other factors affecting first impressions include grooming and body cleanliness, appropriateness of clothing and accessories, hairstyle, and other characteristics of personal style. Although occupational therapists and other health professionals might consider self-care tasks to be solitary activities of daily living, the social context within which they are performed cannot be denied. Teenagers in high school often go to great pains to dress and wear their hair exactly like their peers in an attempt to fit in with specific social groups to which they wish to belong. Cultural norms dictate dress guidelines for specific social occupations or events, such as uniforms and athletic shoes for participation in sports, acceptable dress for attending religious events, weddings, funerals, concerts, or dining out in a restaurant. Members of social and cultural groups usually have a keen awareness of these unwritten codes of dress and appearance. They can also create barriers for people in some situations. For example, in the novel *Blindsided*, a renowned journalist and news producer returning to work after a difficult episode of multiple sclerosis refused to carry a cane, fearing the negative judgments of coworkers and supervisors (Cohen, 2005).

Additionally, people who choose to socialize outside of their usual culture need to think about what changes they should make in their personal style to avoid standing out, or worse, offending other members. Appearance and style guidelines usually include both positives (what to wear) and negatives (what not to wear). For clients who need assistance in making these judgments, therapists may need to discuss some of the specific requirements for their typical cultural events in order to facilitate social participation. For practice, fill in the style guidelines within your own culture in Table 3-6.

Asking Initial Questions

People ask questions in many situations and for many reasons. As people who watch the game show *Jeopardy* know, the key to winning is to ask the right questions. In many ways, the same is true in life. As a starting point, asking questions in order to meet one's needs and gain information requires two steps: (1) identifying the most likely source of information—the right person to ask—and (2) formulating the right question to get what you want or need.

Table 3-6

STYLE AND APPEARANCE WORKSHEET

EVENT	APPROPRIATE CLOTHING	STYLE FACTORS TO AVOID
Attending class		
Pizza party		
Wedding reception		
Religious event		
Grocery shopping		
Dinner at Grandma's		
Playing basketball		

Meeting Basic Needs

"Where can I get something to eat? Where is the rest room? How much does a bowl of soup cost?" The answers to these questions help to meet basic needs. The skill is not complicated, and adults take it for granted in familiar social environments. Yet, anyone who has traveled to a foreign country appreciates the importance of being able to make these simple questions understood. Even without the language barrier, emotions can get in the way of asking basic questions. Everyone remembers the joke about men who refuse to ask for directions while driving, even when hopelessly lost, or the woman in a designer clothing store who pays too much for a sweater because she's embarrassed to ask its price.

Getting Information

Teachers in public school recognize that children who ask questions have a natural curiosity that motivates them to learn. Outside of the classroom, learning what we want to know requires that we first identify who might have the right expertise to know the information we seek. For an allergic reaction, we might ask a doctor or pharmacist what medication to take. To fix a leaky faucet, we'd call a plumber or visit a local home improvement store. When the question involves beliefs or values as well as information, the social implications become more complicated. For example, a teenager new to his or her community might ask, "What can I do for fun around here?" Mom might suggest baking brownies or playing Frisbee with the dog in the backyard. A high school classmate might prefer sexual adventures or drug experimentation at a weekend party across town. Thus, the same question could have a very different answer depending on whom we ask.

Closed and Open Questions

Two types of questions are *closed* questions and *open* questions. Closed questions, which can be answered with a "yes" or "no," are most appropriate when seeking specific information. *Can you play tennis? Are you open for business? Will you vacuum the apartment this morning?* Questions requiring a brief, specific answer also fall into this category. *When can I make an appointment with the doctor? What is your telephone number or e-mail address? What time is the next train to New York? How old are you?* Closed questions, when used in conversation, tend to discourage communication because they do not require a detailed response. When speaking with strangers, this may meet the basic need for information, but when speaking with friends, open questions are preferable.

An open question cannot be answered by "yes" or "no," but requires a longer, more detailed answer. Therapists use open questions to encourage self-disclosure with clients. A friendly conversation may begin with, "What's new with you?" "How's the situation at work?" or "What are you going to do for your next vacation?" All of these questions require description and elaboration. Follow-up questions that ask for further detail or clarification serve to keep the conversation going. Building the skill of asking open questions will be addressed in the next section on social participation in a basic cooperative group.

Social Participation in a Basic Cooperative Group

School-age children often engage in cooperative groups that are organized by teachers, parents, coaches, and recreational leaders. Some examples

---

Table 3-7

SAMPLE SOCIAL EXPECTATIONS IN A BASIC COOPERATIVE GROUP

COOPERATION IN GROUPS—MEMBERS:

- Exhibit eagerness to play with and agree with other members on activities

GROUP NORMS—MEMBERS CAN:

- Act fairly in interaction with others

COMMUNICATION—MEMBERS CAN:

- Begin to express ideas and to problem-solve together

GROUP ROLES—MEMBERS CAN:

- Experiment with a variety of task roles

ACTIVITY BEHAVIORS—MEMBERS CAN:

- Sustain interest in longer projects, across days, then weeks

POWER/LEADERSHIP OF GROUP—MEMBERS CAN:

- Attempt to take on initial roles of leadership when encouraged by leader

MOTIVATION FOR THE ACTIVITY AND ATTRACTION TO THE GROUP—MEMBERS:

- Try to interest peers in preferred activities

Adapted from Donohue, M. V. (2008). *Social profile goals.* Unpublished manuscript.

---

might be playing board games, participating in team sports, singing in a choir, putting on a Christmas pageant at church, or performing in a school play. Each of these requires group members to perform different roles in order to reach an end goal as a group or compete to produce a winner. Participation in these basic cooperative groups is structured by the group activity, with occupational roles coordinated to produce a unified product, such as a concert, a performance, or a team competition with another group.

Groups of students within a classroom may be asked to work together on specific learning tasks that require them to interact with one another, divide up the work, solve a problem, or reach a consensus or a group decision. These groups provide excellent opportunities for social learning; modeling or imitating one another; and trying out roles of initiator, recorder, information seeker or giver, harmonizer, opinion seeker or giver, and other roles that relate to task accomplishment (Benne & Sheats, 1948, 1978).

Adult groups at the basic cooperative level can be found in many work settings, such as a business that must be operated by individuals with different job titles and tasks, communicating in structured ways, or interacting together to solve problems to keep the business running smoothly and to reach specific goals. Consider how these different businesses operate: a restaurant, a clothing store, a travel agency, a car dealership, or a bank. Some community organizations structure groups in similar ways in order to accomplish specific tasks or to perform specific services (e.g., volunteer committees following pre-set guidelines for neighborhood fundraising or voter registration). Social interaction may occur informally while performing tasks, but, at this level, task accomplishment takes precedence over socialization (Table 3-7).

Asking another person questions about him- or herself lays the groundwork for forming meaningful relationships. When meeting someone for the first time at a social gathering, we might ask general questions with the purpose of finding something in common with him or her. The best conversation starters are open questions that cannot be answered with just one word. If Bob asked his new neighbor, "Where are you from?" then "Florida" might be the single word answer. Instead, Bob could ask, "How did you come to live next door?" This open question can lead in many different

Table 3-8

ASKING OPEN QUESTIONS

Directions: For each situation listed in the first column, write an open question that further defines or explores the main concern being expressed.

The hostess, near the end of a dinner party, sighs, "It looks like I'll be up all night cleaning up this mess."	
Your next door neighbor, pointing to a tree close to his property line, "If we get a hurricane, which way do you think that dead branch will fall?"	
A classmate gets a paper back in class, rips it up, and throws the pieces in the trash on his way out the door, "What's the point anyway?"	
A fifth grader comes home with bruises on his face and arms, "I hate school! I'm never going back there."	
A neighbor you happen to meet in line at the grocery store, "Why do they charge so much more for organic products?"	
A new person at after-church coffee hour, "There aren't many places to socialize around here if you're single."	
A co-worker declines an invitation to join you for a drink after work, "I hate bars. Too noisy—you can't even hear yourself think."	
A fellow high school soccer player, who has just invited you to go out for ice cream after losing the game, "Do you think there's any justice in the world?"	

directions: family history, work issues, values, and preferences. The answer will reveal much more about Bob's neighbor as a person and will give Bob a better opportunity to listen and to find common ground.

Social and cultural norms determine what topics of conversation are appropriate and what topics to avoid. For example, with people just introduced at a party, they should avoid asking personal questions, such as about their intimate relationships, their political views, their religious beliefs, or their finances. Maintaining the appropriate social distance can be difficult for people joining a new group or attending a meeting for the first time.

Asking the right questions can be the key to getting to know more about another person. When meeting someone new, closed questions tend to end communication, while asking open questions that further explore the topics that seem important to someone can help to form beginning connections. There are several reasons why this works: (1) your questions show that you are interested in knowing more about someone, (2) further elaboration of an issue allows you to better understand another's point of view, (3) following up on a topic of concern increases the chances of finding common

beliefs and values with which you can empathize, and (4) learning more about someone encourages him or her to reciprocate with curiosity about you. There is no doubt that asking open questions plays an important part in forming relationships and friendships with others. For practice in the skill of asking open questions, try the exercises in Table 3-8.

As a group exercise, try role-playing the situations in Table 3-8, following up each with two more open questions and answering with creative storytelling. A good open question will compel the responder to create new details or directions for the conversation. After each role-play, discuss the results, and ask the group to suggest alternative directions for the conversation. If these were real social situations, the open questions would encourage responders to reveal deeper, more personal or emotional factors that could form the foundations for establishing trust between you.

Awareness of Social Identity

Some people naturally like to converse and feel comfortable interacting with almost anyone they meet. They have no trouble finding things in common with others to talk about and might be viewed as the "life

Table 3-9

DEFINING YOUR SOCIAL IDENTITY

Directions: Part 1—List five social roles you consider to be a part of your identity:

1.

2.

3.

4.

5.

Part 2—Write a short quote you would use to introduce yourself in each of the scenarios listed below, incorporating one or more social roles you listed in Part 1.

Guests you have never met, sitting at your table at a relative's wedding reception _____

The parents of a friend who is hosting a birthday party _____

Someone sitting next to you on a train or plane _____

A customer or client at your place of work _____

A cousin you have not seen in several years _____

An attractive classmate whom you would like to ask on a date _____

Someone interviewing you for a job _____

A sports team you have joined, on the first day of practice _____

A new roommate on move-in day in a college dorm _____

of the party." Such people have a keen sense of social awareness about the prevailing social and cultural norms in group situations. But what helps them most in social situations is a clear sense of their own social identity, which includes a wide range of social roles within their life experience.

Social Roles

According to Bandura's (1977) social learning theory, people learn to engage in more or less adaptive behavior through observing and assuming the behaviors of others. An older sister watches Mom and imitates caregiving behaviors with a baby brother. The sum of these imitated and learned behaviors eventually consolidate into the social role of "mother's helper" or "babysitter." As further discussed in Chapter 7, the adolescent peer group provides teen members with multiple opportunities to try out different social roles and to incorporate the reactions of others when building their social identity as adults. Friendships in adolescence and adulthood form when people have things in common, cross paths regularly, interact with increasing self-disclosure, and reciprocate one another's overtures (alternately sharing problems, listening, and responding) (Fehr, 1995; Karbo, 2006).

However, the critical element in a lasting friendship is "social identity support," the way in which a friend understands and then supports our sense of self in society and the group (Weitz & Wood, 2005).

Social identity includes the important life roles you play with others, such as son or daughter, sibling, student, friend, boyfriend or girlfriend, and worker. People hold multiple roles at any given point in time, and these roles expand and change over the course of a lifetime. The primary role with which you identify also changes with each situation, as becomes evident when filling out the worksheet in Table 3-9.

Once people feel comfortable with their social identities, it becomes easier to find others who play similar roles and to find topics of common interests associated with shared roles. New mothers meeting at a park or playground, for example, might naturally discuss caregiving issues such as feeding schedules, formulas, initial behaviors, or the cheapest place to purchase diapers.

Occupational Roles

Nearly all social roles involve associated sets of tasks or occupations. Participating socially with others who have similar roles often centers around

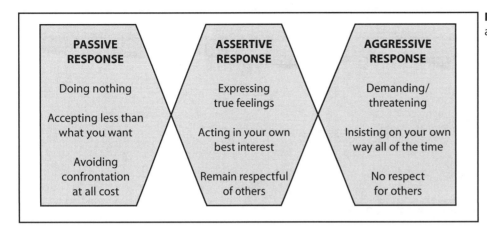

Figure 3-3. Passive, assertive, aggressive behavior continuum.

common occupations, such as co-workers going to a lunch meeting, parents carpooling their kids to baseball practice, mothers supervising play groups for their toddlers, and friends shopping for gifts for a mutual friend's wedding.

Leisure and recreational activities provide many opportunities for social identity, such as being a good golfer, bridge player, or skier. Many workers use childhood talents and interests as hobbies throughout their adult lives, such as playing in a band on weekends, exhibiting handmade quilts at a quilt show, or driving a vintage Corvette in a 1950s auto rally. In this way, even solitary recreational activities become the basis of conversations with others who share similar interests.

Assertiveness Training

Assertiveness as a social characteristic empowers people to stand up for themselves. The concept and methods of assertiveness training date back to the women's movement in the 1970s when women, entering graduate education and the workforce in increasing numbers, believed they needed to behave more assertively in order to effectively compete and succeed in those environments. As a basic part of any communication training program, assertiveness can be found in schools, corporate boardrooms, and psychiatric hospitals for programs as diverse as substance abuse treatment, social skills training, vocational programs, and responding to harassment (*Encyclopedia of Mental Disorders*, 2009). Using assertiveness, people act on their own behalf to satisfy their needs, accomplish their intentions, and achieve their goals while remaining respectful of the needs, rights, and opinions of others. The techniques have a broad application and can be tailored to meet the learning needs of specific groups or situations.

Assertiveness training programs begin by defining three basic types of behavior in social situations: passive, assertive, and aggressive. These behaviors

can be understood as a continuum, as depicted in Figure 3-3. When people begin to correctly identify assertive behavior and distinguish it from passive and aggressive behaviors in themselves and others, they are ready to begin practicing the assertive response techniques described in the next section.

Standing up for Self and Others

Acting on one's own behalf or in one's own best interest means taking an active approach to self-determination, a feeling of being in control of one's own life course. Assertiveness has been associated with positive outcomes for many personal choices related to health, such as avoiding risky sexual or safety situations, refraining from abuse of drugs or alcohol, assuming responsibility for self-care, managing stress levels, and controlling one's time and energy. As a wellness strategy, assertiveness can be useful when other people or circumstances put pressure on you to do something or commit to something that you believe might have negative consequences for your own health or well-being.

Consider the following case. Diana, a 17-year-old high school graduate, married a man 2 years older and a junior in college. She worked as a bookkeeper on the college campus to pay their rent while her husband attended classes. Soon, Diana got pregnant and gave birth to twin boys. Her boss gave her 6 weeks maternity leave but insisted she could not work part-time or have any flexibility in her hours. As a passive person, Diana accepted her fate, continued to work, keep house, care for the twins, and pay the bills. She did not complain about getting only a few hours sleep each night; lacking the focus to perform her job; feeling overwhelmed by housekeeping tasks; and having no time, money, or energy even to take reasonable care of herself much less socialize—until her husband, who never volunteered to help her with anything, came home late one night and threw the plate with his dried out

Table 3-10

PRACTICE IN MAKING "I" STATEMENTS

Directions: Hand out index cards and pencils. On the front, each member of the group writes a brief description of a social situation in his or her own recent life, in which he or she failed to respond assertively or which did not produce satisfying results. Identify the person to whom an "I" statement should be addressed, preferably the person responsible for the unsatisfactory outcome. On the back of the card, write three feeling words that best describe how you felt in this situation. Shuffle the cards and hand them out randomly, so that everyone has someone else's card.

Take turns reading the card you drew and fill in the blanks in the following statement:

"When you, _____ I feel _____."

Members discuss each situation and statement and suggest alternative feeling words as needed. *As homework, try making an "I" statement in a real-life situation during the next week.*

---

dinner across the room, hitting Diana in the face. When she screamed, he slapped her, knocking over her chair, and she hit her head on the edge of the table. In the hospital, Diana learned of an assertiveness training program at the counseling center at the college where she worked.

As an exercise, list 5 situations in which Diana might feel that she did not act assertively:

1. _____
2. _____
3. _____
4. _____
5. _____

These situations may be used to envision the training strategies to follow. In an assertiveness training group, each member would make a similar list of real situations from his or her own life.

The techniques to be learned include owning your own feelings using "I" statements, identifying the specific characteristics of the situation to which the feelings are related, and asking directly for a specific change on the part of the other person or people.

Making an "I" Statement

Identifying one's own feelings in a social situation requires practice in self-awareness. Passive people often deny their own feelings in order to please or appease someone else or to avoid a confrontation. For these people, the best time to explore their own emotions is through reflection upon a difficult situation while in the company of a group of people who can actively listen and provide a safe emotional environment. *For example, how do you think Diana felt when her boss told her she had to come back to work full-time? Disappointed? Angry? A bit desperate? How did she feel when her husband threw the plate at her? Shocked? Terrified? Furious?* When people don't typically think about their own emotions, they may

not have a very good feeling vocabulary. Therefore, at the beginning of an assertiveness training group, members would participate in a group exercise such as that described in Table 3-10.

Making a Direct Request

After expressing one's own feelings about a situation, assertiveness involves asking for a change in the other person's words and behavior. In preparation for making this request, further self-analysis may be necessary to clarify what specific changes would result in the desired outcome. For example, Diana might ask her husband to apologize for throwing the plate at her. While that might make her feel better initially, it will not assure her that the aggressive act might not be repeated. When thinking about the situation, she might ask instead that her husband express his anger with words rather than actions or to make a promise to her that he will never again endanger her physically in anger or otherwise. Assertive requests for change from an offending individual do not always guarantee a positive outcome, but they do clarify which social behaviors are acceptable and which are not. For practice in making assertive requests for change, try role-playing the situations you listed in the case of Diana, or make your own list of situations in which you have felt the need to be more assertive.

People with passive patterns of response sometimes need assistance in becoming aware of their basic rights. Assertiveness programs sometimes begin with a discussion of the legitimate rights of people.

You have a right to:

- Put yourself first sometimes

- Make mistakes

- Be the final judge of your feelings without having to justify them

- Have your own opinions and convictions
- Ask for help and emotional support
- Say no, or choose not to respond to situations
- Receive credit and formal recognition for your achievements

A discussion of legitimate rights can be tailored to specific groups or situations. For example, assertiveness training has been used to address stress on the job. Clear and direct communication can significantly reduce job stress by better defining what is expected and specifying the behaviors upon which workers' performance will be judged. Periodic feedback about performance can also reduce stress by clarifying problem-solving procedures, identifying the need for additional training, or taking steps to correct problems before they become serious enough to terminate employment. Assertive responses are especially helpful in resolving conflicts at work, using a four-step process: (1) state the problem from your point of view, (2) express how it makes you feel, (3) identify how the conflict affects your productivity and motivation, and (4) suggest win-win solutions in which each side gains something positive (Alberti & Emmons, 2001; Davis, Eschelman, & McKay, 1988).

Managing Aggressive Tendencies

Opposite passiveness on the assertiveness continuum is aggressive behavior. People who respond aggressively use power, strength, and control to get what they want, without regard for the rights or feelings of others. Aggressive people usually get their way but find that others do not enjoy being around them. In childhood and adolescence, aggressiveness may take the form of bullying, intimidation, or unfairly holding the spotlight or taking credit away from team or group members. Aggressive tendencies also relate to the appropriate expression of hostile emotions. Without learning and conforming to social norms, some people use their size and strength to overpower others, or may abuse their power and position to treat others unfairly or to ignore their rights as human beings. As such, aggressiveness exceeds the bounds of social acceptability and highlights a need for social skills interventions addressed in later chapters.

Choosing Your Battles

Clearly, there are social situations in which assertiveness may not be the best response. When threatened with violence from a stranger, the obvious choice would be avoidance or aggressiveness, depending on the context and availability of assistance. When learning assertive behavior, practicing in the least confrontational situations allows people to experiment with assertive statements and behaviors with minimal negative outcomes. In everyday life, even the most assertive individuals make many decisions about which issues are important enough to invest their effort and which situations are least likely to result in a positive outcome. Some people and circumstances may be unlikely to change no matter how assertive the participants, and some potential conflicts do not seem to warrant the energy it would take to resolve them. Part of assertiveness training is to get people thinking about different response choices and what might be the consequence in each unique social situation.

Lessons in the use and practice of assertiveness may well be learned in basic cooperative groups in which the group's task accomplishment often depends on the members' ability to cooperate, compromise, and contribute equally to the group's or team's success. For example, consider the skills necessary for participating in a high school marching band.

Forming Basic Attachments and Trust

While attachment begins in infancy, the maintenance of more reciprocal relationships in adolescence and adulthood requires a reliable pattern of responding to one another in ways that are satisfying to both (couples, spouses, friendships) or all members (families, teams, social peers) of a group. As reviewed in Chapter 6, children gradually move away from dependency on parents or caregivers as they develop more independence and confidence in their own ability to participate in larger social groups outside their immediate family. At the basic cooperative level, children can choose friends and activities on their own on the playground and in afterschool and neighborhood games. They can select friends and tasks they like to pursue in scouting badge goals, in hobby groups at friends' homes, and in trips in groups on bikes to destinations they choose together. There is an organizational and personal choice of kids and activities at the basic cooperative level (Figure 3-4).

Social Participation in Supportive Cooperative Groups

By junior high and high school, teens become motivated by their need to belong to peer groups with characteristics they admire or wish to emulate and that offer them support for the development of the social roles that eventually make up their identity as adults. During the teenage years, friendships become close, and peer group members learn the social skills and competencies that help them form and sustain friendships and intimate relationships

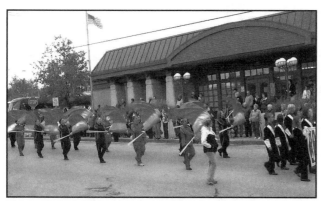

Figure 3-4. A high school marching band performs for the community at a Memorial Day parade down Main Street—A good example of a basic cooperative group.

throughout their lives. Those skills include the expression of empathy and the ability to give and receive social and emotional support (Table 3-11).

Expressing Empathy

Empathy is an emotional and intellectual understanding of another person's feelings, thoughts, and behaviors (O'Toole, 1997). As a personal response directed toward the speaker, empathy conveys understanding and appreciation of another's experience. It is a form of validation and confirmation of the other person, conveying nonjudgmental understanding but not necessarily agreement. Sympathy and empathy differ in this respect. A listener can only share sympathy when similar or like feelings are expressed. When we sympathize with someone, we agree with their point of view and perhaps see ourselves in the same situation feeling and behaving in a similar way. When a relative dies, we sympathize with other family members, grieving together for a lost loved one. Sympathy includes the desire to relieve our own suffering by conveying a feeling of belonging. In contrast, empathy offers understanding while remaining within our own boundaries of feelings and beliefs.

Young children begin to learn empathy when they recognize the emotions and moods of their parents or caregivers and can differentiate themselves from others. Adults encourage children to empathize when they ask, "How would you feel if someone did that to you?" The ability to fully empathize typically emerges around late childhood and adolescence, accompanied by higher level cognitive and moral development. Individuals need a well-differentiated sense of self in order to have a true appreciation of another person.

As a therapeutic skill, empathy requires the therapist to temporarily imagine what it is like to enter the "feeling" world of the client. For a brief moment, therapeutic boundaries become diffuse. The therapist then steps back and thinks about the client's experience. Clear boundaries are restored. The listener must oscillate between feeling the speaker's experience and then thinking about its meaning.

Empathy is a counseling technique that is used in professional as well as personal relationships. First, the therapist listens for the feelings behind the words being said, then makes a statement of understanding by accurately naming the emotional as well as the informational content of the speaker. Therapists call this primary accurate empathy, a way to encourage continued exploration of thoughts, feelings, and behaviors by reflecting or mirroring the meaning behind the client's statements (Egan, 2009).

A good way to learn this technique is to fill in the blanks of the following sentence: "You feel ＿＿＿＿＿＿ because ＿＿＿＿＿＿." After "you feel," choose the most accurate word to describe the speaker's verbal and nonverbal emotional messages, looking for the right level of intensity as well. After "because," offer a brief summary of the situation about which the feelings emerged. For example, "You feel devastated because you think your husband is having an affair," or "You feel annoyed because your roommate left dirty dishes in the sink."

In everyday life, the expression of empathy naturally flows from the process of active listening. By consciously suspending judgment, we can listen more openly to the feelings and thoughts of our friends and family members, our neighbors, and our coworkers without feeling compelled to agree with them. This is a skill that can save friendships and marriages by allowing us to offer understanding and acceptance without compromising our own, often different, points of view. Furthermore, when people establish the habit of expressing empathy first, before any statement of disagreement or criticism, they automatically reassure the other person that having different perspectives about something will not change the closeness of their relationship. For example, parents can learn to use empathy statements with their adolescents who smashed the car or came home drunk, conveying their continued parental love and understanding, while still vehemently rejecting their unacceptable behavior. Practice your empathetic responses by completing the learning exercises in Tables 3-12 and 3-13.

Feelings occur in layers. Usually one emotion stands out, while others may be more subtle. Initial empathy recognizes the strongest emotion first. The other feelings, both yours and theirs, should wait for a later conversation. In personal situations, such as those listed in Table 3-13, you should expect to have a feeling response of your own, which can sometimes

---

Table 3-11

SUPPORTIVE COOPERATIVE LEVEL:
SAMPLE EXPECTATIONS FOR SOCIAL PARTICIPATION

COOPERATION IN GROUPS—MEMBERS':

- Spirit of camaraderie can influence environment.

GROUP NORMS—MEMBERS:

- View group cohesion as (somewhat) more important than task achievement.

GROUP ROLES—MEMBERS CAN:

- Actively encourage peers to express themselves.

COMMUNICATION—MEMBERS:

- Satisfy others' needs through verbal interaction.

ACTIVITY BEHAVIORS—MEMBERS:

- Solicit suggestions of peers for their preferred activities.

POWER/LEADERSHIP OF THE GROUP—MEMBERS:

- Assume a variety of leadership roles reflecting their talents and preferences.

MOTIVATION AND ATTRACTION TO THE GROUP—MEMBERS:

- Enjoy emotional exchange and sharing of opinions and experiences.

Adapted from Donohue, M. V. (2008). *Social profile goals.* Unpublished manuscript.

Table 3-12

EMPATHY LEARNING ACTIVITY

Directions: Groups or individuals can try this exercise as practice in expression of empathy. Cut out pictures of people's faces from magazines and paste them on blank paper. Try to choose unfamiliar faces with a variety and range of facial expressions. Each person in the group takes one picture and identifies words and phrases that describe how this person may be feeling based on his or her facial expression and body position. In a short paragraph, invent a situation that may have caused the person in the photograph to feel as you have identified. Share and compare impressions with the group.

---

interfere with your ability to listen and empathize. In doing this practice exercise, the goal is to put aside your own emotional responses and to focus only on the words and emotions of the speaker. However, your own response can give you some important clues about what the speaker is not saying, what he or she is not ready to admit, or what he or she does not want you to know. When you consistently convey empathy in a relationship, trust develops to the extent that these emotional barriers usually disappear.

Giving and Receiving Social and Emotional Support

Expression of empathy represents one important means of offering emotional support to another person. This type of social support uplifts, assists, and gives others a sense of connection and belonging. Most people understand the support of friends and family to involve both sharing of good times and giving and receiving help through the rough times. In

Table 3-13

RESPONDING WITH FEELING AND CONTENT EMPATHY STATEMENTS

Directions: For each statement, construct a "You feel _____ because _____ " response.

A co-worker, following a review with the boss, "He's going to fire me, I just know it. What am I going to do then? No one else is hiring."	You feel: because:
Your teenage sister, coming home from the hospital with her leg in a cast, "It'll take years before I can play softball again. My friends on the team will forget all about me."	You feel: because:
Your fiancée gets the high-paying job she'd been hoping for, she laughs, "Gee, I hope you're not jealous!"	You feel: because:
Your grandmother, when you visit her in the nursing home, "I miss seeing you more. Being here is not the same." She smiles but her eyes are sad.	You feel: because:
Your friend rushes over holding a bank notice, "They will foreclose on my condo if I don't come up with a lot of money very soon."	You feel: because:
Your supervisor at work who is also a friend, "I've been told I have to fire two of my employees. It won't be you, but I'm afraid you'll have to pick up some of the slack."	You feel: because:
You found ½ oz of pot in your 18-year-old son's backpack, "But Mom, it isn't mine. Why don't you believe me?" He avoids your eyes.	You feel: because:

this respect, social support networks are nurtured by patterns of reciprocation, both giving and receiving over the course of a lifetime.

In fact, social support is a multidimensional concept, including different types of support coming from different levels within social systems. Following Bronfenbrenner's (1993) systems theory, social support comes from four levels, which can be envisioned as broadening circles of distance from the center:

1. *Immediate*—Person or self and members of household, family, roommates, caregivers

2. *Proximal*—Life settings such as schools, classrooms, workplace environments

3. *Community*—Local social networks or groups such as churches, clubs, recreational areas

4. *Societal*—National, political, economic, institutional (i.e., policies, influences, attitudes)

For example, Frank, an older adult with Alzheimer's dementia, may receive daily home care from an adult daughter and, occasionally, a home health aide. His daughter might ask an occupational therapy consultant for assistance in safeguarding her home or in applying for home health assistance from a visiting nurse. While the daughter works, Frank may attend a community adult day care program. His medical needs might be paid for by Medicare, a national agency, and his daughter might visit the state or national Alzheimer's Association Web site to obtain useful information or advice about caring for her father.

The above case description suggests several different types of social support. Three types of support are practical, informational, and emotional. Practical support includes things like providing meals, transportation, home cleaning and maintenance, assistance with self-care, and financial assistance. This type of support may come from neighbors, friends, or family members outside of the household and is often a temporary measure to get someone through a crisis situation. Informational support includes education, training, advice, and connecting with needed resources such as health agencies, sources of adaptive equipment, or support groups. Emotional support, often perceived to be the most needed and helpful for those in crisis, offers esteem, encouragement, validation, empowerment, and a sense of belonging and that one is not alone. In the case of Frank and his daughter, they were able to obtain practical and informational support from the community, state, and national resources, but emotional support may still be lacking. Emotional support must come from personal social networks—friends and family who care enough to become involved at a more intimate level. Everyone needs to cultivate his or her own personal social support network.

Research suggests that social support becomes more available to those who have given support to others (Bowling, Beehr, & Swader, 2005). To assess your own support system, Berrett (2009) suggests drawing it on paper (see Learning Activities at the end of the chapter) to determine whether it is adequate and what is missing. When people who have not often helped or supported others suddenly experience adversity, they may find themselves without an adequate source of social support. People who pride themselves on their own independence may find it difficult to accept help from others, even when it is obviously needed. Therapists often find clients with acquired disability in these predicaments and may need to assist them in building and nurturing social networks. Berrett (2009) offers the following guidelines for building and nurturing social support networks by giving and receiving support.

Giving Support to Others

× Write down some of the names of people whom you consistently give support.

× List some of your own talents, skills, and resources that can support others.

× Find three people you could support now or in the near future.

× Offer the following to at least one of these people every day for a week: a phone call, a letter sent, a kind act, a smile, an expression of gratitude, or encouragement.

× Choose someone with whom you would like to become closer, and let him or her know your hopes in that relationship. Begin to share with him or her.

× Spend more time giving support and love and less time trying to get it.

Receiving Support from Others

× Write down names of people from whom you could ask for help right now.

× Decide what you need to do to encircle yourself with others who support you.

× Find opportunities to ask for help, and then ask directly for what you need.

× Teach your loved ones how to give you the specific type of support you need.

× Allow yourself to accept the help others offer and then show gratitude.

× Reach out and be a friend. Keep at it with patience—relationships take time.

While these guidelines were originally intended for clients with eating disorders, they can assist anyone who may have difficulty identifying an adequate social support network. Berrett (2009) suggests that those with eating disorders also do the following: take responsibility for their own recovery, learn to take good care of themselves, act assertively to obtain needed help, and, after mistakes, refrain from self-judgment or punishment—instead, build self-respect by making and keeping promises to yourself. Both therapists and people in recovery recognize the need for such advice; the barriers of depending too much on the same helpers until they become overburdened or give up, or on the flip side, recovering individuals feeling unworthy of being supported or too ashamed to ask for support.

The Learning Activities at the end of this chapter help people become aware of their own social and family networks, as well as determine their adequacy in harder times and identify gaps on both the giving and receiving side. People with larger and closer social networks typically have less difficulty with obtaining support when the need arises.

Development of Group Cohesiveness

When the same group of people meet regularly, whether at a religious-based youth group, a senior memoir writing group, or an adult community service club, the members often develop a feeling of closeness and trust, sometimes called group cohesiveness. Cohesiveness means attraction to the group; it implies that members of the group enjoy being together no matter what they are doing and that the importance of social and emotional support surpasses the choice of occupation or activity. In therapeutic groups, leaders encourage members to self-disclose—actively listen to and empathize with one another in equal measure in order to facilitate the development of cohesiveness. When a new person joins, the group does not have the same level of trust with that person and needs to build trust through ongoing interactions. The concept of cohesiveness is central to participation in a supportive cooperative level group, as described in Table 3-13.

Acceptance and support for one another forms the foundation of supportive cooperative groups. Friendships from childhood and adolescence have the potential to reach a level of intimacy that can be maintained for many years into adulthood when groups of friends reconnect at social events such as school reunions or homecomings, weddings, holiday celebrations, or other events of common interest.

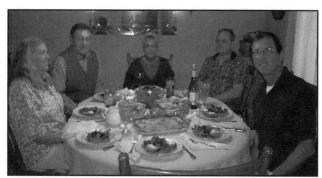

Figure 3-5. Couples' gourmet group dinner—everyone brings one or two dishes to make a delicious meal, but enjoying each others' company is the main focus, exemplifying a supportive cooperative group.

Family relationships also change and deepen as children grow up to become coequal adults with their parents, siblings, aunts, uncles, and other relatives, functioning as reciprocal social support networks for each other even when living great distances apart.

For adults, extra-work socialization may take the form of many such groups, buddies playing golf, tennis, poker, or bridge on a regular basis; couples entertaining each other in their homes; and clubs and organizations meeting together where the same people rotate leadership while continuing to enjoy each other's company. Informal supportive cooperative groups may also be found at local salons, diners, fitness centers, or coffee shops frequented often by the same individuals. An example of building socialization around a leisure occupation is pictured in Figure 3-5. Four couples who share an interest in gourmet cooking each prepared different parts of the dinner shown in the photo, which they take turns hosting four times each year. While the task (the dinner) is important for this group, the members' enjoyment of each other's company overshadows the task, making the couple's gourmet group a good example of an adult supportive cooperative group.

Social support groups, organized by communities, health professionals, religious organizations, and other government or nongovernment agencies for people coping with a variety of disabilities or life stressors, have the purpose of facilitating group members in providing one another with social and emotional support. Some examples are widow bereavement groups, Weight Watchers, Alcoholics Anonymous, Alzheimer's caregiver support groups, and Parents Without Partners. Such groups work best when facilitated by a trained leader who can model the techniques of active listening and expression of empathy and establish positive social norms, such as nonjudgmental acceptance and the development of group cohesiveness. Specific support groups will be further discussed in later chapters (see Table 3-13).

Learning Activities

Social Support: Personal Network Map

Using a blank sheet of paper, write your name in the center. List 10 people close to you whom you rely on for social and emotional support, and briefly describe the special talents and attributes of each. Draw lines from your name to theirs, indicating the approximate distance from you in terms of trust and intimacy. Draw a circle around these 10 people. This is your inner circle. Now, list 10 people who rely on you to give them some type of social support. Add these names to your network, either inside or outside the inner circle. Sometimes, support can be given or received from whole groups of people. Use small squares to identify these groups, and also place them inside or outside the circle. Finally, identify community agencies, local or national organizations, and other distant people or groups from whom you receive or give some type of support. Write these organizations or entities near the outer margins of the page.

Working from the completed personal network map, identify individuals from whom you could elicit social support, and briefly discuss reasons for your answers or give an example of a real situation, if applicable.

Personal Network Map: Template

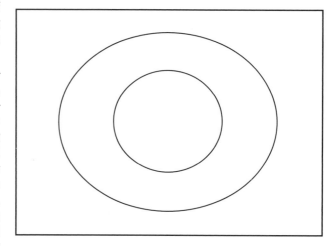

Practical Social Support

- ✗ Who would you call if you needed to borrow money?

- ✗ Who could you count on to help you move to a new apartment?

- ✗ When you get sick, who do you count on to give you personal care?

- ✗ If you are planning your wedding, who would you ask to be members of your wedding party? (*choose 3 or 4 individuals*)

- ✗ If you were arrested while traveling out of state, to whom would you place your one telephone call?

Informational Social Support

- ✗ Who would you ask to help you choose or shop for an outfit for a special occasion?

- ✗ If you had questions about a research project for school, from whom would you request help and guidance?

- ✗ If you had an opportunity to plan a trip to Florida for spring break, who would you consult in making the specific arrangements?

- ✗ Whom would you call to help you find a summer job in your hometown?

Emotional Social Support

- ✗ Who do you count on to give you a sense of belonging? (*can be more than 1 person*)

- ✗ If you are upset about a personal issue, who could you call to discuss it?

- ✗ If someone bullied or harassed you, who could you look to for help and support?

- ✗ When something wonderful happens to you, who is the first person you would tell?

- ✗ If something terrible were to happen to you, which individuals could you turn to?

Family Support

- ✗ Looking at your drawing, underline in red the names of all blood relatives.

- ✗ What members of your family are included, and which are missing? Why?

- ✗ List the people you would invite to an important event, such as a wedding or funeral.

- ✗ If you had to contact a family member for an emergency message, where would you look for their contact information? How would you go about contacting these individuals?

- ✗ If family telephone numbers, e-mail, or home addresses are out of date, make a list on your computer or in a notebook and keep it where you can easily find it when needed.

Script: Sorority and Fraternity Group Negotiation

Seating Chart

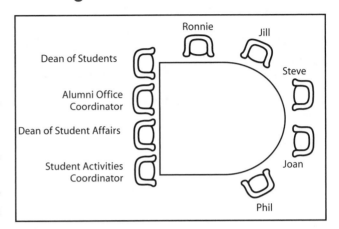

Characters and Situation Overview

The scenario is set in an American college that has active sorority and fraternity groups on campus. The members of the sorority and fraternity are required by school policy to participate in community service of some sort on- or off-campus; however, participation on sports teams is not considered by the college to be service to the school. This policy exists despite huge amounts of time devoted to sport practice, games, and travel to games. So, sorority and fraternity members who participate in sports must also carry out other college or community services in addition to their studies. The result is a stressful and Spartan schedule. Representatives from two sororities and three fraternities have chosen to jointly meet with the administration because they believe that sports greatly contribute to school spirit and that too heavy of a schedule removes the fun from sports and the satisfaction from service participation activities.

Jill: Tall, blonde, and tan; her sports are volleyball and swimming. Currently a junior, she represents her sorority sisters' viewpoints regarding the college community service policy.

Steve: A senior who holds the position of fraternity president and captain of the college football team. He is tall and well-built and has come as spokesperson for other fraternity members who also participate in sports.

Dean of Student Affairs: Designated chairperson of the meeting, he tries to remain impartial.

Dean of Students: Still single in his early 30s, this administrator can still remember what it felt like to be a student with the pressures of grades, sports, and service in addition to upholding the social status of his fraternity.

Alumni Office Coordinator: Age 54, he has had this position for almost 30 years and acts as historian for college traditions; holds the "official" position regarding the issue at hand.

Ronnie: An engineering and business major, he has come prepared with an organized alternative plan to illustrate how a different policy regarding sports and service might work.

Phil: College senior who spent part of his junior year studying marine biology in Australia. He currently holds the position of captain of the college swim team.

Joan: New sorority member attending college on a track-and-field scholarship. Her intended major is elementary education, a 5-year program ending with a master of arts in teaching.

Student Activities Coordinator: In her 40s and married; she represents the service organizations for which students volunteer. Her job is recruiting students for volunteer jobs and scheduling volunteer hours so that the needs of intended recipients are met and tasks accomplished within time limits set by the organizations.

Action Begins Here

Jill: *(to college administrators and faculty)* Thank you for meeting with us today to discuss our issues with the campus participation expectations.

Dean of Student Affairs: We have heard of your concerns and are willing to meet with you to discuss our policy.

Steve: We want you to know that we are very devoted to the college here and wish to collaborate with you to promote school spirit in the organizations we participate in.

Alumni Office Coordinator: We have had these policies for 30 years now, and we feel that they have worked very well. Some athletes would never realize that there is a real world out there, like Meals on Wheels and Habitat for Humanity, and needs on campus, like staffing the school newspaper, if we did not have the current policy of requiring students to carry out service participation.

Ronnie: Most of us who have come to meet with you today are involved in competitive sports that play on- and off-campus. The role of sports has changed in the past 30 years. Sports have expanded, including girls' sports, and are now taken more seriously, requiring a lot of practice and travel time. For

us to also keep our grades up and do community service, we feel spread too thin; and we are not doing justice to any of these areas. Ideally, we'd like to do everything, but are finding it stressful.

Jill: Also, we believe that sports make a contribution to the spirit of social participation on-campus. So really, sports could be counted as a community service.

Student Activities Coordinator: You all are young and have a lot of energy. We believe that participation in the school newspaper staff, the band, the chorus, and peer counseling will help to keep you away from drugs and other distractions to completing your education.

Phil: We'd like to do it all, but some students feel so pressured that they can't wait for their junior semester abroad to get away from the combination of what we have to do. There are only so many hours in a day. Here on campus, we find it tempting to take drugs just to stay awake long enough to meet all these expectations.

Dean of Students: Well, we'd like to keep the combination of studies, sports, and service participation. So, how can you problem solve and find a solution? Can we compromise here?

Joan: Well, we were wondering if we could try an experiment next year, since most sports are seasonal, to participate in school or community volunteer work in the off season?

Alumni Office Coordinator: Wouldn't that break up the continuity of our campus organizations?

Ronnie: We'd be willing to meet with the Student Activities Coordinator to lay out spread sheets and schedules to cover the organizations for both semesters. We could use the college Web site to advertise and organize the positions that are available and need to be covered. In business these days, there is more allowance made for flextime... so why not here?

Dean of Students: You have an interesting proposal that sounds feasible. We need time to think it over to see what the ramifications are in terms of fallout in campus activity groups. Thank you for bringing this issue to our attention and for this productive discussion. We were all students once too, so we'll deliberate on your concerns.

Dean of Student Affairs: How about if we set up another meeting for 2 weeks from now? We need some time to discuss this with faculty. But, we also don't want to lose sight of taking action, if we go in that direction, as soon as possible. Is this same time in 2 weeks good for you all?

Joan: I can't attend on that date due to a sports event, but I think that everyone else can...

(Nods from Steve, Phil, Ronnie, and Jill)

Dean of Students: So we'll see you all then.

Steve: Thank you for your time and for considering our ideas.

The End.

Discussion

1. What perspective does the college administration have about sports and those who participate in sports?

2. How do sports promote school social participation? Should participation in sports qualify as community service? Why or why not?

3. Who were the leaders for each side of the issue? What are the social circumstances of participants, and how did these attitudes influence the problem-solving process?

4. What type of conflict does this interaction represent (refer to Chapter 1)?

5. What conflict-resolution principles can you identify, and how well did they work?

6. What level of interaction does this group represent and why?

7. In what sense does this group discussion demonstrate the interaction of peer group members, and what behaviors represent support for one another during the conversation?

References

Alberti, R., & Emmons, M. (2001). *Your perfect right: Assertiveness and equality in your life and relationships* (8th ed.). Atascadero, CA: Impact Publishers.

Bandura, A. (1977). *Social learning theory.* New York, NY: General Learning Press.

Baum, C. M., & Christiansen, C. H. (2005). Person-environment-occupation-performance: An occupation based framework for practice. In C. H. Christiansen, C. M. Baum, & J. Bass-Haugen (Eds.), *Occupational therapy: Performance, participation, and well-being* (3rd ed.). Thorofare, NJ: SLACK Incorporated.

Benne, K., & Sheats, P. (1948). Functional roles of group members. *Journal of Social Issues, 4,* 41-49.

Benne, K., & Sheats, P. (1978). Functional roles of group members. In L. Bradford (Ed.), *Group development* (2nd ed., pp. 52-61). LaJolla, CA: University Associates.

Bernieri, F. J. (2005). The expression of rapport. In V. Manusov (Ed.), *Beyond words: A sourcebook of methods for measuring nonverbal cues.* Mahwah, NJ: LEA.

Berrett, M. E. (2009). Social support: The cradle for growth and recovery. Social support with eating disorders. Retrieved March 27, 2009 from www.eatingdisorderhope.com/social-support.nt.html

Bowling, N. A., Beehr, T. A., & Swader, W. M. (2005). Giving and receiving social support: The roles of personality and reciprocity. *Journal of Vocational Behavior, 67,* 476-489.

Bronfenbrenner, W. (1993). Toward an experimental ecology of human development: Research models and fugitive findings. In R. H. Wozniak & K.W. Fischer (Eds.), *Development in context: Acting and thinking in specific environments* (pp. 3-44). New York, NY: Erlbaum.

Cohen, R. M. (2005). *Blindsided: Lifting a life above illness, a reluctant memoir.* New York, NY: Harper.

Davis, M., Eschelman, E. R., & McKay, M. (1988). *The relaxation and stress reduction handbook.* Retrieved March 27, 2009 from www.uvm.edu/-uvmeap/stress8.html

Egan, G. (2001). *The skilled helper* (5th ed.). Monterey, CA: Brooks/Cole.

Egan, G. (2009). *The skilled helper: A problem management and opportunity development approach to helping* (9th ed.). Belmont, CA: Brooks/Cole.

Encyclopedia of Mental Disorders. (2009). *Assertiveness training.* Retrieved March 27, 2009 from www.minddisorders.com/A-Br/Assertiveness-training.html

Fehr, B. (1995). *Friendship processes* (Vol. 12). New York, NY: Sage Publications.

Karbo, K. (2006). Friendship: The laws of attraction. *Psychology Today, Nov-Dec,* 91-95.

Laidman, J. (2009). It's all over in 30 seconds. *The Toledo Blade.* Retrieved June 8, 2009 from www.cjonline.com/stories/062501/pro_impressions.shtml

Nichols, M. (1995). *The lost art of listening.* Guilford, CT: Guilford Publishing.

O'Toole, M. (1997). *Miller Keane encyclopedia and dictionary of medicine, nursing, and allied health* (6th ed.). Philadelphia, PA: W.B. Saunders.

Reich, N., & Wood, J. (2003). Sex, gender, and communication in small groups. In R. Hirokawa, R. Cathcart, L. Samovar, & Henman, L. (Eds.), *Small group communication* (8th ed., pp. 218-229). Los Angeles, CA: Roxbury Publishing.

Robertson, K. (2005). Active listening: More than just paying attention. *Australian Family Physician, 34,* 1053-1055.

Rogers, C. (1961). *On becoming a person: A therapist's view of psychotherapy.* Boston, MA: Houghton Mifflin Co.

Weitz, C., & Wood, L. (2005). Social identity support and friendship outcomes: A longitudinal study predicting who will be friends and best friends 4 years later. *Journal of Social and Personal Relationships, 22,* 416-432.

Additional Resources

Donohue, M. V. (1999). Theoretical bases of Mosey's group interactions skills. *Occupational Therapy International, 6,* 35-51.

chapter 4

Social Capital:
A Systems Perspective

Mary V. Donohue, PhD, OTL, FAOTA

"Behold, how good and how pleasant it is for brethren to dwell together in unity." (Psalm 131:1).

It is valuable for professional leaders, whether teachers, therapists, politicians, lawyers, or businesspeople, to become aware of the potential for professional growth in knowing how to participate in groups, networks, and civic society. It is also productive for these professional leaders to encourage their pupils, clients, voters, and customers to learn about the benefits of social bonding and bridging as they develop their own knowledge, expertise, judgment, and emotional understanding of themselves and others. Earlier chapters have focused on social participation broadly as a construct; this chapter aims to increase the reader's understanding of the resources and assets of various types available through networking and building professional, political, and economic interpersonal relationships.

Overview

There are many perspectives on social capital, and there continues to be much disagreement as to how to define it (Bordieu, 1986; Coleman, 1994; DeFilippis, 2001; Dekker & Uslander, 2001; Field, 2003; Fukuyama, 1999; Putnam, 2000; Putnam, Feldstein, & Cohen, 2003). A number of these theorists come from sociology and others from economics, so their viewpoint is colored by their background in related fields. Capital, in general, relates to monetary resources. Related and overlapping resources include social capital,

human capital, physical capital, cultural capital, and political capital. These relationships can be depicted by a Venn diagram (Figure 4-1).

Human capital consists of human work abilities, skills, and expertise available for a job. *Political capital* consists of connections in political systems, such as voting parties, assemblies, councils, committees, coalitions, associations, and courts. *Physical capital* consists of equipment, supplies, buildings, and real estate owned by individuals, groups, companies, and governments. *Cultural capital* refers to the status and selection of the art, music, dance, architecture, dress, schools, and clubs of an individual or group of people.

Various theorists have a focus or a perception of social capital as leaning toward or heavily influenced by one of the other types of capital, especially toward economic, cultural, and political capital aspects.

A definition, assembled from various sources, depicts social capital as independent of these other capital areas, but still related to them. *Social capital* consists of networks of interaction among similar and diverse people, developed through norms of trust, shared values, and reciprocity of assets. In Figure 4-1, social capital has the potential to overlap with economic capital in the center and political and cultural capital on the periphery. In fact, DeFilippis (2001) argues that the centrist view of social capital should have more of an economic focus while opposing others who would like to see more political emphasis within traditional social capital. Bordieu (1984) emphasized the concept of cultural

Cole, M.B., & Donohue, M.V. *Social Participation in Occupational Contexts: In Schools, Clinics, and Communities* (pp 67-80).
© 2011 SLACK Incorporated

capital as emanating from family circumstances and the educational status of schools attended.

The term *social capital* began as a metaphor for the exchange of benefits through mutual interactions. Gradually, it has become a construct with a variable meaning ranging from social political or cultural capital to social economic capital. In this spectrum, the notion of "connections" as facilitating political power, cultural contacts, and economic prosperity are seen as embedded in social interaction (Community Foundation of Silicon Valley, 2008).

There has been agreement upon two subdivisions of this construct, consisting of two concepts: *bonding social capital* and *bridging social capital.* Bonding social capital consists of interactions among people of like-minded norms, such as family members, neighbors, sports teams, and other organizations of people with common interests, such as religious and small professional groups. In contrast, the concept of bridging social capital refers to interactions or organizations of heterogeneous, diverse groups, for example at work, in civic movements, and ecumenical religious associations. At the extremes in society, it is possible to find people who are antiparticipation for a number of reasons, while at the other extreme it is possible to find people who never bond but are involved in manic networking seemingly without a purpose. This range or continuum is depicted by Figure 4-2.

Major Theorists of Social Capital

The three major theorists who have developed the construct of social capital are Bordieu (1980, 1984; Bordieu & Wacquant, 1992), Coleman (1988, 1991, 1994), and Putnam (1996, 2000; Putnam et al., 2003).

Bordieu

Bordieu (1980, 1984) began his study of social capital with an emphasis on cultural capital as indicating that the taste of people's choice of concerts, theater, musicians, artists, and way of life reflected a status or position of individuals in society. He was a French sociologist who saw people's cultural background from elite schools, clubs, and family history of nobility resulting in social inequality in the community. He believed that inclusion in cruises; soirees, receptions, dances; and sports such as tennis, golf, and sailing replaced the influence of families as to whom their children married. Meanwhile, Bordieu (Bordieu & Wacquant, 1992) began to shift his perspective toward social capital as he did not accept the notion of social inequality as an inescapable disparity among people at various

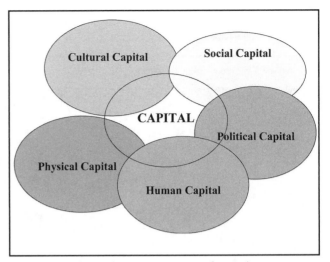

Figure 4-1. Relationships among types of capital resources.

economic levels. He began to examine the social capital of professional people who employ their accumulation of economic and political connections to win the respect of clientele in high society, thus adding to their educational credentials. Bordieu indicated that keeping up a network requires labor to sustain the relationships as durable, in terms of reciprocal obligations and investments in mutuality in multiple directions. He perceived sociability as an underpinning of maintaining connections.

Bordieu has been criticized as believing in a static structure of societal hierarchy, yet he acknowledged the impact of human agency in influencing unequal conditions. At times, Bordieu perceives that social capital can hide the financial profit-seeking or desire for superiority of its façade, and he points out that people can accumulate social capital to enhance their status. For people working with children, adolescents, adults, and seniors in educational, clinical, and community settings, reflecting on the importance of social capital for themselves, for their interventions with their clients, and for their clients' own future immersion in society can enlighten them on the motivation of their altruistic practice.

Coleman

Coleman (1994), a renowned educational sociologist, studied America's economically marginalized neighborhoods. His work indicated that social capital was not just limited to financially advantaged groups. Coleman perceived social capital as a resource that included the awareness of reciprocity, trust, and similar values within people's networks. His focus was to expand the study of social capital as an interdisciplinary science that would span economics and sociology. His emphasis was on social capital being expanded through rational action in pursuing

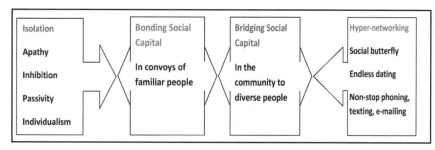

Figure 4-2. Spectrum of social capital participation.

individual interests with others with similar interests. He also thought of social capital as a form of exchange explaining how people interact with cooperation. This approach of rational choice theory was designed to indicate the underpinnings of collective economic action. This line of thinking supports the contention that cooperation results through pursuit of individual interests that require joint efforts.

With his interest in education, Coleman researched relationships between social inequality and school achievement. He noted the influence of peer groups shaping adolescent views more strongly than a parent's or teacher's influence (1961). His studies validated that family and community conditions are stronger than the school itself in influencing scholastic results. These studies demonstrated that community norms' impact on parents, and students tended to ameliorate the influence of social and financial deprivation stemming from the family (Coleman & Hoffer, 1987). Coleman also wished to distinguish between social capital and human capital and to simultaneously highlight their relationship. Finally, Coleman indicated that social capital is a practical asset that can be used through an individual's social relationships; while seeking an individual self-interest, cooperation is an essential, integral component (1988).

Coleman was criticized for presenting social capital as uniformly beneficial for society (Field, 2003). He is perceived by some to have an overly optimistic stance in his view of social capital. He is similar to Bordieu in seeing social capital as an asset for educational progress. He also placed great value on the contribution of the family to social capital, expressing regret at the decline in family life as diminishing the expansion of social capital for the individual and for society. Some critics believe that Coleman valued bonding social capital to the detriment of developing bridging social capital. Coleman's theory and research provides opportunity for reflection on the balance between bonding and bridging social capital in the work of educators, clinicians, and community organizers, and in the goals they tend to emphasize with the children, adolescents, adults, and seniors they serve.

Putnam

Putnam may currently be the best known of these three theorists of social capital with his popular books. As a political scientist, he began his work on social capital in Italy, comparing civic regions of northern and southern Italy and their impact on democracy (1993). He is famous for his book, *Bowling Alone* (2000), a metaphor for the change in American society where people moved from bridging bowling in leagues to bonding bowling with family and friends. Putnam aligns the decline of social capital with the spread of television.

Putnam defines social capital as social organization with aspects of "trust, norms and networks, that can improve the efficiency of society by facilitating coordinated actions" (1993, p. 167). Subsequently, he also emphasizes that one of the norms of social capital is reciprocity within the networks, which can influence the productivity of individuals and groups (2000) (Figure 4-3).

It is Putnam who introduced the distinction between bonding and bridging social capital. He points out four rationales related to trends and activities causing the decline of social capital in the United

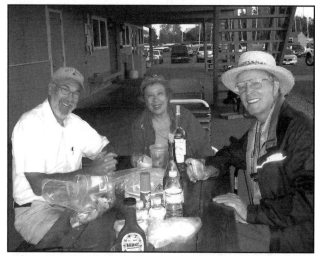

Figure 4-3. Two sailors off a boat share a picnic with their disabled friend who arrived by land to join them, enjoying the social capital encouraged by a sailing club.

States. First, the stress of two-career families has minimized the time parents can devote to the community (Putnam, 2000). Second, community sprawl diminishes the people in networks who are spread out geographically. Third, electronic home entertainment like television, computer games, and the internet limit social interaction. Fourth, generational differences in reading the newspaper, in voting, and in belonging to community associations manifest themselves with older people being more active in civic participation (2000).

Putnam has more recently published a book, *Better Together* (2003) with Feldstein and Cohen. Here, he sets forth a number of case studies of American communities that are restoring their social capital through neighborhood initiatives, labor groups, dance interaction, bringing seniors into schools, letting young people lead, and virtual communities.

Critics point out that Putnam does not acknowledge the influence of economic aspects in his discussion of social capital. In fact, DeFilippis (2001) points out incongruities in Putnam's discussion of affluent people in suburbs who are disconnected and isolated despite their financial assets. In contrast, he reflects that it is people in low-income areas who are told to become interactive socially as a way to improve their economic situation. DeFilippis sees a disjuncture in these two environments' needs in moving toward community economic development to solve opposite problems with a single solution.

Putnam provides a new perspective now through the Saguaro Seminars (2008) on civic engagement in America and topics such as diversity, immigration, and social capital. Based at Harvard, www.hks.harvard.edu/saguaro and www.bettertogether.org are Web sites to which teachers, clinicians, and community leaders can go to connect with others, build trust, and get involved in civic life. Putnam includes criticisms of his own work and points of view on his Web site, so readers can examine his research, look at his measurement tools, and blog their inquiries and responses on the Saguaro Web site.

Negative and Weak Aspects of Social Capital Theories

While these theorists for the most part present the desirable aspects of social capital, they have also pointed out the downside of negative social capital situations where trust and cooperation are undermined. Bordieu (1986) pointed out that some people try to disguise the economic aspects of social capital, especially those social networking aspects that can be manipulated to favor elite individuals, in situations

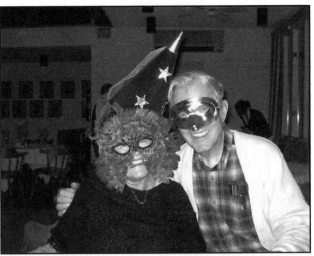

Figure 4-4. Mardi Gras masks team up to celebrate Halloween. In other contexts, masks can also hide identities when making a social statement.

such as aggressive profit seeking. This aggravates inequality rather than promoting positive social interaction as it sustains connections for the purpose of maintaining class superiority over others.

Social capital connections established through elite schools can also have a negative outcome for fostering equality, as Coleman indicated (1994). Peer group pressure, especially disapproval of others' social behaviors, is a powerful motivator and an example of negative social capital. Economic deprivation in some families can negate the usual positive influence of bonding social capital when parents and children perceive themselves as outside of the average circle of success due to being in a lower class. Some critics have pointed out that Coleman's premise that self-interest will lead to cooperation among people because collaboration pays off in the accomplishment of personal goals may not work out in real life (1990). Coleman's reliance on family and religion for stability in providing bonding social capital as an argument for development of children's futures is diminishing gradually in both areas that were formerly pillars of the community. Another weakness of Coleman's stance is in emphasizing bonding social capital over bridging social capital. Here, he undervalues the importance of loose ties in favor of close ties. Both are needed in adult life (Figures 4-4 and 4-5).

In 1999, Fukuyama used the example of negative groups, such as the Mafia and the Ku Klux Klan, who have strong social capital in order to illustrate weaknesses in the theory. Other examples of negative social capital have been provided by history in Marxist circles and Nazi Gestapo organization. Hate groups and inbred organizations, bureaucracies,

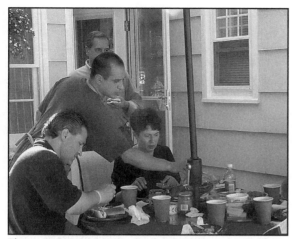

Figure 4-5. Everyone in the family helps to make this a special occasion, enjoying the outdoors and the social capital of each other's comfortable company.

and departments have strong bonding social capital, but no sympathy to reach out with bridging social capital to others.

Xenophobia generally creates tight circles of bonding as a result of fear of bridging. In some cultures, clannish families teach their children not to trust anyone outside the family and that it is not unethical to attack outsiders in order to uphold family power, finances, and status (Fukuyama, 1999). Professionals working with people in these cultures find that the norms of the family often do not allow for bridging to people in the next village despite being in the same country, which results in mistrust passed on from generation to generation.

It can be seen that organizations or businesses, with far-reaching bonds that promote lobbying to legislators, can undermine democracy as they pit groups against each other in vying for funding for pet projects. The development of powerful interest groups can vitiate the general public good by emphasizing the political aspects of bridging social capital to the detriment of prioritizing the village, state, or country's best interest (Fukuyama, 1999). Some degree of coordination and regulation of social capital strengthens the economic infrastructure of political entities.

Putnam (2000) included a chapter on "the dark side" of social capital. In it he mentions the distortion of social capital to achieve what is "good for business" despite the violation of social norms. In another example, Putnam indicates how tight community norms can restrict the freedom of the individual who becomes subjected to the tyranny of neighbors in culturally enforced conformity. Putnam reiterates some of the negative points made by Fukuyama. On the other hand, Putnam asks if society has become more

tolerant in areas of race, gender, and civil liberties of "outsiders" while simultaneously becoming less connected to each other. These trends would appear to belie the premises of social capital, thus weakening its theory of the value of shared norms, reciprocity, and cooperation. These changes could speak to the need for some space in society to allow for the growth of bridging social capital to balance bonding social capital.

Research on Social Capital

Coleman was interested in relationships between social inequality and academic success in school. In a study of high school students in 1961, he found that they were more influenced by their fellow students than they were by parents and teachers. A few years later, Coleman was asked to undertake a study commissioned by the U.S. Office of Education to examine educational access and achievement among six different cultural groups. This study indicated that a student's family and community background was more influential than the nature of the school itself (1961). Coleman regretted that some politicians and community officials tended to downgrade the importance of the schools themselves. In some areas, this Coleman report led to enforced racial segregation, busing, and "white flight" from some neighborhoods, thus increasing inner city racial ghettos.

In the 1960s, Coleman organized a series of empirical studies designed to compare the achievement record of private and public schools. Collecting demographic data, Coleman and his collaborators studied thousands of high school students in parochial and public schools. He reported that students in parochial schools, even in the inner city, had higher performance scores, less absenteeism, and lower dropout rates (Coleman & Hoffer, 1987). Coleman attributed this to the community norms of parents and pupils, which reinforced teachers' norms in these private schools, indicating that social capital worked in a positive manner in the network of parents, students, and teachers despite disadvantaged cultural and socioeconomic settings.

In 1999, Fukuyama asked, how do you measure social capital? In his article titled "Social Capital and Civil Society," he proceeds to build a formula incorporating factors such as the sum of the membership of all groups, the size of groups, the measure of cohesion in the groups, and designation for the radius of trust and distrust of the organization's collective action. He then points out that structuring such a formula is an impossible effort because the factors are so complex, numerous, and difficult to measure. Fukuyama points the reader to using the National Opinion Research

Council's General Social Survey for the United States and the University of Michigan's World Values Survey for international data.

This is exactly what Putnam did, using the General Social Survey, the DDB Needham Life Style Survey, and the Roper Social and Political Trends as his major archives (2000). Putnam identified four limitations of these surveys: problems with comparability of data among the databanks, reliability of data with only one panel of time measured, inability to gather additional comprehensive information because the questions are not designed by the researcher, and variance produced by the noncurrent timing of data collection. Putnam, nevertheless, proceeded to see how he could triangulate the results of the surveys. He structured an *Index for Measuring Social Capital in the American States* containing 14 indicators (2000, p. 291). They are organized under five headings: measures of community organizational life, engagement in public affairs, community volunteerism, informal sociability, and social trust. He found that the 14 indicators of formal and informal community networks and social trust were inter-correlated, pointing toward a single underlying dimension, measuring related but distinct aspects of community social capital.

Using a map of the United States, similar to a weather map, Putnam shaded the states as very high, high, moderate, low, and very low social capital. Northern states bordering Canada had very high social capital; plains states above the Mason Dixon line had high scores; Mid-Atlantic states, Illinois, California, and New Mexico, had average scores; and southern states and Nevada are low and very low in social capital (2000). Then, Putnam presented a series of data plots using the Social Capital Index, spreading out the states' initials as data points across the plots. He found correlations of states with higher social capital scores were associated with the following:

- × Kids being better off
- × Lower mortality
- × Better working schools
- × Lower tax evasion
- × Kids watching less TV
- × Higher rates of tolerance
- × Violent crime being rarer
- × Economic equality
- × People being less pugnacious
- × Civic equality
- × Better public health

Putnam found age cohort differences among adults in his study. People born earlier in the 20th century were more engaged in groups but less tolerant of others. Gradually, over the years, people become more tolerant but less engaged in community activities (2000). Putnam currently provides a paper titled, "Social Capital: Measurement and Consequences," where his map of the United States and the scatter plots of social capital trends mentioned above are illustrated at the site for the Organization for Economic Cooperation and Development at www. oecd.org/dataoecd/25/6/1825848.pdf. In this article, his major graphs show decline in average membership in voluntary associations, active organizational involvement, club meeting attendance, trust, and philanthropic generosity. In Table 4-1, Putnam's 14 indicators of his five-part index are modified for individual ratings.

Social Capital Measurement Activity Based on Putnam's Indicators

To evaluate yourself and your class/group, it is suggested that you rate yourself here on these 14 items:

a. Using the following Likert scale, rate yourself on items 1 and 2:

   0: Never; 1: Sometimes; 2: Frequently; 3: Regularly

b. For items 3 through 12, indicate the number of times per year you participated in the activity

c. For items 13 and 14, indicate your degree of agreement with the statement using the following Likert scale:

   1: Strongly disagree; 2: Disagree; 3: Sometimes agree; 4: Agree; 5: Strongly agree

d. Add all of the numbers for 1 through 14 on your individual assessment

e. Add all of the totals for individuals in your group or class to obtain a total of totals

f. Divide the total of the totals by the number of people in your group or class

g. Announce the average score

This is a quick and rough assessment; however, it will enable you to examine your own level of social capital building activities on a personal level beyond just scanning these items. If you have been very busy this year, select an earlier year to rate yourself. Analyze your weakest area of the five component areas. Share results in a class discussion.

- × Were you encouraged by your family or friends to participate in clubs, volunteer, or socialize in groups?

Table 4-1

PUTNAM'S SOCIAL CAPITAL INDEX MODIFIED FOR RATINGS OF INDIVIDUALS

A. MEASURES OF COMMUNITY ORGANIZATIONAL LIFE

1. Served on committees of local organizations in the past year.

2. Served as officer of some club or organization in past year.

3. Memberships in social organizations.

4. Number of club meetings attended last year.

5. Number of group memberships in past year.

B. MEASURES OF ENGAGEMENT IN PUBLIC AFFAIRS

6. Number of times voted in elections last year.

7. Number of times attending public town, political, or school meetings.

C. MEASURES OF COMMUNITY VOLUNTEERISM

8. Number of nonprofit organizations volunteered in.

9. Number of times worked on a community project, walk, race.

10. Number of times did volunteer work in the past year.

D. MEASURES OF INFORMAL SOCIABILITY

11. Time spent visiting friends or relatives last year.

12. Number of times entertained at home in past year.

E. MEASURES OF SOCIAL TRUST

13. Degree of agreement on statement: "Most people can be trusted."

14. Degree of agreement with statement: "Most people are honest."

Adapted from Putnam, R. D. (2000). *Bowling alone. The collapse and revival of American community.* New York, NY: Simon & Schuster.

× Would you say that your neighbors are friendly?

× Do people in your neighborhood walk to school, the post office, market, or library?

× In your earlier school years, were you involved in extracurricular activities?

× Were your favorite activities attractive because of the people present, the nature of the activity itself, or both?

× What is your current attitude toward social capital participation?

× Will social participation assist you with your professional career?

× Do you think that your students, clients, and group members can use an understanding of social capital in their development and recovery?

× Do you encourage your students, clients, and group members to search the web for information and support groups related to their spectrum, disability, or disorder?

× Do you facilitate an exchange of telephone numbers or e-mail addresses with other people they can relate to as they are being discharged?

× In general, can the Web facilitate connections, or is it an escape from real social life?

× Do you know anyone who has/is an avatar character?

× Do you plan to participate in a professional organization or to make presentations at professional conferences in the future?

This is an example of your collaboration in participatory action research.

Relationship of Social Capital to Health

Poortinga (2006) asks a question concerning whether social capital is an individual or collective resource for health. The European Social Survey data from 22 countries were used. Results indicated that individual levels of social trust and civic participation were strongly associated with good health in individuals. In contrast, social trust and civic participation aggregate scores were not associated with people's health at the national level. Countries with low levels of social capital have individuals with good health ranking at lower levels of subjective health than countries with higher levels of health ratings.

The Social Capital of Health Care "Without Borders"

Can professionals in education and health fields move these caring professions beyond the restrictions of insurance systems to expand their scope of service to those most in need? A number of "without borders" groups have moved into international sites to work with marginalized people with basic health needs. Social aspects of enlarging the outreach to those who are excluded and disaffiliated come under the scope of social capital. In the larger sense, aspects of marginality, exclusion, and disaffiliation touch on a lack of social integration in every country, despite its designation as a developed or developing country (Galheigo, 2005). This perception can arise from a perspective of poverty or disaster stricken people as disposable. This standpoint of bias in developed areas can even permeate the mission of caring professionals.

Within borders of developed countries, immigrants, the mentally ill, and homeless are groups of people who become socially invisible, incarcerated, or placed into dangerous "shelters." Social change in the status quo of developed countries may be considered as upsetting to social order and equilibrium. Social exclusion may be perceived as part of the capitalist lifestyle (Galheigo, 2005). This perspective regarding exclusion is in conflict with the mission of caring professions in teaching and treating people at all levels of societal incorporation. In assisting people who are underserved in health domains, professionals need to assist students and clients in realizing that they can become social actors capable of taking care of their health needs (Galheigo, 2005).

Professionals can consider local needs in their area to set up social support networks for those who are socially or politically excluded from the health care system. Other avenues that can bring about change in health care provision include newspapers, television, and computer networks. The social field is perceived by some authors as a context for teachers and health service professionals' interventions (Barros, Ghirardi, & Lopes, 2005). For example, social aspects of occupational therapy practice can move interventions to the common sites of everyday life into collaborative support programs designed for and with participants (Swarbrick, 2009). The role of the therapist should be delineated by his or her social vision as a health professional dedicated to reaching out to people in the community; for example, psychiatric patients who no longer fit into the institutionalized or penal system (Barros et al., 2005; Swarbrick, 2009). These authors perceive occupational therapists as having the social capital required to move social services into the community.

Tolerance Can Expand

Social psychologists Elaine and Art Aron developed a program with four interactive sessions. Half of the group was told that there were prospects of a new relationship developing with someone of another culture, and the other half was not given any future expectations. They call this work a self-expansion model of motivation and cognition in bonding relationships in which they predict that the outcome will be developing a relationship with people of other ethnic groups. Their experiment and study showed that when the likelihood to develop a relationship was previously expected within pairs, there was a greater attraction between them than in pairs not expecting anything. This research revealed that intergroup prejudice can be reduced with a program of specific intervention (Aron et al., 2004; Aron, Steele, Kashdan, & Perez, 2006). Details of the program will be presented in a later chapter. From this research, it appears that mutual trust between people of varying cultures could develop with cultivation to offset the usual reaction of suspicion.

Social Capital and Use of Online Social Network Sites

Steinfield, Ellison, and Lampe (2008) carried out a longitudinal analysis of social networking on the Internet with the online social network Facebook, examining the relationship between degree of use, measurement of psychological health, and bridging social capital development. Survey data collected at the beginning and end of 1 year of Facebook use by college students indicated the outcomes for development of bridging social capital. Self-esteem and satisfaction with life improved more in students with initial lower self-esteem than higher self-esteem students in the area of bridging social capital. The researchers interpret these results to indicate that Facebook use assists lower self-esteem students in reaching out to experience forming large, heterogeneous networks that are associated with bridging social capital.

Centers for Disease Control and Prevention

The Center for Disease Control and Prevention (CDC) Department of Health and Human Services maintains a homepage on social capital on its Web site, www.cdc.gov/healthyplaces/healthtopics/social.htm.

On this Web site, they define social capital as the "fabric of a community and the community pool of human resources" (CDC, 2010). They expand their definition by explaining that time and energy devoted to community improvement, social networking, civic engagement, and personal recreation create social bonds among individuals and groups. They recommend facilitation of extracurricular activities for children, recreation time for adults after work, involvement in neighborhood improvement projects and events, and time for family members to spend together. Their premise is that the health of individuals and families will be affected if circumstances prevent or limit social capital in a community.

United Nations Development Programme

The United Nations Development Programme (UNDP) has organized a Human Development Index that can determine the level of well-being in a country. NYU Wagner's Women of Color Policy Network of the Wagner Graduate School of Public Service carried out a 4-year study in New York City examining its neighborhoods (Heinlein, 2007). The districts were rated high, medium, and low in human development by examining residents' longevity; education; standard of living; health; income; environment; race; achievements; and access to medical facilities, parks, and public transportation. One large goal of UNDP is to provide employment programs in countries needing support in job skills training (UNDP, 2010).

World Health Organization

As described in Chapter 2, the World Health Organization (WHO) has published the *International Classification of Functioning, Disability and Health (ICF)*

(2001). In a section on Activities and Participation, Chapters 7 and 9 titled "Interpersonal Interactions and Relationships" and "Community, Social, and Civic Life" indicate how social capital reflects the importance of social participation on general health. This WHO guide in Chapter 7 emphasizes the importance of social relationships, in general and in particular, in the family, between couples, and in informal settings. In *ICF* Chapter 9, the focus is on community life, recreation, leisure, religion, spirituality, human rights, political life, and citizenship. In general, WHO aims to fight global disease, provide medications internationally, control tobacco, intervene in disease after disaster, and research chronic diseases (2001; see Appendix).

The World Bank

The World Bank and the Organization for Economic Cooperation and Development (OECD) (World Bank, 2001) accept the integration of social capital theory with economic theory by way of becoming a proponent of sustainable development in economically disadvantaged countries. In the Bank's poverty reduction programs, community improvement, village problem solving and decision making, group designing of civic projects, and building up local organizations were linked to monetary funding. Both perceive the need for social capital development in the projects they undertake.

Governments that the Bank aims to assist also request a participatory, bottom-up approach to support local organizations in a manner sensitive to cultural contexts, such as micro-financing programs and micro-lending to small businesses in women's cottage industries (Field, 2003). Unfortunately, sometimes local groups have been taken advantage of by powerful bosses, such as in Mexico where patronage practices slowed down development of social capital for deserving poor people, thus reflecting the dark side of efforts to promote positive growth of local government (Field, 2003). Globally, the World Bank concerns itself with agriculture, energy, governance, and sustainable cities (2001).

International Monetary Fund

The International Monetary Fund (IMF) deals with macro-financing of countries internationally who have concerns of liquidity and whose markets are in crisis. They provide funding through loans in order to assist governments in developing a sound financial base (Fukuyama, 1999).

The Social Capital Foundation

In its mission statement, the Social Capital Foundation (TSCF, 2002) explains that it is a nonprofit organization that pursues the promotion of social capital and social cohesion. This group perceives social capital as a resource with a set of mental dispositions and attitudes fostering cooperative behaviors in communities. Its orientation focuses on the dimensions of market economy, the central role of the middle class in democratic societies, the strengthening of civic responsibility and social partnership, and the preservation of cultural identity in communities (TSCF, 2002). This group publishes a journal called *The International Scope Review.*

Discussion

Have you ever witnessed a scenario like this? (Table 4-2). In business settings, do women have less social capital than men? When women give good suggestions, do they sound confident? What is going on here? What is your theory?

What components of social capital do you see surfacing in this poem (Table 4-3)?

Table 4-2

"A group of 10 professional staff members have gathered with their boss for a monthly planning meeting. After some initial explanation of a new dilemma mentioned by one of the staff, one member makes a suggestion to solve the problem in a manner she hoped would make it easy for people to understand and accept. No one picks up on this idea, but the discussion goes forward. After several minutes, the boss says, 'You know, I've been thinking, we should do X.' And the woman is sitting there thinking, 'Unbelievable, I just said that.' But no one had heard her, and no one corrects this impression. It was as if, when the woman spoke, a television was on with the sound turned off. This has happened to every woman I know" (Daum, 2008, p. 74).

Table 4-3

COMMUNITY BUILDERS

Untitled Poem:
Problem-Solving by a Student Living in a 'Hood'
By Anonymous

Listen my children and you shall hear about,
How we live and what we fear,
Other kids don't feel the shame, kids in our hood,
Fear violence and gangs.
Hobos, prostitutes surrounded by trash,
With drunk, broken bottles and dealers making cash.

The people say, "We're so cute."
Try to pat our heads and say "Now shoo."
They say they'll help,
Then give us the boot.
They tell us something, but don't tell us the truth.
Would you like living around this abuse?

There is only one way to come to school,
That's past 13 liquor stores, and that's not cool.
When we walk past the stores, what do we see?
Boarded up buildings and drunks who are obscene.
We're a team, we work together,
To move those stores, now and forever.

Community helpers want to picket,
Hey the MOVE team does it the legal way.
We've worked hard to get where we're at,
But we're not quite finished yet.
We want future kids to grow up safe,
Not knowing the abuse that we had to take.

We don't care what people say,
We're not going to quit till those stores
Are out of our way,
Stores, out of our way
Stores, out of our way
Stores, out of our way.

Adapted from An anonymous poem mailed by S. Mason, May 25, 1994, St. Louis, MO. In W. F. Tate (Ed.), *Educational Researcher, 37,* 409.

Other community builders include book clubs where neighbors who never spoke to each other come together to discuss, argue, reveal themselves, and experience each other's humanity (Hernandez, 2008). Members of this group admit that they have commonalities that they are surprised about. The promotion of communication and conversation is good for the community.

A cardiac club is described by a self-confessed loner and couch potato who discovered the good in groups. The group convinced this man after open-heart surgery that exercise would not cause him to collapse and die on the gym floor (Edwards, 2006). The author admits that his fellow rehabbers supplied a boost to him to get engaged. Support groups are another way to build community. When people have health problems, they can learn from each other and find empathy.

Community building came as a surprise for five friends who found the recipe for financial success in a financial support group (Pesce, 2008). One member had been a freelance writer who spent years covering personal finance in *Newsweek*. However, her own fiscal situation was not up to par. This imaginary scenario presents a meeting of the five women.

Script: Financial Support Group

April: I did everything wrong for a while in my 20s. I cashed out a 401(k). At that time, I owed $30,000-plus in credit card debt. I was living from one paycheck to another.

May: I'd like to talk about my finances, but I hope that what we say here is confidential.

All: *(nods of agreement)* We agree. It will be.

Jane: I need some sympathy and support, but usually talking about money is more personal than talking about sex.

Sue: I saw this Oprah special on finances, and it made me think that we could help each other.

Kim: It's a good idea, but I don't want to end up having to cut out my social life or trips.

Jane: Let's try to meet once a week for a while, and see what happens.

Sue: What I like about this group is that you all know what my life and lifestyle are like. If we went to a financial advisor, that aspect might be ignored.

April: I agree, and we have somewhat similar lifestyles, and no one has a personal or commercial stake in anyone else's financial investments.

Kim: April, I've gone through a period of reckless spending like you. It used to be so hard for me not to go to clothing sales when I'd see them on TV.

May: Let's bring in our numbers next week and all bring calculators. Bring in your salary numbers and outstanding loans like school and car loans, as well as what you pay for rent.

Jane: Should we have one chairperson or rotate chairpeople?

Sue: Let's rotate chairpeople. Who would be willing to go first?

April: If we also rotate apartments, I'll go first if it can be at my apartment next time.

Kim: Next week, we can crunch our numbers and figure out how much we need to save for IRAs and if we want to buy a condo.

May: Once we get started, let's also take turns researching topics such as online bill paying, IRAs, retirement plans at work, stocks, savings accounts, and health and insurance plans.

Sue: Also, if we pick the same night of the week from now on, we can make our other plans around it.

April: Shall we have food to make it fun?

All: *(nods of agreement)* Yeah, that sounds like a good idea.

Jane: How about if everyone brings something to share?

The End.

One group in Canada (Pesce, 2008) who followed this format said that they became financially solvent, paid off debts, and became fiscally literate. They figured out their individual preferences in spending, established retirement accounts, and improved their credit scores. They also set long-range goals for the future. Together, they found areas where they could save money. They were so successful that they developed a television program on the topic and wrote a book guiding others (Baxter, Self, Dunsworth, Gunn, & Hanna, 2000). *What types of capital and principles does this financial support group demonstrate? Give examples.*

Social Networking Guidelines Online

For social networking sites online, some people use a pseudonym as an online name. It also is sometimes advisable to create an additional e-mail account for forwarding social network messages. Later, this account would be easier to cancel if it is kept as a "spare" account. Never use the same login/password on more than one site. Do not be afraid to say no or stop contact with someone encountered online. If meeting an online friend for the first time or conducting a transaction generated online, meet in a public place (Symantec, 2010).

Combining Social Capital and Political Capital to Find Peace

Terrorism gave way to cooperation when two men with a great deal of political capital used their social capital to shift from aggression and strife in Northern Ireland to a desire for economic improvement. Unionist leader Ian Paisley and Sinn Fein President Gerry Adams met in March 2007 to iron out plans for economic collaboration between the two "religious" groups. The threat for Protestants had been that the larger numbers of Catholics could outvote them in union negotiations. Their popular leaders saw the success of open markets in southern Ireland and convinced their people through social and political capital to find peace and economic improvement through collaboration in unions, shipyards, offices and cottage industries, glassware, tool and dye, and communications equipment manufacturing (Mulvaney, 2007).

Development of Social Capital and Political Capital Network in National Election

The presidential election of 2008 illustrated the possibilities present in building a grassroots network online through a national Web site developed by Barack Obama, www.barackobama.com. Through this medium, he recruited new and old voters, published speeches, advertised his proposed legislation and positions on national issues, and raised funds (Barack Obama Official Web Site). Teachers, practitioners, and community leaders can use the Web to develop networks of information about educational topics; possible interventions for health and psychological conditions; as well as suggestions for organization of community activities, events, projects, and improvements.

Summary

Members of service professions in education and health have the luxury of having enough social capital to extend their caring reach through and with their students and clients. Students and clients need to see themselves as participants in society through service to each other and to the larger community. In this way, social capital is shared, and students and clients perceive themselves as making a contribution to society. Thus, they feel like they belong to the communities of school; clubs; teams; and civic, spiritual, and support groups.

Script for Analysis: Sailing Club Meeting

Seating Chart

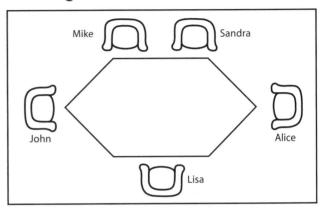

Background

The monthly sailing club meeting is gathering at a local restaurant in a side room. The major goal of this meeting is an educational presentation on weathering storms on the water. Before the meeting begins, members socialize, moving from table to table. The membership consists of roughly half and half boat owners and crew members. The boat owners connect with crew at these meetings, and the crew are looking for skippers who would be glad to have them on board. Members rely on their social capital to enable them to collaborate on plans to sail together in a sociable setting. In addition, sailing together in a cooperative environment builds social capital for the participants and for the club. Five club members sit down at a restaurant table.

Characters

John: A successful architect who is a great sailor and loves to be on the water. He always carries two of every mechanical boat part on board in case of emergencies on his medium-sized boat or on others' boats. He is generous in sharing his expertise and supplies.

Sandra: A stage lighting director for a troupe of Shakespearean actors who travel around the country. She is an expert sailor, having taken a number of Power Squadron courses on navigation, weather, and seamanship. She prefers cruising to racing.

Mike: Crew person who has taken many sailing courses, as well as having experience on cruising to Maine, on the Long Island sound, and in the Caribbean. He is an engineer in a village of an affluent suburb and has crewed for John for years. They win many races.

Alice: Loves to cruise and provide galley gourmet provisions for the boats she sails on. She has taken several water and classroom courses from the Red Cross Safely Sailing program. Alice and Sandra love to swim off boats together while at anchor or mooring.

Lisa: Owns a medium-sized boat and is able to sail calmly without barking orders. She is also a great chef and generous provider. She is the Commodore of the sailing club this year. She is a computer Web site operator by profession.

Action Begins Here

John: Are any of you going on the cruise this year? Mike and I will be going together. The fleet captain is suggesting we go to Maine for a 2-week cruise.

Sandra: I'm available to be a crew on the cruise, if you are looking for more crew.

Lisa: Did anyone check the tides in terms of the best time and day to leave?

John: The fleet captain did go over that at the skipper's meeting.

Alice: Lisa invited me to join her on her boat, so we'll be eating up a storm!

John: We'll be rafting up with your boat whenever we can. Sandra, I'd love to take you on my boat, but I need to check with my first mate to see if she has invited other people, too.

Sandra: One week would be enough for me. I could meet up with you at a port halfway.

Alice: That's what I'm doing, too. Just 1 week is a good amount of time to be on the water. Lisa, would you like me to bring lunch and appetizer supplies?

Lisa: That would be good because we'll eat on shore most nights, until we get to Oldport where we can barbeque on their grill.

Alice: Great. The crew would like to treat you to dinner one night.

Mike: How many boats are going this year?

Lisa: Five, I think, but you know how it is. Boats converge in and out of the planned itinerary.

John: We'll keep in touch by monitoring channels 16 and 72.

Mike: Has the assistant fleet captain made reservations for us at yacht clubs along the way?

Lisa: Yes, he took care of those calls about 2 weeks ago.

Alice: I'm looking forward to the cruise. It's always an adventure.

Sandra: It looks like the guest speaker is about to be introduced.

To be continued...

Discussion

1. How does the club promote social capital building as a process?

2. How does the current planning process facilitate social capital?

3. How does the focus on sport and travel provide capital to grow social participation?

4. Which members here demonstrate leadership?

5. Which member intervened to reassure Sandra?

6. What other clubs or groups develop social capital among members?

7. What other aspect of this script would you like to discuss?

References

Aron, A., McLaughline-Volpe, T., Mashek, D., Lewandowski, G., Wright, S. C., & Aron, N. (2004). Including close other in the self. *European Review of Social Psychology, 15,* 101-132.

Aron, A., Steele, J. L., Kashdan, T. B., & Perez, M. (2006). When similars do not attract: Tests of a prediction from the self-expansion model. *Personal Relationships, 13,* 387-396.

Barros, D. D., Ghirardi, M. I. G., & Lopes, R. E. (2005). Social occupation therapy: A socio-historical perspective. In F. Kronenberg, S. S. Algado, & N. Pollard (Eds.), *Occupational therapy without borders* (pp. 140-151). London, England: Elsevier Churchill Livingstone.

Baxter, A., Self, A., Dunsworth, K., Gunn, R., & Hanna, S. (2000). *The smart cookies' guide to making more dough.* New York, NY: Random House.

Bordieu, P. (1980). Le capital social: Notes provisoires. *Actes de la rescherche en sciences socials, 31,* 2-3.

Bordieu, P. (1984). *Distinction: A social critique of the judgment of taste.* London, England: Routledge.

Bordieu, P. (1986). The forms of capital. In J. G. Richardson (Ed.)., *Handbook of theory and research for the sociology of education.* New York, NY: Greenwood Press.

Bordieu, P., & Wacquant, L. (1992). *An invitation to reflexive sociology.* Chicago, IL: University of Chicago Press.

Coleman, J. S. (1961). *Adolescent society: The social life of the teenager and its impact on education.* New York, NY: Free Press.

Coleman, J. S. (1988). Social capital in the creation of human capital. *American Journal of Sociology, 94,* 95-120.

Coleman, J. S. (1990). *Equality and achievement in education.* Boulder, CO: Westview Press.

Coleman, J. S. (1991). Prologue: Constructed social organisation. In P. Bourdieu & J. S. Coleman (Eds.), *Social theory for a changing society* (pp. 1-14). Boulder, CO: Westview Press.

Coleman, J. S. (1994). *Foundations of social theory.* Cambridge, MA: Belknap Press.

Coleman, J. S., & Hoffer, T. (1987). *Public and private high schools: The impact of communities.* New York, NY: Basic Books.

Community Foundation of Silicon Valley. (2008). *The Social Capital Benchmark Survey.* Retrieved from www.cfsv.org/communitysurvey

Daum, J. H. (2008). Lessons from the front lines. *Newsweek, October 13,* 74.

DeFilippis, J. (2001). The myth of social capital in community development. *Housing Policy Debate, 12,* 781-806.

Dekker, P., & Uslander, E. M. (Eds.). (2001). *Social capital and participation in everyday life.* London, England: Routledge.

Edwards, M. (2006). My cardiac club. *AARP Bulletin,* May, 12.

Field, J. (2003). *Social capital.* London, England: Routledge.

Fukuyama, F. (1999). *Social capital and civil society.* International Monetary Fund (IMF). Retrieved April 1, 2008 from www.imf.org/external/pubs/ft/seminar/1999/reforms/fukuyama.htm

Galheigo, S. M. (2005). Occupational therapy and the social field: Clarifying concepts and ideas. In F. Kronenberg, S. S. Algado, & N. Pollard (Eds.), *Occupational therapy without borders* (pp. 87-98). London, England: Elsevier Churchill Livingstone.

Heinlein, S. (2007). For richer or for poorer. *NYU Alumni Magazine, Fall,* 21.

Hernandez, C. (2008). One book, one community. *Newsday, March 9,* 22, 24.

Mason, S. (1994). Untitled poem. Problem-solving by a student living in a 'hood. In W. F. Tate (Ed.), *Educational Researcher, 37,* 409.

Mulvaney, J. (2007). Two reasonable men find the path to peace. *Newsday, April 8,* 39.

Pesce, N. L. (2008). 'Dough' girls. *Daily News, October 16,* 42.

Poortinga, W. (2006). Social capital: An individual or collective resource for health? *Social Epidemiology, 62,* 292-302.

Putnam, R. (2008). Diversity and social capital work. *Saguaro Seminar: Better Together.* Retrieved October 16, 2008 from www.bettertogether.org

Putnam, R. D. (1993). *Making democracy work: Civic traditions in modern Italy.* Princeton, NJ: Princeton University Press.

Putnam, R. D. (1996). Who killed civic America? *Prospect, 7,* 66-72.

Putnam, R. D. (2000). *Bowling alone. The collapse and revival of American community.* New York, NY: Simon & Schuster.

Putnam, R. D., Feldstein, L. M., & Cohen, D. (2003). *Better together. Restoring the American community.* New York, NY: Simon & Schuster.

Saguaro Seminars. (2008). *Diversity, immigration and social capital.* Retrieved October 16, 2008 from www.hks.harvard.edu/saguaro/

Social Capital Foundation. (2002). Retrieved May 2008 from www.socialcapital-foundation.org/

Steinfield, C., Ellison, N. B., & Lampe, C. (2008). Social capital, self-esteem, and use of online social network sites: A longitudinal analysis. *Journal of Applied Developmental Psychology, 29,* 434-445.

Swarbrick, M. (2009). Collaborative support programs of New Jersey. *Occupational Therapy in Mental Health, 25,* 224-238.

World Bank. (2001). *The Organization for Economic Cooperation and Development (OECD).* Retrieved October 2008 from www.worldbank.org/

World Health Organization. (2001). *International classification of functioning, disability and health.* Retrieved Ocober 2008 from www.who.int/

Additional Resources

Barack Obama Official Web site. (n.d.). Retrieved from www.barackobama.com/

Better Together. (n.d.) Retrieved from www.bettertogether.org

Centers for Disease Control. (May 18, 2010). Retrieved from www.cdc.gov/healthyplaces/healthtopics/social.htm

Community Foundation of Silicon Valley. (2010). Retrieved from www.cfsv.org/communitysurvey

Interntional Monetary Fund. (2005). Retrieved from www.imf.org

Organization for Economic Cooperation and Development. (n.d.). Retrieved from www.oecd.org/dataoecd/25/6/1825848.pdf

Saguaro Research. (2007). *About Social Capital.* Retrieved from www.hks.harvard.edu/saguaro/research/saguaroresearch.htm

Symantec. Retrieved from www.symantec.com/norton

United Nations Development Programme. (2010). Retrieved from www.undp.org

chapter 5

Social Participation in Professional Education

Mary V. Donohue, PhD, OTL, FAOTA

Overview

Classes, labs, joint projects, and study groups provide invaluable opportunities for the development of professional social participation. Aspects of cooperative learning, leadership, research, group session, and programmatic organization will be included so that students begin to plan now for continuous experiential professional development to be ongoing during their career. This chapter will focus on the processes of social participation in professional education: interaction in groups, the characteristics of individual professionals, modeling in graduate education, opportunities for exchange of social capital aspects of classmates, and social emotional learning through class projects. Additional topics will include fieldwork supervision groups, group presentations, study groups, research partnerships, and collaborative field meetings. Finally, this chapter will address problem-based learning, volunteer opportunities, participation in professional organizations as a student, and the potential for problem-solving teamwork in business group decision making. During this discussion, topics related to professional skills such as cognitive, psycho-emotional, analysis, and decision making will be emphasized as they can be developed by social participation in classes and in carrying out joint assignments.

Social Participation and the Individual's Professional Characteristics

No two clinicians, teachers, or therapists are the same. *What are the appropriate social parameters of being a professional? What is the range of acceptable interpersonal interaction? Do the role models seen in soap operas and medical shows on television subliminally influence the formation of professionals in educational and clinical arenas today?*

To answer these questions, this section will consider the traits of sociability, social presence, and socialization into roles as they relate to the process of individual professional socialization (Gough, 1957). Taken as a composite, these characteristics provide a foundation for establishing a professional identity. Chapter 2 provided general definitions of these three characteristics.

Sociability (Gough, 1957) varies across environmental settings. In informal settings, people may manifest sociability through a gregarious personality, an outgoing friendliness, and a relaxed appearance of having expanses of time to interact with others. In study groups of professional students, this affability may be moderated while focusing on learning content. However, in educational and clinical settings, the professional's friendliness needs to be general in the sense of being as impartial as possible

Cole, M.B., & Donohue, M.V. *Social Participation in Occupational Contexts: In Schools, Clinics, and Communities* (pp 81-96).
© 2011 SLACK Incorporated

toward individual children, clients, and community group members. The emerging professional needs fieldwork settings in which to practice becoming comfortable with listening to others and spending adequate amounts of time in assessing and treating them.

In the hallways of work settings, the professional needs to learn how to greet staff, children, and clients in a brief, friendly manner, taking care of their immediate needs, such as where to find an office or a therapist. All professionals need some "downtime" for socializing informally with peers in appropriate areas such as staff lounges. Professionals of all types need to curtail discussion of clients or children in public areas.

The first time a practicing professional student, new clinician, or teacher experiences the attraction and potential of friendship with a child, adolescent, adult student, client, or consumer, the developing professional may experience conflict in wishing to be friendly, yet being aware that it is necessary to remain in a professional role stance. Whether a new or seasoned professional, relationships between students, clients, and patients need to remain focused on the benefit desired by professionals for those in their care. Spending an inordinate amount of time, energy, and emotion on one student, one patient, or one client confuses the recipient and deprives others needing care of the attention they deserve. It also establishes a relationship outside of the boundaries of the professional role, which both caregiver and recipient of care may emotionally desire but is outside of the parameters contracted within the norms of a professional relationship. The caregiver needs to keep in mind that he or she is in a superior position of power, which should not be used to gratify an emotional attraction with a care recipient.

Likewise, the reverse instance, where patients are ignored while professionals discuss or indulge their own personal interests is unethical. In supervision, the clinician, teacher, or professional can obtain support and guidance for awkward situations and relationships that may arise during fieldwork or later while on the job.

Social presence (Gough, 1957) of a professional nature requires assessment of the individual and group population. The degree of social assertiveness in a professional setting is dictated by time constraints in working with each individual child or client. This is the area where the individual traits of the professional are most in evidence. For example, some therapists can provide therapeutic support for the clinical climate by using their sense of humor tailored to the client and his or her current condition. Other

therapists' efforts at humor might fall flat. Feedback received during and after classroom practice presentations can be helpful indicators about one's professional/personal style. In group situations in classrooms or hospitals, the professional needs to consider whether the particular group has a sense of humor, is being regulated on medication on an inpatient service, or is living in the community while attending a day hospital or clubhouse because of a chronic condition. All of these considerations are part of developing a therapeutic relationship with patients (Figure 5-1).

Gradually developing experience as a professional over time from practice situations with other students in groups to initial and advanced fieldwork exposure in clinics, schools, and the community is the usual path to understanding and becoming capable of entering into a therapeutic relationship. As students come into early contact with children, patients, and groups in the community, they need to focus, as they develop their social presence with clients, on the needs and goals of those they serve. In this way, they will be less self-conscious as well as on target with who they are as professionals. During this process, the ability of the student to assess the personal, social, and cultural aspects of individuals and groups as entities will also enable him or her to form his or her professional social persona. These clinical judgment processes are essential to incorporating the values of the profession to which the students aspire. These developmental professional processes prepare the student for entering into therapeutic relationships with the children, patients, and clients in the community.

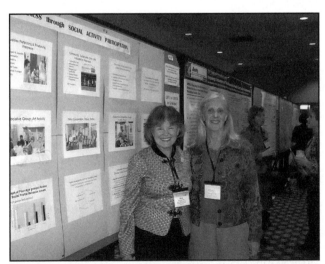

Figure 5-1. Two colleagues collaborate at a CDC conference to share perspectives in a poster designed to explain the concepts and research findings of social participation.

Table 5-1

STRATEGIES TO PRACTICE PROFESSIONAL SOCIALIZATION

Professionals who are perpetual "people-pleasers" can undertake a number of strategies to change their high level of social participation. Practice some of these strategies in class or on your own time with a friend:

1. Postpone a reponse to a request until you check your calendar and your goals.

2. Examine your motivation for acquiescing to a request to make certain it fulfills your goals and not someone else's goals.

3. Role play to practice asserting your needs. Practice saying no to unreasonable requests until your responses begin to feel natural.

4. If you say yes initially and then regret it, return to the individual and say that you had to reconsider for reasons that relate to your work.

When leading inpatient activity groups on a locked unit in a psychiatric hospital with newly admitted, newly medicated, and sensitive individuals, the therapist may need to moderate an assertive self-presentation as patients may be in a sensitive state of response. On the other hand, while being supportive of chronic outpatients who are somewhat lethargic or lacking in motivation, the therapist can present him- or herself with energy and hope for the future of their well-being. Cultural aspects of encounters with some children, adolescents, adults, and seniors need to consider their social developmental setting, attire, and customs. In some cultures, male patients would be expected to avoid shaking hands with a female therapist. The therapist needs to be accepting of these circumstances, while pointing out to the client that in some job search situations, he may be expected to shake hands.

In classroom settings, a substitute teacher cannot expect to have the same rapport with a new class that he or she has with the usual class group. Calling on the class or group to assist with social interaction between the teacher and the students can assist a new teacher in being "him- or herself" so as to be most efficacious in working with the class or group members. At the same time, appropriate classroom and clinical norms of behavior by the therapist or teacher need to be expected to be achieved.

Socialization (Gough, 1957) into one's profession varies according to the role of the professional in any given setting and within certain sets of activities. Norms for dress may depend on whether the professional is a sports coach, child sensorimotor therapist doing floor activities, college professor, or the head of a department. Requirements of the style of intervention demand various types of social participation on the part of the teacher, coach, therapist, or nurse in order to engage the child or client. New therapists require time to meet the expectations of both the clients and the other staff and supervisors. When working on a team, the professional should represent his or her own profession and not feel constrained by the norms of other professions if they are not appropriate to one's own role. In some settings, all professionals are expected to dress more formally for a team meeting, in contrast to the attire for teaching kitchen activities of daily living or for playing baseball later in the day.

In the process of socialization, professionals need to learn how to say no on occasion to children, patients, and colleagues. Otherwise, becoming a "people-pleaser" to accommodate the requests of others can cause stress, burnout, and maladaptive intervention. Responding to the needs of others is an essential part of normal social functioning, but people-pleasers are so invested in outside approval that they may set their realistic professional needs aside, becoming overwhelmed by day-to-day activity. As a result, these therapists or teachers have no time to advance their own professional careers, for example, by not being able to undertake a research project related to developing evidence-based practice for their work. These behaviors exact a heavy toll not only on the individual, but on the profession's progress in building its theoretical base upon an empirical foundation (Table 5-1).

Social Participation and Professional Development in Various Group/Class Levels of Interaction

The five levels of group interaction of Parten (1932) and Mosey (1968, 1986) can be employed by faculty and students for the students' experiential learning of professional participation skills and intervention methods. While originally the five levels are learned at age-appropriate intervals, they can be used throughout the human lifespan to achieve a variety of goals and methods of intervention.

Parallel level (Parten, 1932; Mosey, 1986) instruction occurs in didactic classroom presentations by the faculty or during student presentations when students sit parallel in chairs and spend most of the time listening to information on a topic. Some students prefer this type or level of setting for learning. It is valuable in providing lengthy instruction through educational videos, which can then be discussed. When faculty organize discussion by eliciting viewpoints and information from students as they sit in parallel chairs, there is opportunity for participation, which greatly adds to the vitality of the learning experience. In this way, students provide each other with the opportunity to get to know the knowledge base, cultural background, and cognitive philosophical viewpoint of others in the class. This forum provides students with the opportunity to venture into a sphere of public speaking in order to become accustomed to hearing their own voice in a larger gathering. Taking that risk is an important professional skill that requires practice in order to increase the student's comfort level in larger discussion groups, such as grand rounds in a hospital, faculty meetings in a school, or meetings with parents in a school open house event (Figure 5-2).

Associative level (Parten, 1932) interaction occurs in dyadic pairings or small groups of three to four students assigned to work together for brief periods of time (e.g., reading or arithmetic instruction by one-on-one coaching, practice in making splints, fitting for wheelchairs or crutches, or experiential interpersonal exercises with randomly assigned partners who briefly discuss their reactions with each other at the end of the activity). Students may be assigned to one-on-one role playing of a therapist and child relating around balance activities, refocusing interventions, and repeated guidance to engage an autistic child in an activity of the child's choice.

There are multiple opportunities for associative-type participation practice during curriculum or

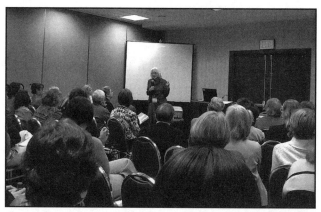

Figure 5-2. An expert in the area of the Well Elderly Studies explains interventions and research findings to interdisciplinary colleagues at a Centers for Disease Control conference, enhancing her own and the audience's professional socialization.

professional preparation of one-to-one or small group activity interaction for working with children, clients, and community members. It is very advantageous for future professionals to experience various levels of social participation so as to understand the impact of close one-on-one contact in working with others. Some children and clients greatly enjoy this amount of attention; however, others may be intimidated by the closeness. It is the professional responsibility of teachers, therapists, clinicians, and social workers to develop the ability to assess the reactions of people they are working with in close proximity and adjust their approach to children and clients accordingly.

The *International Classification of Function (ICF)* (World Health Organization [WHO], 2001), in the section on Activities and Participation, Chapter 7, "Interpersonal Interactions and Relationships," points out the need for brief interactions in social participation in some public settings, which is also apropos in some aspects of professional roles (e.g., in greeting clients, patients, or children in the treatment facility or school during the change of classes or sessions).

Basic cooperative level (Mosey, 1986; Parten, 1932) course participation is built into many curriculums when small groups of 4 to 10 graduate students are asked to first plan an activity that will achieve a certain goal, and then to carry it out. This type/level of group is used as part of teacher preparation in fostering social participation to guide students in working in small project groups in the future, as well as part of therapists' practice for coaching clients to interact socially in therapeutic activity task groups, such as cooking, movement, sports, or artistic expression. Students need to practice how to coach such a small ongoing group, allowing members as much latitude as possible to problem-solve their choices, make some mistakes, consider other options, and bring the task to completion in one or multiple sessions, as is appropriate to the activity.

Students being professionally prepared will also have opportunities during fieldwork to guide actual ongoing groups of children, teens, and adults who may need some facilitation or coaching to achieve social interaction appropriate to the activity but who should be given as much autonomy as possible. As they experience a variety of groups, professional students need to learn how their style warrants moderation: whether they are too controlling to permit the group enough space to interact, or if they are too passive to engage the group with evocative interaction. In addition, students preparing themselves to lead groups need to learn to assess if the group needs more or less guidance and support depending on the group's personality.

Supportive cooperative level (Mosey, 1986) course participation introduces a new dimension into the professional students' group interaction by encouraging the expression of feelings during and after an activity is completed. Professional students who will be working with groups as teachers, therapists, and guidance counselors need experience in demonstrating emotion to others at a moderate level of sharing. They can use feedback in such courses as group therapy, activity group process, guidance, or rehab counseling groups as to whether their style of reaction and interaction is suitable, passive, sarcastic, impatient, or overemotional in nature. Often, practice with assertiveness activities can assist groups of professional students to evaluate what is called for in situations that may arise. Role playing such scenarios, as may arise in afterschool coaching or club moderator settings, is needed so that future leaders of groups come to understand how they may react on the spot in actual situations.

Future professional group leaders can benefit greatly by being in interactive simulated situations so as to come to know their own emotional range and responses. Some professional students may over-identify with adolescents, and others may tend to dominate a group of teens in a parental manner. Teens and adults whose activity has the potential for group interaction with the expression of emotions need teachers, therapists, and counselors who can permit the group to explore possible emotions, share cultural and political differences of life and opinion, and create a temporarily challenging environment that can evolve into a positive experience. Professional students need to incorporate social emotional learning so that they may pass it on to their clients, students, and patients (Cohen, 2006; Zins, Weissberg, Wang, & Walberg, 2004).

Mature level (Lifton, 1966; Mosey, 1986) course participation can occur in professional programs after students have had the opportunity to become comfortable with supportive cooperative group interaction and are ready to integrate this ability with task or basic cooperative goals, so as to function as a mature productive group. This level of group participation combines the basic cooperative task and supportive cooperative levels of group performance. In some programs, this occurs in joint research project groups where the task is an essential goal needing expedited accomplishment in a brief period of time, perhaps over two semesters. Emotions can arise during the process of deciding on a subject to research, dividing up the tasks, experiencing an uneven level of participation by some members, or experiencing the temptation to cut corners in the research process. Other courses often require assignment of a professional/political/community project to be undertaken by groups of graduate students where similar dilemmas demand working together under time-limited circumstances.

Professional students usually pull together to accomplish their task in these groups that demand mature participation levels. A few groups may fail to form as cohesive entities or may fail to organize clear-cut goals. These groups can usually self-identify their deficits and need to express emotional concern to each other about their lack of progress in completing their tasks in a timely manner with all members participating. Their communication to each other can be facilitated by as simple a statement as, "We need to..."

In other instances, a reorganization of roles assumed may need to take place for the ultimate good of all, even if one student is not pulling his or her weight. Sometimes, unforeseen events occur in the life of a graduate student group member who needs to share with the group the disruption of the usual routine and the predicted inability to carry out the shared role or responsibility. At that point, a truly mature group would rearrange tasks so that the group as a whole could complete their goal and obtain a desirable grade. The experience of such social participation in graduate education is applicable to many future life situations when working in a group and needs to be shared to bring high school and college students along in the developmental progression of achieving a similar mature result in their groups (e.g., in ethical dilemmas in sorority, fraternity, or sports groups).

Process of Applying Social Learning Theory to Professional Socialization

Bandura would be pleased with the type of methods available in most professional courses designed as they are for the development of socialization of caregiving professionals in education and health. The question is, "Do graduate students fully appreciate and take advantage of these opportunities for social modeling and self-efficacy?" When other professional students are presenting material in public speaking opportunities using Power Point and videos, do the students in the audience analyze these live models and symbolic models for imitation of their strategies and style as in Bandura's (1977) participant modeling? These same student presentations provide a setting for relating to and experiencing the performance exposure and performance desensitization Bandura speaks of through the multiple sessions of observation of presentations and subsequent experience of presentations.

Bandura (1977) also encourages self-instructed social skill performance, which can be carried out when education and health professional students are expected to teach a social skill to themselves or to each other, such as a joint computer game or a joint art project. In this manner, they may experience how to approach this learning mode so as to make it part of their learning repertoire. This process can teach future professionals what the experience of social skill instruction might be like for the children, clients, or community members with whom they will work. Professional students can also provide themselves with social skill instruction when they try out various methods of affirmation and role playing to determine what works best for them. Sensory arousal and relaxation techniques (Bandura, 1977) carried out in groups or individually can also promote self-efficacy learning.

Professional students need to learn how to commend a fellow student on a good presentation and how to give feedback suggestions to coach a peer toward better performance in the future, in an objective manner without hostility or condescension. These skills need to be integrated by students into their profile of professional socialization. In a more formal situation, a compliment can be accompanied by a handshake. Bandura (1977) would refer to these methods as attribution and exhortation. There are many opportunities to work on these skills in classes practicing assertiveness, in role playing, and in group therapy labs.

Experiences of identification of emotion following an activity of symbolic desensitization, exposure to an unfamiliar travel experience, and self-control of breathing teach future professionals that they can regulate emotional arousal (Bandura, 1977). Later, these professionals can assist future clients, students, and group members in desensitizing themselves so as to tolerate unexpected and stressful situations. Knowledge of these approaches can restore someone's social participation, which was stymied by fear of travel or agoraphobia. Seeing a video about how someone conquers a fear or overcomes an obsession can enable future professionals to become convinced about how therapeutic and educational interventions can be efficacious.

Professional Socialization

Most professions have guidelines for practice that present the scope of that profession's domain. These guidelines include areas of practice for the professional, client factors considered, performance skills and patterns of the profession, contexts and environments for that profession, and the process of assessment and intervention for that profession. The professional socialization of students and practitioners consists of knowledge and acceptance of these parameters in order to become identified with a specific profession and be considered an ethical and competent member. Educators in the professions are directed and guided by such frameworks to develop their students along these lines. One example of a composite of directives is the *Occupational Therapy Practice Framework: Domain and Process* (American Occupational Therapy Association, [AOTA] 2008). Within these guidelines, the Framework speaks to the topic of this book that the occupational therapy practitioner is expected to work in the social context and environment composed of relationships with individuals, organizations, and populations of people with disabilities. In treating individuals, the practitioner is directed to incorporate spouses, friends, and caregivers in the treatment's scope. The practitioner also needs to acknowledge the groups and organizations important to the individuals in their past and current life. Likewise, the practitioner is guided to assist individuals in interfacing with social systems such as political, legal, economic, and institutional contexts in their recovery process. The practitioner attempts to enable individuals to recognize social norms, role expectations, and routines that they will encounter in society (AOTA, 2008).

Table 5-2

ACTIVITY EXAMPLE

An activity that can elicit positive personal characteristics of others in groups consists of the leader asking each group member to write down, on three small pieces of paper, three positive attributes that he or she possesses. The papers are then folded and put in a box. The box is placed in the middle of the table or floor. Each group member takes a turn selecting a piece of paper and reading the trait aloud to the group. The group then guesses to whom the characteristic belongs. Usually, the group identifies a number of people in the group who have this positive strength of character, which is a morale builder for the group in general. The leader can ask for examples of when the individual manifested that trait. After three people have been named as exhibiting the trait, the leader asks, "Who was the writer of the trait?"

The professional student leader then can lead a discussion of this activity, asking how the group felt in sharing their opinions of traits of strength in themselves and in others. Comfortable? Awkward? Sincere? The student leader can next ask the group how they perceive that they interacted among themselves during the process of the activity. Cooperatively? Generating individual and group satisfaction? Next, the student leader can ask where and when the group can apply this experience, in a social setting, in order to generalize the process in the outside world. Congratulating others? Giving complements? Encouraging a team member?

Professional Socialization Through the Social Capital of Professors and Class Groups

One of the greatest values of professional education is that both the experience of professors' lives and the lives of fellow students can be a broadening factor in professional socialization and career development. These contacts can be far reaching, providing students with a spectrum of domains of culture, personality, knowledge, and life experience.

Among all of the social capital experiences promoting professional socialization, one with great potential for the expansion of therapeutic use of self is learning to be a group leader. When practiced in small groups such as in courses like group dynamics, activity group process, professional practice classes, and fieldwork occupational therapy groups, students can follow the guidelines for formatting a group and use activities in which they have expertise to practice leadership (Cole, 2005). They then have the setting for encouraging members' group and individual goals in the process of carrying out the activity. Modeling leadership styles and skills, students can express empathy for others and facilitate emotional expression in group members ready to interact at a supportive cooperative level.

Social participation is encouraged when the students in the leadership role conduct a discussion after the activity, sharing experiences, processing emotional reactions and interactions, and generalizing the application to the future and to the outside world. Then, getting feedback from fellow students after the leadership experience deepens the value of this learning opportunity. Observing other students leading the group is an example of social capital class group participation with great potential for professional social growth (Table 5-2).

Another opportunity for the development of joint leadership skills can be found in the collaboration of students who put together study groups. A study group is a small group of students organized by themselves to better understand subjects they are studying and to support each other in learning. Here, the students can ask questions more freely, admit what they do not know, and seek input and assistance from other students. As a result, students are better prepared for tests, papers, and discussions in class. These groups offer alternatives to studying alone. Cooperative learning as a supplement to studying alone is recommended by several learning centers: www.muskingum.edu/~cal/database/general/group. html; www.how-to-study.com/studygroups.htm.

Do professional students adequately take advantage of the background knowledge of a peer's previous jobs, undergraduate education, travel, and cultural settings, thus amplifying the social capital knowledge they can derive from the class or group of people? While having a base of friends in a class is valuable for study and social emotional exchange, the opportunity to expand one's comfort zone is available when professors vary group composition across assignments, projects, and lab groups. Fellow students often provide information about fieldwork experiences that can influence job-making choices in the near or distant future. Peers from other communities and cultures can expand perspectives and provide insights that otherwise might not be achieved. If a student believes he or she knows everything about everyone in the class, he or she needs to expand his or her curiosity in an appropriate manner. *When were you last surprised by new information about a fellow student or professor?*

When students are not enamored with certain professors or peers, practicing how to relate to them provides an opportunity again to develop the professional profile necessary to become a broader thinker and colleague. Shutting down or closing fellow students out of a group, unless it has become too large, does not lend itself to a good management style, which will be needed in future career situations where cooperation and coordination of teachers, therapists, and staff is required. Helping to problem-solve a situation that can accommodate each associate in some way, regardless of personal incompatibility, facilitates a positive, democratic-style environment, enabling social participation among colleagues.

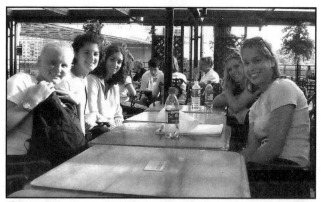

Figure 5-3. Occupational therapy students from Quinnipiac University discuss group process while on field visits in London, England.

Problem-Based Learning Programs in Professional Studies

Problem-based learning (PBL) programs are curriculum models and a system of education designed to be used in problem-solving processes through setting up students in a proactive situation as decision makers in health, educational, and business cases. These cases are arranged to reproduce reality-based problems with material presented in an unorganized fashion with the expectation that students will analyze, organize, and propose solutions for the person. First applied in the 1960s in the health sciences at McMaster University in Canada and in the School of Medicine at Case Western Reserve University, it was further used at Harvard Medical School and at Maastrich University in the Netherlands (Garcia-Famoso, 2005). Theoretically, it may be perceived as a pairing of cognitive and social constructivist approaches of Piaget and Vygotsky (Figure 5-3).

The purpose of PBL is to develop critical-thinking and decision-making skills for real life problems. It is expected that students will assume more responsibility for their own learning and will develop lifelong learning skills, as well as a self-motivated attitude. There is also a social dimension to PBL as students are expected to work in teams, which is similar to the manner in which they will work eventually in the field (Savery, 2006; Wood, 2003). In initial work with a PBL approach, it may be advisable for a faculty facilitator to provide an overview of possible resources

and learning patterns, as well as to be a part of the small group discussions to guide clinical and educational reasoning steps (Sweller, 2006). In advanced work in a PBL model, groups can be responsible for scheduling their meetings, discussing the time needed for tasks, and selecting roles they wish to assume (Schmidt, Van Der Arand, Moust, Kokx, & Boon, 1993; Song, Grabowski, Koszalka, & Harkness, 2006). During groups, students may assume the role of leader, facilitator, recorder, or team member. In problem-stimulated PBL, there is more guidance from instructors as resource people to the teams. In student-centered PBL, students who are more advanced have more latitude in directing their own projects.

What are some of the advantages and disadvantages of PBL? Would you like all or some of your curriculum to be designed for PBL?

Social Emotional Learning in Professional Education Settings

Participation in career growth needs to be based on self-knowledge. While social emotional learning has been a part of professional courses in group process, activity group process, and management courses for some years, social emotional learning programs as a means of teaching motivation and self-regulation have now been introduced at the early childhood level (Cohen, 2006; Zins et al., 2004). As occupational therapists work more frequently with children in school systems, they need to be acquainted with these programs so as to collaborate with the classroom teachers. This will be expanded upon in Chapters 4 and 10.

For their own professional personal preparation, occupational therapy and teaching students need to begin with their own social emotional learning if they have not been exposed to such programs earlier in their schooling. At the graduate level, students have feelings, attitudes, and behavioral patterns in response to life situations that will influence their interactions with clients, children, parents, and adults in clinics and in schools. Being open to social emotional learning and consolidating a foundation in this personal professional preparation before going out into these fields is a distinct advantage for the new therapist, teacher, or clinician. Social emotional learning has been described as learning values and skills that improve our capacity to understand ourselves and others in order to become creative and flexible decision makers (Cohen, 2006). These goals are urgent for professional students as well as for elementary school children.

One of the major programs in designing social emotional learning, the Collaborative for Academic, Social, and Emotional Learning (CASEL) (Zins et al., 2004; Zins, Elias, & Maher, 2007), emphasizes five competencies in their core program that are invaluable for professionals working as educators and caregivers: self-awareness, self-management, social awareness, relationship skills, and responsible decision making. Other similar programs focus on communication, collaboration, and the formation of a realistic, while positive, self-image (Elias, Zins, Graczyk, & Weissberg, 2003; Greenberg, Kusche, & Riggs, 2004). In general, CASEL programs aim to assist children in becoming capable of self-regulation by listening, thinking before acting, and focusing on cognitive education until emotional responses can be attended to (McCabe, Cunnington, & Brooks-Gunn, 2004). Professional graduate students who have not mastered these skills have plenty of opportunities in graduate courses and fieldwork to practice these intra- and interactive emotional skills. *In the last week, what situations have enabled you to practice social emotional learning skills?*

In addition to in-class group projects, class meetings designed to stimulate class spirit, and select community projects such as in fundraising, walks, clothing and holiday gift drives, and fixing up and painting an elementary school provide ample opportunities for reflecting on social emotional learning skills. These are out of class, nongraded meetings of civic and democratic undertakings, and events that provide practice settings for expansion later into mature, professional services for local, state, and national contributions. *Does your class have regular class meetings devoted to outreach in the community?*

Social Participation and Socialization in the Field Through Professional Research

One of the most challenging courses in graduate education is the undertaking of relevant research that reaches out into the community clinics and schools to examine the value of teaching and therapeutic interventions for the public served by professionals. These courses demand that the developing professional pull together earlier knowledge learned about collaborating with others and apply it to working with a graduate student group or alone. In both cases, working with community schools, agencies, hospitals, and clinics to develop empirical skills and apply objective methods to confirm the value of educational and health services is part of professional development.

Coordinating with Institutional Review Boards (IRBs) as part of the process of research clearance for relating to human subjects requires flexibility and cooperation with outside philosophies and policies in order to receive research project approval. Sometimes, the process is frustratingly slow, but it needs adept social-professional skills to achieve a balance in the language and research approaches requested by the review board.

If your research experience is designed to be accomplished in a small group of professional graduate students, your mission will be achieved only within the realm of working in tandem with other students. Jointly selecting a researchable topic, dividing up tasks, sticking to deadlines, and assisting others when the need arises demand a combination of supportive cooperation and mature focus on goals. The ideal research group cannot always be achieved. However, it is hoped that these groups can experience some degree of camaraderie as they carry out their serious assignment. *What types of cooperation have your research group achieved together?*

At times, professors set up studies in schools, clinics, or communities in courses other than their research courses. Collaborating with your course faculty to add to the knowledge base of your field and provide evidence-based practice information is an exciting opportunity. You may be asked to carry out observations, gather data on forms, and request that study participants sign Institutional Review Board permission forms. Whether the research work is part of your class assignment or you are being paid by the hour or case, you can enhance your professional

Table 5-3

PROFESSIONAL COMMUNICATION

When the public is asked what qualities they look for in an educational or health professional, they invariably say that the individual "must communicate well," by which they mean "a willingness to answer questions." How are you currently practicing these skills of social participation with fellow students so as to prepare yourself for an appropriate public professional persona?

social participation skills in how you relate to staff, faculty, or study participants around this undertaking, with consideration and respect for all of your contacts regardless of cultural background, language abilities, or cognitive functional levels (Table 5-3). *Can you collaborate with personnel in community sites to carry out your research design?*

Social Participation in Professional Fieldwork

Professional preparation includes the challenge and excitement of fieldwork where students interact with multiple professionals related to their future work. Whether that would be in the health field working with physicians, psychiatrists, psychologists, social workers, nurses, physical therapists, speech therapists, occupational therapists, and rehabilitation counselors (Figure 5-4), or in education working with teachers, principals, parents, and classroom aides, professional students need to develop their own professional role unique to themselves and their perception of being in a helping profession. Many students enjoy this team-oriented clinical and educational collaboration. Others may be anxious about their professional and individual roles.

Fieldwork settings with the guidance of supervisors provide the emerging professional with a great opportunity to learn how to do joint clinical and educational reasoning for clients as individuals and in groups. Supervision can take place in groups in moving "rounds" bedside or in grand rounds reviewing patient and child cases for mutual assessment and planning. Practicing how to best problem-solve and carry out clinical reasoning with fellow students and other professionals requires in-depth participation for the development of professional socialization.

Individual supervision in health and educational settings in a dyadic arrangement may at first be intimidating for beginning teachers, therapists, and health personnel; however, it is an unusual opportunity for basic task cooperation, mutually supportive teamwork, and mature mutual planning for the child

and patient, whose care and education must always be primary. The ability to work collaboratively in this manner at this level, with an experienced professional teacher or therapist by placing the needs of the patient and student first, is precisely what constitutes professional role behavior. The social participation in group and individual supervision provides the new professional with a venue in which to practice new professional reasoning, behaviors, and roles.

Working with children and clients in educational and health settings during fieldwork presents additional opportunities for expansion of social participation abilities in emerging professionals. Altruistic motivation is certainly a part of the reason for choosing the fields of education and health as career paths. These fields provide ample interactions for students practicing skills of encouraging and coaching children and clients in a style appropriate to their age and abilities. In working with children, students may find themselves in a type of parental role that can foster a therapeutic alliance if mixed with creativity and fun as part of their social participation with the child or children. Students in fieldwork need to gradually bring children along

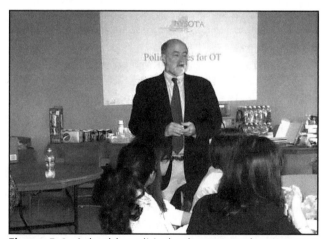

Figure 5-4. A health political advocate updates a state conference audience about the current issues regarding professional legislation.

as they reveal the potential for growth and development by permitting their interactions to mature to a higher level of social participation. In working with adolescents, students need to exhibit a stance of older peer who expects cooperation and elicits joint problem-solving interactions with knowledge of current cultural developments. Students need to make the adolescents feel comfortable, point out positive strengths, and demand maturing behaviors, indicating that the adolescent is capable of rising to the occasion of nearing adult development. Helping to meet their growing esteem needs, exploring their interests, and assisting them in imagining future potential can enable teens to sustain their need to study and practice skills for the long haul.

In working with adults with disabilities, students need to appeal to the interests and strengths of the individuals, along with finding out what is important to them in their cultural background. Adults with disabilities may find themselves feeling that they have returned to an adolescent stage of exploring what they can do in the future and need supportive guidance in searching for their new identity. All of these social interactions require a willingness to participate in a relationship with the child or client, by the therapeutic use of self, in a professional manner combining challenge and support simultaneously.

One method of learning new roles, in the transition between students roles and community leadership roles, is to pair students as activity group leaders in schools, hospitals, and community groups. The social interaction between the students enables them to learn from each other and provides support in situations needing joint problem solving (Donohue, 2001).

Fieldwork Examples of Projects of Learning and Developing Programs

Collaborative planning (Costa, 2007a, 2007b, 2009a, 2009b) within fieldwork with supervisors, staff, and program participants has been encouraged to enable students to develop innovative interactions within new activities and programs. Costa indicates that the questions a fieldwork supervisor asks, in supervision with students, can be transformative because of their collaborative participation around the case profiles and details of treatment planning discussed together. She also indicates that there is a need for research on fieldwork education related to supervision models, clinical program

changes, problem-based learning, values, and learning styles (Costa, 2009b). In the service of the participants, students can then perceive themselves as change agents (Coppola et al., 2009). Examples from gerontology practice settings with students have included working with a wellness department on a falls prevention program in a retirement community, with a focus on lighting. In a skilled nursing facility, students interviewed residents sitting in the hallways about their past occupations and linked their descriptions with photographs of the residents that were then displayed on the walls in the facility. Residents were enthusiastic about collaborating with students in this photo voice-type activity (Wang & Burris, 1997). Horticulture occupations were initiated with people interested in gardening as a project in a long-term care setting (Coppola et al., 2009). The students approached a botanical garden where they had led therapeutic groups previously for support with this project. This focus facilitated interaction among people who had been hesitant about participating, and group members identified the activity as fun (Coppola et al., 2009).

Discuss these social situations of interaction with children, clients, and other professionals with your professor in this course:

- You are working with a client in a rehab center who was in a serious automobile accident and is awaiting surgery. He can tell fabulous stories and comes across as an interesting cowboy. You feel physically attracted to him. What do you do?

- You are observing children in a preschool class of 5 year olds. There is a very outgoing, flirtatious child who plays with the guitar as if he is serenading all of the girls. During clean-up time, he comes behind you and swats you on the derriere with the broom. What do you do?

- You are working with a client in a task group who is very clumsy with his hands. You know of his interests in a particular musician and in cars. What can you do to elicit his participation with other group members?

- You are coleading a large group, and your co-leader begins to favor one client over others by playing games only with her and ignoring the rest of the group. What can you say to her? If her behaviors do not change, should you talk to your supervisor about your partner's behaviors?

- You are co-owner of a private practice in hand therapy with several hand surgeons. You feel that the doctors who are making referrals to your practice are not paying you adequately. What do you do? If they refuse to change their policies, what do you do?

Problem Solving and Decision Making in Educational, Clinical, and Business Groups

Learning to work in groups to problem solve cases in order to make decisions with children, adolescents, adults in educational and clinical settings, and clients and colleagues in business settings spans a lifetime of professional learning situations. From the first time future professionals are exposed to working in groups in grade school, high school, college, and in employment environments through to a graduate course in activity group process, problem-based learning classes, small study groups, student government, community committees, joint research classes, to professional team meetings and postprofessional workshops, problem solving and decision making are linked in groups. Whether these meetings are generally positive in their process, are able to proceed with constructive conflict, or are derailed by destructive perspectives and interactions, may depend on the short-range sharing of agendas for a meeting or the long-range preparation of learning about group process participation. Gouran and Hirokawa's chapter on effective decision making and problem solving in groups has been cited as an excellent source on this topic (2007).

Historically, the "standard agenda" for systematic procedures for problem solving has included six steps (Mosey, 1986; Napier & Gershenfeld, 1998):

1. Problem identification

2. Problem analysis

3. Solution criteria

4. Solution suggestions

5. Solution evaluation and selection

6. Solution implementation

Any and all of these steps can include brainstorming. Unfortunately, some groups circle repeatedly through these steps, while others head immediately to propose solutions. The group can discuss its sequence of steps and, for example, may want to vote on a selection of a solution in a subsequent meeting. Guidelines for brainstorming include not critiquing ideas or asking for clarification during brainstorming, encouraging creative ideas, and fostering participation to include all group members.

There are other decision-making methods that can be investigated, such as the Program Evaluation Review Technique (PERT) (Meade, 2009). The Holden Leadership center indicates the multiple types of decision making: unilateral rule, majority rule, minority rule, rule by clique, or consensus (Holden Leadership Center, 2010). This center warns participants not to let discussion be cut off by someone who says, "Now we are all agreed, right?" They denote this as a type of "baiting." Some groups, if they are large, prefer to work in subgroups first, then report back to the large group.

Tropman (1995), in his book on effective meetings, provides reality-based rules:

× The Rules of Agenda Integrity:

    1. Deal with all the items on the agenda

    2. Do not deal with any items that are not on the agenda

× The Rules of Temporal Integrity:

    1. Start on time

    2. End on time

    3. Keep a time order within the meeting

Within his book, he also explains rules for proportion of old, present, and future items on the agenda. He recommends making an important decision at a second meeting, if possible. Tropman (1995) points out how essential it is that the participants have the agenda in advance of the meeting. He notes that the last part of a meeting may deteriorate into, "What's for lunch?" He also recommends that there be an Angel Advocate at each meeting to counterbalance the Devil's Advocate (Tropman, 1995).

Decision making in health care has been described to include the BRAND mnemonic:

× **B**enefits of the action

× **R**isks in the action

× **A**lternatives to the prospective action

× **N**othing (i.e., doing nothing at all)

× **D**ecision

In contrast, decision making in business and management includes a number of types of processes. However, in general, it is recommended that business and management systems be set up to permit decision making at the lowest possible level. The business approaches include a SWOT analysis by the organization consisting of a discussion of strengths, weaknesses, opportunities, and threats. Other approaches in business decision making include the military-originated operations research, grid analysis, cost-benefit analysis, decision trees, game theory, Analytic Hierarchy Process, stepladder techniques, force field analysis, and impact analysis. Hyperlinks to these terms for effective decision making in financial, business, and management techniques can be found at the Mind Tools Web site at www.mindtools.com. Professionals interested in these approaches can examine books on operations research, take online courses (Stanford University Center for Professional Development, 2009), obtain software titled "Make Better Decisions (Decision Lens, 2009), and visit "Because it's everybody's business" at www.micro-soft.com/everybodysbusiness (Microsoft, 2009).

Script: Professional Socialization—Student Research Planning Meeting

Seating Chart

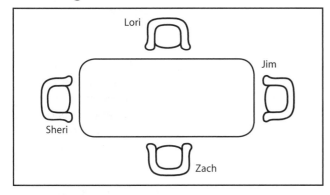

Background

This group of graduate students in a health and educational research course is meeting for the second time to follow up on the assignments they gave themselves in their first meeting. They plan to continue a study begun the previous year in a psychiatric hospital using the Sensory Profile for adults.

Action Begins Here

Sheri: For our updated review of the literature, I searched the web and the university library and came up with 11 new references. Here's a copy of the list for everyone. This coming week, I'll insert them into the reference list from last year.

Zach: I contacted our liaison for this project at the hospital. She gave me four possible dates that fit into our schedule that we could go out for our initial visit. Which date would be best for all four of us? February 7, 14, 21, or 28?

Jim: Any of those would be good for me because they are all Fridays.

Zach and Sheri: Same for me…and me.

Lori: My mom has been getting cancer treatments, and I arranged on Fridays to take her to the clinic so I would not have to miss class…

Sheri: I wish that we could all go.

Zach: Well, maybe, due to circumstances, the three of us could represent the group.

Jim: I made copies of last year's students' study results from the hospital, so we can review and add to their data. Here they are…

Zach: Can all three of us go on the 14th?

Sheri: I can drive, or do you want to go on the train and then take a taxi?

Zach: If you could drive, that would be great. Okay?

Sheri: Yeah!

Lori: This week, I printed out the Institutional Review Board Human Subjects forms, and I began to fill them in about the facts of our group and study, but I thought that we should select the rationale together.

Sheri: Okay, let's look at last year's study first and check their rationale.

Jim: They said that they wanted to look at the relationship between affective disorder and border-line personality disorder, and the four quadrants of the Social Profile.

Zach: They were only able to collect data for 18 participants, so their results are too small to analyze. We can only say that there is a trend for both groups to be sensory avoidant, so we need to collect additional data from about an equal number of participants to arrive at a total of at least 30 people.

Sheri: It sounds like this group could be considered sensory sensitive compared to most people.

Jim: Yes, but at this point, we cannot draw any conclusions. Even with 30 people, we can only say that the findings "suggest" certain trends.

Zach: The design from last year looks good—a quantitative descriptive correlational research design.

Sheri: …Yes, with its main purpose to establish a relationship using aspects of the Sensory Profile.

Lori: So, how shall we word the rationale for the IRB form?

Jim: We could say that our rationale continues to be to see if the Sensory Profile can give us the information needed to detect an association between borderline personality disorder and bipolar disorder, and the para-suicidal behavior of self-mutilation, which they were all involved in.

Zach: We can also say that this is the second year of the study and that part of our rationale is to collect more data during this semester.

Sheri: When we go out to the hospital with the list of people our liaison will give us, we need to get permission to check the charts for the diagnosis and the self-mutilation behaviors. Then, we can make appointments with the willing participants for them to fill in the Sensory Profile.

Lori: I wish I could go, too, but I appreciate that you all will represent us as a group. I'll fill in the IRB form this week with the rationale we developed and send a copy to you all.

Sheri: I'll write up the additional literature entries and send you copies for next week.

Zach: *(pulls out planner and pen)* When can we meet next week? Same time?

(all nod yes)

Jim: Wait! Do we need to meet next week, or can we just send all these reports to each other online? Then, we'll save time for our trip to the hospital...

All: Sure...okay...yeah.

The End.

Discussion

1. In this student group research meeting, what could have derailed the process?

2. Is it typical that graduate students would achieve this high level of basic and supportive cooperation and mature group level of participation?

3. Have you had experiences in student group planning sessions that have gone awry? Would you like to review and discuss them? Or would that violate past group confidentiality, if the students in the other group are recognizable? If so, where else could you review this past situation, if it feels unresolved?

4. Is there a balance of leadership here?

5. Do you believe Lori's excuse and situation?

6. Is it "fair" for three people to carry the responsibility of the hospital visit for the group?

References

American Occupational Therapy Association. (2008). Occupational therapy practice framework: Domain and process (2nd ed.). *American Journal of Occupational Therapy, 62,* 625-683.

Bandura, A. (1977). *Social learning theory.* New York, NY: General Learning Press.

Cohen, J. (2006). Social, emotional, ethical and academic education. Creating a climate for learning participation in democracy and well-being. *Harvard Education Review, 76,* 201-237.

Cole, M. (2005). *Group dynamics in occupational therapy* (3rd ed.). Thorofare, NJ: SLACK Incorporated.

Coppola, S., Darwin, A., Bagby, M., Carlson, C., Cox S. B., Gunnigle, C., ... & Warrick, T. B. (2009). Fieldwork projects with older adults: Stories of learning and contributing. *Special Interest Section Quarterly, Gerontology, 32,* 1-4.

Costa, D. M. (2007a). *Clinical supervision in occupational therapy: A guide for fieldwork and practice.* Bethesda, MD: AOTA Press.

Costa, D. M. (2007b). The collaborative fieldwork model. *OT Practice,* January 22, 25-26.

Costa, D. M. (2009a). Transformative learning in fieldwork. *OT Practice,* January 19, 19-20.

Costa, D. M. (2009). Call for research on fieldwork education. *OT Practice.* Retrieved June 29, 2010 from www.findarticles.com/p/articles/mi_7687/is_200903/ai_n32205241/

Donohue, M. V. (2001). Group co-leadership by occupational therapy students in community centers: Transitional learning. *Occupational Therapy in Health Care, 15,* 85-98.

Elias, M. J., Zins, J. E., Graczyk, P. A., & Weissberg, R. P. (2003). Implementation, sustainability, and scaling up of social-emotional and academic innovations in public schools. *School Psychology Review, 32,* 303-319.

Garcia-Famoso, M. (2005). *Problem-based learning: A case study in computer science.* M-ICTE, 2009. Retrieved from www.formatex.org/micte2005/196.pdf

Gough, H. G. (1957). California Psychological Inventory. (CPI). *Administrator's Guide.* Palo Alto, CA: Consulting Psychologists Press.

Gouran, D. S., & Hirokawa, R. Y. (2007). Effective decision-making and problem-solving in groups: A functional perspective. In R. Y. Hirokawa, R. S. Cathcart, L. A. Samovar, & L. D. Henman (Eds.), *Small group communication: Theory and practice.* Oxford, UK: Oxford University Press.

Greenberg, M. T., Kusche, C. A., & Riggs, N. (2004). The PATHS curriculum: Theory and research on neurocognitive development and school success. In J. E. Zins, R. P. Weisberg, M. C. Wang, & H. J. Walberg (Eds.), *Building academic success on social and emotional learning: What does the research say?* (pp. 170-188). New York, NY: Teachers College Press.

Lifton, W. M. (1966). *Working with groups: Group process and individual growth.* New York, NY: John Wiley.

McCabe, L. A., Cunnington, M., & Brooks-Gunn, J. (2004). *The development of self-regulation in young children. Handbook of self-regulation: research, theory, and applications* (pp. 340-356). New York, NY: Guilds.

Mosey, A. C. (1968). Recapitulation of ontogenesis: A theory for practice of occupational therapy. *American Journal of Occupational Therapy, 22,* 426-438.

Mosey, A. C. (1986). *Psychosocial components of occupational therapy.* New York, NY: Raven Press.

Napier, R. W., & Gershenfeld, M. K. (1998). *Groups. Theory and experience* (6th ed.). Boston, MA: Houghton Mifflin.

Parten, M. B. (1932). Social participation among pre-school children. *Journal of Abnormal and Social Psychology, 27,* 243-269.

Savery, J. R. (2006). Overview of problem-based learning: Definitions and distinctions. *The Interdisciplinary Journal of Problem-based Learning (IJPBL), 1,* 1.

Schmidt, H. G., Van Der Arand, A., Moust, J. H., Kokx, I., & Boon, L. (1993). Influence of tutors' subject matter expertise on student effort and achievement in problem-based learning. *Academic Medicine, 68,* 784-791.

Song, H. D., Grabowski, B., Koszalka, T., & Harkness, W. (2006). Patterns of instructional-design factors prompting reflective thinking in middle-school and college level problem-based learning environments. *Instructional Science, 34,* 63-87.

Sweller, J. (2006). The worked example effect and human cognition. *Learning and Instruction, 16,* 165-169.

Tropman, J. E. (1995). *Effective meetings. Improving group decision making* (2nd ed.). Newbury Park, CA: Sage Publications, Inc.

Wang, C., & Burris, M. A. (1997). Photovoice: Concept, methodology, and use for participatory needs assessment. *Health Education and Behavior, 24,* 369-387.

Wood, D. F. (2003). ABC's of learning and teaching in medicine: Problem-based learning. *British Journal of Medicine, 326,* 328-330.

World Health Organization. (2001). *International classification of functioning, disability, and health (ICF).* Geneva, Switzerland: Author.

Zins, J. E., Elias, M. J., & Maher, C. A. (Eds.). (2007). *Bullying victimization, and peer harassment. A handbook of prevention and intervention.* Binghamton: Haworth Press.

Zins, J. E., Weissberg, R. P., Wang, M. C., & Walberg, H. J. (Eds.). (2004). *Building academic success on social and emotional learning: What does the research say?* New York, NY: Columbia University, Teachers College Press.

Additional Resources

Decision Lens. (2009). Group decision making. Retrieved from www.decisionlens.com/

Holden Leadership Center, University of Oregon. (2010). Leadership exercises & tips. Retrieved from leadership.uoregon.edu/resources/exercises_tips

CAL Learning Strategies Database. (n.d.). Retrieved from www.muskingum.edu/~cal/database/general/group.html

Meade, L. (2009). Communications. Retrieved from www.comp.uark.edu/~lmeade/Communication/Communicationhome.htm

Microsoft. (2009). Because it's everybody's business. Retrieved from www.mricrosoft.com/business/peopleready/en-us/#poid

MindTools. (2010). Retrieved April 19, 2009 from http://www.mindtools.com/pages/article/newTED_00.htm

Stanford University Center for Professional Development. (2009). Stanford strategy decision and risk management. Retrieved from www.strategicdecisions.stanford.edu

Professional Development Strategies: Study Groups. (n.d.). Retrieved from webserver3.ascd.org/ossd/studygroups.html

Theories of Social Participation Across the Lifespan

chapter 6

Social Development in Infancy and Childhood

Mary V. Donohue, PhD, OTL, FAOTA

"It takes a village." (Clinton, 1996; Cowen-Fletcher, 1990)

This chapter on theories of infancy and childhood social development spans pre-preschool, preschool, primary, and middle school years. It also considers environmental aspects of groups in families, in the community, and on the World Wide Web. Positive and negative aspects of social participation in these arenas will be considered and discussed as they have been set forth in social development theories.

Theories that will be presented include Vygotsky's general social development theory, Bowlby's attachment theory, Mahler's separation-individuation theory, Erikson's stages of psychosocial development theory, and Parten's group social participation development theory. This chapter will also include a discussion of impediments to social development and roles assumed in childhood.

Family Beginnings

There are myriad configurations for family formats; however, when a baby enters this world, one of its first social interactions occurs in looking up at his or her mother's face and hearing his or her mother's voice, familiar from uterine life, even before vision is mature. This interaction is hopefully reinforced multiple times beyond this preliminary dyad. Social participation expands as the infant responds to seeing and listening to other family members: its father, siblings, grandparents, aunts, uncles, cousins, and caregivers. Infant social participation is extended through listening to cooing, singing, talking, infant games, nursing, rocking, and meals with the family members. Being washed, dressed, and carried around involves social interaction as the infant is dependent on adults for these activities.

Many motor and sensory responses of an infant consist of reaching out to communicate. Arm and leg movements, as well as cooing and crying, can express emotion and messages designed for social participation with other humans. Being cuddled, lifted, spun, and swung about in delight can elicit satisfaction and trust in social interaction with others in the family. Styles and degrees of social participation can be observed and imitated or shunned, depending on the infant's personality and environment. Infants with autism and learning disabilities do not fit this pattern of human interaction, so additional activity on the part of family members is required to encourage them to engage in social participation with others.

Gradually, infants are included in the family circles at the table, in cars, on the floor, and in front of the television. Facial expressions, peek-a-boo, pointing, and crying are early efforts to become involved in social participation. When their minds recall words and their tongues are sufficiently mature, infants begin to imitate sounds. *When nonverbal infants pick up a phone, do they imagine that this device will enable them to talk?*

Cole, M.B., & Donohue, M.V. *Social Participation in Occupational Contexts: In Schools, Clinics, and Communities* (pp 99-108).
© 2011 SLACK Incorporated

Professionals can carefully and intently watch infant occupations and speculate and imagine what emotion or communication is desired or expressed. Baby language and nonverbal communication can persist in family settings and carry over into nursery settings. The degree of language communication for each infant is dependent on the individual child's personality as well as upon the amount of interaction expressed in the family group. Beyond the family, the school and community members play a part in social development, which is why it can be said that it takes a village (Clinton, 1996; Cowen-Fletcher, 1990) to raise a child who is able to participate as fully as possible in social life.

Vygotsky's Overview of Social Development

In his theory of social development, Vygotsky's (1978) perspective of social interaction provides for a basic function in learning. He believes that the process begins between people socially, through the observation of behaviors of adults or peers by infants or children, and then crystallizes inside of the infant or child. Relationships between individuals that encourage and enable formation of social, cultural, and cognitive concepts elicit attention and enhance memory. Vygotsky contends that social behavior with adult guidance or peer role modeling fosters a range of skills, which exceeds what the child could achieve alone; the first step in development, he maintains, is interpsychic between people and the second is intrapsychic within the infant or child.

As an example, Vygotsky's theory of the internalization of language development by which we recognize and organize inner speech intellectually begins with attempts to imitate and communicate with adults in a social interaction. This theory of language learning in children is dependent on social stimulation outside of the child (Vygotsky, 1962).

Bowlby's Attachment Theory of Social Development

With Vygotsky's theory in mind, it is not surprising to find Bowlby's attachment theory emphasizing maternal interaction with the infant as primary for social development. Bowlby (1951), in fact, considered attachment as a motivational system within an evolutionary need for survival. He believed that attachment behavior is a primal strategy for protecting infants from danger. In a pattern of social development, Bowlby saw the mother as having a profound

influence on who the infant becomes as a reflection of the mother's perception of her child. The infant's range of feelings and behaviors mirror what is recognized, expressed, and emphasized by the mother in their social interaction (Bowlby, 1969).

Bowlby perceived the dyad of mother and infant as essential to the development of social participation. Furthermore, he thought that the infant also in part becomes who he or she is by responding to or coping with the mother's personality. In addition, he conjectured that if the mother did not recognize an aspect of the child's personality, the child also would fail to perceive this aspect of him- or herself (Bowlby, 1988). Bowlby emphasized that the mother provides a secure base from which social growth of the child can occur. Because of this belief, he called for joint treatment of the child with the mother present, even in the case of hospitalization of the child.

Biographically, it is interesting to note that Bowlby's significant initial caregiver, a well-loved nanny, departed from the family when he was 4 years old, leaving him bereft. His own mother was distant from him in a belief that a child should not be spoiled at home, but instead sent off to boarding school, which in fact occurred when he was 7 years old (Bowlby, 1973; Coates, 2003).

Mahler's Separation-Individuation Theory of Social Development

In typical social development patterns, separation-individuation would follow the attachment stage. Mahler's conceptualization of the ability to separate from the mother and develop individually was embedded deeply in her belief in the mother-infant dual unity occurring first (Mahler, Pine, & Bergman, 1975). Within that unity, she perceived that the child adapts to the mother because of its capacity for pliability. She referred to the infant's attachment behavior as part of the process of the infant's social development. In a clinic where she worked, she witnessed firsthand the failure to thrive syndrome, which can occur with the rupture of separation from a primary caregiver (Mahler, 1977). In an earlier paper, Mahler had written about the significance of the deep emotional bond of the mother and child (Mahler, 1963). Later, Mahler and colleagues described *The Psychological Birth of the Human Infant* (1975) as based first on a symbiotic-type relationship that provides the foundation for individuation as developmental growth in social relationships. If a child does not risk separation, he or she cannot become an individual who can interact socially with other people. Mahler and McDevitt (1982) refer to the infant's internalization of the mother's interactive social behavior, such as soothing the infant, thus learning that skill. Like Bowlby, Mahler believed in the active participation of the mother during the treatment of the child.

Furthermore, like Bowlby, Mahler had a mother emotionally removed from her, but fortunately she had a father who related to and believed in her capacity as an individual. His support of her career validated her goals and desires, insulating her somewhat from her exposure to maternal rejection (Coates, 2003).

Erikson's Stage Theory of Psychosocial Development

Erikson built his stage theory of psychosocial development on the three psychosexual stages of Freud, extending the continuum into adulthood with eight stages (1950, 1967). He perceived each stage as a crisis of growth that needed to be worked on, understood, and resolved in order to move on to the next stage. Erikson visualized the need at times for individuals to remain at a stage level for a period of time in order to consolidate gains before moving on to the next stage.

In the first stage, trust versus mistrust, the social ability to rely on others when needed is experienced. The child is initially dependent on his or her mother for everything because she can anticipate an infant's needs, but gradually the infant begins to trust that when mother is out of sight, she will return. Erikson (1950) indicates that a lack of development of this perspective can cause paranoia later in life and a lack of trust with suspiciousness in social interactions. Hope in the basic goodness of others with a realistic foundation will help to prevent mistrust of the motivations of others encountered over the years. A lack of resolution of this stage can lead to isolation, preventing social development through a lack of interaction. Or, the other extreme can occur, in depending too much upon one's parents or becoming too possessive of life in the family, with an accompanying inability to move out and move on to participate in wider circles of new acquaintances. In each of these stages, opposite extremes of reactions to the dilemma or crisis can be stifling of increased social participation. This stage is comparable to Bowlby's conceptualization of the need for a secure base developed through appropriate attachment.

Erikson's second stage (1950), autonomy versus shame and doubt, is the focus of a developmental social struggle of the child for independence from his or her parents, older siblings, and caregivers. Coming to understand that operating in conjunction with others in a cooperative manner is a social skill that does not lead to shame and doubt is the issue of the traditional "terrible twos." The understanding that independence is not in conflict with joint efforts is the work of this critical period. This stage can extend from ages 1½ to 3 years or can develop into a lifetime of social resistance to parents, teachers, and bosses. Mahler called this struggle separation/individuation as the child becomes aware that he or she is a separate person. Adults need to guide the child toward other choices or solutions to situations that arise. If adults shame the child too much when he or she makes mistakes, a defiant outlook develops. It is the work of the adult to enable the child to develop self-control without losing self-esteem so that goodwill and confidence grow out of this stage (Erikson, 1950). The extreme positions that can develop during this stage are lack of self-esteem in interactions with others, stubbornness due to an inability to perceive other possible choices or solutions to life's problems, or insistence on becoming socially independent by emphasizing differences between people rather than grounds of similarity.

The initiative versus guilt stage, Erikson's third stage of social development during ages 3 to 6 years old, brings the child to a crisis of taking on risks—judging what can be safely done, and what can be selected to undertake and plan without confronting opposition in the environment. The child's preferences for activities challenge him or her to enter even more cooperative pathways if the enterprises require interaction with others. Fantasies of who the child is personally emerge and are compared with others at home, in preschool, or in the neighborhood. Guilt at being overly ambitious or invading the initiative desires of others is a new feeling, which parents and teachers need to help the child understand and become comfortable with (Erikson, 1950). Socially, mutual responsibility toward others is undertaken with small tasks at home or school, which contribute to the social fabric of the setting, giving new satisfaction to feelings of initiative. Courage in attempting new tasks needs to be balanced with feelings of frustration by failure or aggressive insistence on the child's ideas or outlook. Children need encouragement in setting goals that are balanced, by the opinion of adults and others, as to how well they are doing in their efforts. At this stage, the two extremes that can emerge are not taking on new projects without much assistance from adults versus taking on overly ambitious projects that cannot be completed. The value of the sense of guilt that develops can guide children toward a reasonable conscience that is not rigid and will shore up their self-control efforts.

Industry versus inferiority as a critical stage moves the child away from pure play toward the undertaking of a spectrum of skills—motor, sensory, cognitive, and psychological—all in a social setting that has broadened out with responsibility to search for success in one's strengths. The child needs to learn the feeling of satisfaction that goes with success in order to stave off feelings of inferiority. Children need to be taught how to learn from their mistakes and from their lack of ability in new tasks. Systematic instruction in an organized manner in a social environment can be a struggle for children with learning disabilities. All children also need to become acclimated to working on achievements in a social setting such as school courses, family babysitting, team sports, and community afterschool activities. These challenges require concentration on longer tasks carried out cooperatively with others over a series of days, which need to be completed satisfactorily. Exploring hobbies, the outdoors, and team groups using rules and safety guidelines is the task of this stage of practice for adult responsibilities at work in the future. Learning the enjoyment of bringing a task to completion is an important satisfaction usually taking place in a public or semipublic forum, requiring participation with others socially. Learning about a number of possible jobs and careers can give him or her glimmers of what he or she might be able to accomplish in society and for society in the future. Lack of success in school, on the playground, or in the neighborhood can cause discouragement, rebellion, and turning to drugs at an early age. The two extremes at this stage are overinvolvement in afterschool clubs and activities versus a drop out, with a disengaged outlook that may elicit bullying or the need to join a gang.

Erikson's further stages, referring to *Identity: Youth and Crisis* (1968) and *Adulthood* (1967), will be discussed in later chapters.

Parten's Theory of Social Levels of Group Participation in Preschool Children

While Parten's theory was introduced in Chapter 2 as the prime example of a theory of social participation, it is presented again here as a developmental theory of social growth. In participation and interaction theory for toddlers, Parten (1932) indicates that tiny tykes initially observe others and explore by smiling, reaching out for toys, and playing

peek-a-boo and patty-cake as preliminary initiatives and responses to people in their family circle and as antecedent to group play. Toddlers also enjoy solitary play behaviors with rattles; mini-bikes; pots, pans, and spoons; scooters; blocks; beads; cartons; paper bags; magic markers; and paper in an exploratory style as preparation for play with others.

Once children can play with toys and materials of their choosing and availability, they initially do so in a parallel manner (Parten, 1932) next to other family members or nursery school companions. At this level of social participation, preschool children through 2 years of age can tolerate the presence of others and can be stimulated by their presence to engage in activities in proximity to others, but without interaction with those present (Parten, 1932). Practice playing alone in parallel mode builds trust and respect for others in the environment (Figure 6-1).

In the next level of participation, preschoolers notice which children like the same activities they do and begin to *associate* (Parten, 1932) with those present who are also ready to interact, briefly or silently, in the same activity. Building blocks, coloring together, rolling balls, climbing slides, looking at picture books together, and swinging on adjacent swings provide opportunity for short associations of social participation. Parten illustrates how early preschoolers explore their social peers through mutually attractive activities, with verbal baby talk, words, phrases, and nonverbal interaction.

As preschool children mature and become comfortable at home and in school groups, their language skills consolidate around wishing to be understood with short commanding and imperative sentences: "Go away," "Come here," "Hey, watch out," and "I want to play." Parents and teachers can coach children

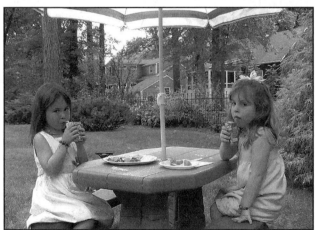

Figure 6-1. Daydreaming as they "hang out" in parallel mode of social interaction. Some associating is probably also taking place off camera.

Table 6-1

AUTHORS AND CONCEPTS IN THE MAJOR CONSTRUCT OF CHILD SOCIAL DEVELOPMENT THEORY

PARTEN, 1932

Parallel play

Associative play

Cooperative play

VYGOTSKY, 1950

Interpsychic observation

Separation/individuation

Intrapsychic internalization

Social relations and cognition

ERIKSON, 1950

Trust versus mistrust

Autonomy versus shame and doubt

Initiative versus guilt

Industry versus inferiority

MAHLER, 1963

Psychological birth

Failure to thrive

BOWLBY, 1951

Attachment

Secure base in dyad

Evolutionary motivation

around these interactions in order to encourage a basic cooperative style (Parten, 1932) of participation among playmates around common activities.

An explosion in social exchange appears at about 3½ years of age (Donohue, 1999) as language develops and fantasy life grows. The consolidation of the basic cooperative interaction increases throughout childhood (Parten, 1932), moving through group participation of imagination: "Let's dress up," "Let's have a tea party," "Let's build a tower," or "Let's play hide and seek, or cops and robbers, or hopscotch." As children mature in learning norms and rules, their sophistication in organizing themselves with basic cooperation expands into forming teams: "Let's play baseball, football, basketball," or "Let's play house, doctor and nurse, board games, video games."

Parten's presentation of her theory, as a construct of social participation and development, incorporates many aspects of the concepts described earlier in the work of other theoreticians. Table 6-1 provides a summary of the theoretical concepts of the social developmental theories in this chapter.

The work of Parten continues to be studied with recent authors wishing to pass on her heritage to student teachers and therapists across the world (Bracken & Nagle, 2007; Dau, 2003; Hughes, 2009; Wellhousen & Crowther, 2004). Bracken and Nagle expand the discussion of Parten's work and clarify the degree to which her concepts are developmental, in initial appearance, versus purely developmental as stages.

Barriers to Social Development in Infancy and Childhood

There are a number of sources or situations that hinder or delay the growth of social development in infants and children. These sources may be inherent in the child, parents, siblings, or the general environment. They may be temporary such as infant colic, prevalent in 1 out of 6 infants for about 3 to 4 months (Springen, 2008), with constant crying, which can prevent the infant/mother social bond from developing. This condition can be alleviated by simulating the setting of the uterus by wearing a sling for the baby, rocking the infant, providing white noise with a fan to sound like blood flow, riding in a car, or using warm baths. These activities relate to Bowlby's attachment theory and may differ from the usual maternal attachment activities but may be soothing.

Some infants have other impediments to typical social development, such as cerebral palsy, mental retardation (American Psychiatric Association [APA], 2000), or sensory processing deficits/defensiveness, which can also interfere with the infant/mother dyad interaction (Champagne, 2008).

Pervasive developmental disorders (APA, 2000), such as autistic disorder, Rhett's disorder, and Asperger's syndrome also disrupt the development of social attachment in families. Regulatory or disruptive behavior disorders (APA, 2000) can prevent the usual progression of social development through attention deficit, hyperactivity, conduct, school adjustment, and oppositional defiance disorders. While the attention deficit and hyperactivity may appear to be neurological in nature, these children need modified activities addressing social development through both attachment and separation/individuation methods. Children with conduct and defiance disorders violate the rights of others in their interactions and ignore social norms of behavior (APA, 2000). Erikson (1950) would perceive their aggression, destruction, and deceit as derailed social interactions in relationships that needed to stimulate trust, support autonomy, and encourage appropriate initiative. Separation anxiety disorder can emerge as a child begins preschool, which is a time period of separation/individuation noted by Mahler and McDevitt (1982). Enuresis, which is not due to a medical condition, can also be disruptive of the social interaction of children and their parents and may relate to Erikson's autonomy crisis (APA, 2000; Erikson, 1950).

Physical deficits in infants and children such as maternal drug-induced syndromes, diabetes, shaken baby syndrome, birth defects, and childhood diseases can disturb the social growth of infants and children because so much energy and time needs to be focused on the ill child, sometimes to the detriment of the social sibling interactions, causing jealousy and resentment in the family. Maternal or paternal physical illnesses can also change the patterns of social development of infants because roles of family members shift due to coping with these ailments.

Severe social developmental damage to an infant's social growth can also occur during a mother's postpartum depression, ongoing depression, schizophrenia, or obsessive and eating disorders (APA, 2000). Alcohol and other substance disorders also center parents' concerns on themselves instead of on their infant, thus impairing their infant's social relationships with them, and subsequently with others. Fetal alcohol syndrome has serious consequences for promoting addiction in the infant, thus stifling social developmental growth by interfering with attachment, separation, and individuation patterns (Bowlby, 1951, 1969, 1973; Mahler, 1963; Mahler & McDevitt, 1982; Mahler et al., 1975).

Personality disorders in parents also set up patterns of social relationships with an infant that can have complex and far-reaching effects subsequently. Parents who are not ready for parenting and lack parenting skills may have anxiety disorders, hypochondriasis disorders, obsessive compulsive tendencies, post-traumatic stress syndrome, borderline personality disorders, and eating disorders. These disorders can permanently impede social development and may lead parents to neglect or abuse their children (APA, 2000).

Given the number of personal and environmental impediments to social development that are sequential and timely according to ideal, typical expectations, it is not surprising that infants and children need outside support and intervention. Therapeutic interventions assisting social development will be addressed in later chapters. This is why it takes a village to foster social development in infants and children because moving outside of the family circle is an essential part of social participation in society.

Roles Assumed in Childhood

Traditional children's roles may have been considered invisible in the past. A child has usually been assumed to be a son or daughter, and perhaps a sister or brother. Being the oldest child often confers a role of junior parent, being responsible for the safety of younger children, keeping them entertained, and maintaining the norms of the family during activities with younger siblings. The youngest child sometimes is placed in the role of being the baby or favorite, perhaps to hold on to the family unit to prevent moving on in life. Other children may develop roles as clown, rebel, mediator, bully, or artist.

At home, it is hoped that parents assist children in developing a self-respect and self-care role, appreciating themselves, cleaning and dressing themselves, and selecting clothing for the day.

Other social roles inherent in families have included being a niece, nephew, cousin, and grandchild. These relationships expand and may disrupt the nuclear family relationships. Cousins can be exciting children who play hide-and-go-seek together. Aunts typically may be just "themselves," while uncles may be intrusive. *Does a youngster know how to relate to an uncle who sings and becomes a little tipsy at family gatherings?* A niece may be confused as to how to relate to the uncle's exaggerated behaviors. Or another uncle, putting himself in the role of entertainer, may greet a niece and nephew by calling her or him "Aunt Jane" or "Uncle Leo," while shaking hands over the child's head with an invisible tall hand. Confusion about the appropriate response in this situation may leave the child at a loss as to his or her role. *Laughing? Or ignoring the behavior?* Another uncle may play coin or card tricks on nieces and nephews. *How do you perceive the roles of response possible in these interactions?*

Early in life, a child is expected to be a "player," one who interacts with things and people in the environment for the sheer joy of the behavior itself. Playing with people can include cooing, language imitation, peek-a-boo, grabbing hair, smiling, and later as a toddler, talking, singing, poking friends and siblings, hide and seek, and playing telephone. As a player with objects, children include balls, boxes, cartons, clothing, magic markers, paper, chairs, tables, and jump ropes that they learn to manipulate, developing as a sensorimotor skill player (Kramer & Hinojosa, 1993). When building, structuring, or creating art, children are in the constructive player mode (Kramer & Hinojosa, 1993).

Another player role or mode involves using and developing imagination, being an "imaginer." In the past, imagining being a father, mother, fighter, policeman, athlete, comic strip character, lion, bull, or cartoon character has been a role of play for children. Today, children identify with avatars and other computer program characters, often playing parallel and in associative interaction with companions working dual controls in video partner roles of pursuit and conquest. In other computer programs, children can imagine themselves buying objects, houses, and cars with money accumulated in their game. Wishing to attract and outshine others, social imaginary interaction can include dressing avatars for various occasions where the child would like to participate.

Student roles for children have become enlarged as children go to school younger and are not only preschool members but also afterschool program members. In preschool, children are perceived as a "toy player" with dolls, carriages, trucks, planes, cars, and pull-along toys. Some children like the role of drummer, later playing other instruments and becoming a child musician (Figure 6-2). In the primary school student role, a child becomes a reader, writer, artist, and class government member. Students become homeworkers and learners. Through school courses, children can become budding scientists, historians, inventors, respecters of the environment, explorers, producers, and cultural participants, some of which

Erikson described (1950). Currently, children have become computer and phone users often with little assistance from anyone. *What other roles did you have as a child? What other roles have you seen in children?*

Playmate Role: Initiation and Invitation

Discussion

1. What roles are represented in the song in Table 6-2?
2. What kind of role play is described?
3. Will the friendship be sustained?

Table 6-2

SONG

"OH, PLAYMATE, COME OUT AND PLAY WITH ME"

Playmate, come out and play with me,
And bring your dollies three,
Climb up my apple tree,
Shout down my rain barrel,
Slide down my cellar door,
And we'll be jolly friends for evermore.
Oh, she couldn't come out to play.
'Cause it was a rainy day.
With tearful eyes and tender sighs,
She heard her cry,
And this is what she'd say:
I'm sorry playmate,
I cannot play with you.
My dollies have the flu
Boo, hoo, hoo, hoo, hoo, hoo
Can't climb your rain barrel,
Can't climb your cellar door,
But we'll be jolly friends, forever more.

(Source: Written by Unknown, Copyright Unknown; 2nd Source: Words and Music by Saxie Dowell, Copyright Santly-Joy-Select, Inc., 1940. For the music, go to www.kids.niehs.nih.gov/lyrics/playmate.htm or www.kiddiddles.com/lyrics/o017.html.)

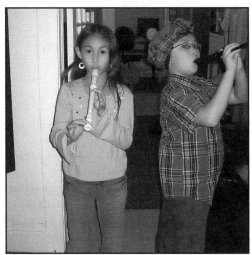

Figure 6-2. Basic cooperative level participation is demonstrated in this musical performance of piping in unison.

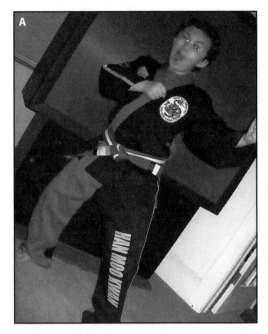

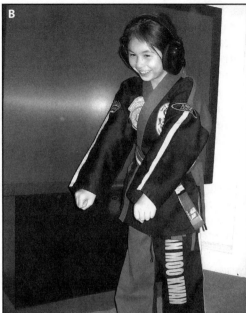

Figure 6-3. Tae Kwan Do: Usually serious, these two young martial artists show their humorous side in mocking their stance to the camera and audience. Normally operating at a basic cooperative level of interaction, here their flash of comedy displays other feelings in a more supportive cooperative mode of participation.

Group Member Roles for Children

While playmates are in a dyadic or buddy role, another social participation role for children is being a group member (Olson, 1993). These roles have been thoroughly analyzed for adults by Bales (1950), whose work is presented in many group process textbooks. For children, Bales' task roles could be described as activity participation roles, and his maintenance or social emotional roles might be described as social participation roles. Children involved in activities express their opinion of the activity, give information and suggestions about how to carry out the activity, and ask for opinions and information; therefore, children can be in the roles of evaluators, clarifiers, confirmers, and questioners.

Among the social participation roles for children, it is possible to observe children in helper roles, supporter roles, and humorous, tension-reliever roles among the positive roles (Figures 6-3 and 6-4). Within a negative focus or outlook, children can also express social participation roles of disagreer, withdrawer, antagonizer, or bully. Learning to cope with these types of roles in oneself and others needs the exposure and practice opportunities of family gatherings, playground opportunities, school recess, and after-school groups during the childhood years to attain readiness for adolescent and adult roles (Williamson, Szczespanski, & Zeitlin, 1993).

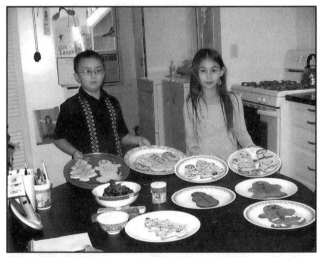

Figure 6-4. Basic cooperative level interaction brought about coordination in using batter, utensils, and the oven while these youngsters competed in decorating these cookies.

Script: Family Support of Children: "It Takes a Village"

Scenario

A family, with divorce between the parents, is meeting in the kitchen of grandpa's house after having lunch together. For economic reasons, the father of the two children lives with his father (Grandpa), and the boys come over for the weekend. The kitchen meeting includes three generations: Grandpa; Aunt Sophie (the father's sister); Grandpa's significant friend, Sue; the father of the two boys; his brother (Uncle) from Missouri; and the two boys, Jason and Eddie, 8 and 11 years of age. It is early June, and the father needs to make plans for how to get the children to day camp every day for 6 weeks starting at the end of June.

Seating Chart

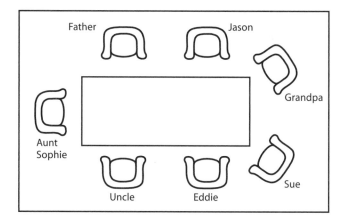

Action Begins Here

Father: We need to figure out a way to get the kids to the day camp every day for 6 weeks for their summer break. Their mother and I are working and can't take them every day.

Grandpa: I'll be out of town for the first week.

Aunt Sophie: I'll be able to come over to take them that week.

Father: I don't want you to have to drive back and forth on the highway each day from Alabama to Louisiana. You could stay here overnight for a few days while Gramps is away.

Aunt Sophie: OK. That will work out…

Father: Dad, you changed your schedule this year to be over at Sue's an extra day per week.

Sue: I wanted to spend more time with your Dad since he makes the interstate trip, too.

Uncle: Well, how about their mother doing it sometimes?

Father: Yeah, she is the mother…

Jason: Supposed to be…

Eddie: *(slumps in seat)* Well, Mom has to work…

Father: This would just be for a few weeks after you return from your trip.

Sue: OK, we can change our weekly schedule for a few weeks so the kids can go to day camp.

Father: I'll work out some details with their mother.

Sue: *(to one boy)* Why are you slumped down? Don't you want to go to camp?

Jason: Mom never shows her ID to go into the camp area. She just barges in past the gate. We have our season passes, but it's embarrassing that she doesn't pay. I think that the guards are afraid of her at the park.

Father: I'll probably have to buy a season pass for her to go into the park.

Sue: Okay. I have to drive back to Alabama. Have a good rest of the weekend.

The End.

Discussion

1. Are there gaps in social development parenting here? And in the community?

2. Are there aspects of attachment, separation, and individuation in this case? How are they made up for by the structure of this extended family?

3. Are the children able to voice their relationship concerns?

4. Is one boy protecting his mother's work hours, or is he trying to avoid embarrassment? Is this usually an issue at this age or in adolescence?

5. Are the children facing advanced social issues because of the divorce situation?

6. Do you feel that some resolution to the caregiving dilemma has been reached in this discussion?

References

American Psychiatric Association. (2000). *Diagnostic criteria from diagnostic and statistical manual–IV–TR*. Washington, DC: Author.

Bales, R. (1950). *Interaction process analysis*. Reading, MA: Addison-Wesley.

Bowlby, J. (1951). *Maternal care and mental health*. Geneva, Switzerland: World Health Organization.

Bowlby, J. (1969). *Attachment: Attachment and loss* (Vol. 1). New York, NY: Basic Books.

Bowlby, J. (1973). *Separation, anxiety and anger: Attachment and loss* (Vol. II). New York, NY: Basic Books.

Bowlby, J. (1988). On knowing what you are not supposed to know and feeling what you are not supposed to feel. In J. Bowlby (Ed.), *A secure base: Parent-child attachment and healthy human development* (pp. 99-118). New York, NY: Basic Books.

Bracken, B. A., & Nagle, R. J. (2007). *Psychoeducational assessment of pre-school children* (4th ed.). Hillsdale, NJ: Lawrence Erlbaum Associates.

Champagne, T. (2008). *Sensory modulation and environment: Essential elements of occupation* (3rd ed.). Southampton, MA: Champagne Conferences.

Clinton, H. R. (1996). *It takes a village*. New York, NY: Simon & Schuster.

Coates, S. W. (2003). John Bowlby and Margaret Mahler: Their lives and theories. *Journal of the American Psychoanalytic Association, 52*, 571-598.

Cowen-Fletcher, J. (1990). *It takes a village.* New York, NY: Grifalconi/Scholastic.

Dau, E. (2003). *A practical guide to working with children.* Croyden, Victoria: Tertiary Press.

Donohue, M. V. (1999). Theoretical bases of Mosey's group interaction skills. *Occupational Therapy International, 6,* 35-51.

Erikson, E. H. (1950). *Childhood and society.* New York. NY: Norton.

Erikson, E. H. (1967). *Adulthood.* New York, NY: W. W. Norton.

Hughes, F. P. (2009). *Children, play and development.* Thousand Oaks, CA: Sage.

Kramer, P., & Hinojosa, J. (1993). *Frames of reference for pediatric occupational therapy.* Baltimore, MD: Williams & Wilkins.

Mahler, M. (1963). Thoughts about development and individuation. *Psychoanalytic Study of the Child, 18,* 307-324.

Mahler, M. (1977). *Psychoanalytic movement.* New York, NY: Columbia University.

Mahler, M., & McDevitt, J. B. (1982). Thoughts on the emergence of the sense of self, with particular emphasis on the body self. *Journal of the American Psychoanalytic Association, 30,* 827-848.

Mahler, M., Pine, F., & Bergman, A. (1975). *The psychological birth of the human infant: Symbiosis and individuation.* New York, NY: Basic Books.

Olson, L. (1993). Psychosocial frame of reference. In P. Kramer & J. Hinojosa (Eds.), *Frames of reference for pediatric occupational therapy.* Baltimore, MD: Williams & Wilkins.

Parten, M. B. (1932). Social participation among pre-school children. *Journal of Abnormal and Social Psychology, 27,* 243-269.

Springen, K. (2008). Colic help. *Newsweek, June 9,* 65.

Vygotsky, L. S. (1962). *Thought and language.* Cambridge, MA: MIT Press.

Vygotsky, L. S. (1978). *Mind in society.* Cambridge, MA: Harvard University Press.

Wellhousen, K., & Crowther, I. (2004). *Creating effective learning environments.* Clifton Park, NY: Thomson Delmar.

Williamson, G. G., Szczespanski, M., & Zeitlin, S. (1993). Coping frame of reference. In P. Kramer & J. Hinojosa (Eds.), *Frames of reference for pediatric occupational therapy.* Baltimore, MD: Williams & Wilkins.

Additional Resources

Erikson, E. H. (1968). *Identity: Youth and crisis.* New York, NY: W. W. Norton.

chapter 7

Adolescent Social Development and Participation

Marilyn B. Cole, MS, OTR/L, FAOTA

Having its biological onset at puberty, adolescence has historically been associated with times of emotional turmoil. As a life stage, it begins with age 13 and ends at 19, otherwise known as the teenage years. Although normal social development does not always follow chronological age, this chapter equates adolescence with the middle and high school years in the United States. First, we will review developmental theories that address this age span, focusing on social development and behaviors. Second, we will describe some social norms, roles, and contexts typical of adolescence, including classrooms, peer groups, roles in the family, and roles in the community. Third, we will identify and discuss some current social problems associated with adolescence, including bullying, hazing, mental health issues, gangs, and school violence. The chapter ends with learning activities, cases, and scripts for analysis.

Theories of Social Development

Earlier theories of the 20th century view adolescence as a separate life stage beginning with pubertal awakening and characterized by "storm and stress, a normal disruption essential for full passage to adulthood" (Seltzer, 1982, p. 17). Anna Freud viewed biological drives as the force behind development of the ego, and its defenses determined the character and social identity of the emerging adult. Erikson (1963) adds a social anthropology perspective, defining the goal of adolescence as the development of ego identity through engagement with a widening social radius. Both Freud and Erikson believed that failure to resolve conflicts of earlier childhood stages could disrupt the development of a healthy, mature ego. Children need consistent recognition for achievements in order to pass from role diffusion to a positive choice of career and sexual identity, based on a continuation of strengths and abilities built during childhood.

Gesell (1933) continued his tracking of physical milestones to age 16, viewing periods of balance and imbalance, organization and disorganization, and regression as a part of growth and adjustment. In concert with Freud and Piaget, Gesell focused on the importance of the process, the development of skill in rebalancing, and adjusting one's self-concept in order to consolidate gains. Revising one's self-perception occurs through interaction with others in a variety of social situations. Socially mature individuals use this ability in order to deal positively with change, loss, stress, and challenge throughout adulthood. Although different cultures define adolescence and maturity differently, the process is believed to occur across cultures.

Attachment theory (Bowlby, 1969) suggests that a secure sense of connection with a primary caregiver (parent) promotes separation, while the teen who has projected parts of the self onto the parent lags

Cole, M.B., & Donohue, M.V. *Social Participation in Occupational Contexts: In Schools, Clinics, and Communities* (pp 109-126).
© 2011 SLACK Incorporated

Table 7-1

KOHLBERG'S VIEW OF ADOLESCENT MORAL DEVELOPMENT

STAGE 2: CONVENTIONAL (AGES 9 to 10)

1. Social conformity—Desires to fit in and therefore internalizes norms of social behavior

2. Law and order—Concerned with fairness, child may be upset to discover that peers, siblings, and parents appear to be "cheating"

STAGE 3: POSTCONVENTIONAL (AGE 11+)

1. Relativistic thinking—Moves beyond obedience to what is right and wrong in different situations

2. Social contracts—Awareness of legal consequences, internalizes societal values relative to own versus different cultures

Adapted from Pownall, S. (2001). Aspects of child development. In L. Laugher (Ed.), *Occupational therapy for child and adolescent mental health* (pp. 48-66). London, England: Churchill Livingstone.

---

behind in attempts to separate and to form a new social identity. The dependency issue may be especially acute in teens with chronic illness or disability, who may need extra support and encouragement from an external source (teacher or therapist) in taking steps toward independence by participating in peer groups outside the family during adolescence.

Bandura (1964) comes the closest to a continuity theory of adolescence, looking at the development of maturity as primarily shaped by environmental reinforcement of social behaviors. Contrary to the biologically enabled storm and stress theories, Bandura's study of middle class adolescent boys in a school setting found that adolescents had internalized the morals and values of parents, and their peer group mainly reflected parental norms. Evidence from this research showed that adolescent independence was more of a problem for parents than teens and that defiance and rebellion represented a deviation from the norm. On the other hand, teens' rebellion against larger social norms could be triggered under certain social conditions: (1) lack of jobs commensurate with their skills and (2) values learned during their upbringing were no longer in harmony with current social reality. This was exemplified by conditions present during the 1960s when a whole generation (hippies) refused to grow up if that meant giving up the more "expressive" aspects of life (Seltzer, 1982, p. 33).

Adolescent Moral Development

Piaget (1972) sees in adolescence the development of higher cognitive ability and the emergence of logical thought, allowing the teenager to move away from ego-centrism toward an awareness and acceptance of multiple realities. The leap to formal operations thinking consequently intensifies the

pressure for interpersonal understanding as the adolescent moves toward physical and emotional separation from parents. This increase in cognitive ability also gives adolescents a clearer view of objective reality, and their place within it, upon which to base decisions and moral judgments. Kohlberg (1970) builds on Piaget's intellectual development theory in creating stages of moral development, each requiring a higher level of cognitive organization. In Kohlberg's view, adolescents experience a "new cognitive world" complete with "an upsurge in feelings of power and a readiness to evaluate and compose new systems for society" (Seltzer, 1982, p. 35). The move from Kohlberg's conventional to postconventional moral reasoning typically occurring during adolescence is outlined in Table 7-1.

Hoffman (1980) summarizes past developmental theories into three categories: psychoanalytic, cognitive, and empathy-based (moral) theory. These three aspects of development interacting together determine social behavior in adolescence. White (1959) noted that as adolescents' more fundamental needs are met, their primary motivation to act becomes social. An effective experience of competence is mainly achieved through social roles within the adolescent peer group, which serves as a basis for adult role effectiveness in larger society.

Role of Self-Concept and Identity

Body image—how adolescents think of their own body appearance—continually changes through puberty, and with it, their sense of self or identity changes. By the end of adolescence, the fully grown body merges with a new identity that considers the continuation of the self in past, present, and future (Garberino, 1992). The emerging identity covers a full range of social and ideological roles: family roles and those concerned with politics, religion, education, and career (Marcia, 1980). Gilligan (1982) altered these categories with her studies of feminine social development, adding also nurturing roles, intimate partnerships, and gender roles incorporating sexual identity. Self-esteem—holding oneself in high regard—has been found to predict the social adjustment of teens (Dumont & Provost, 1999). Of three categories of eighth and eleventh graders, well-adjusted teens had the highest self-esteem, followed by the resilient group. The other discriminating variable found by these researchers was antisocial and illegal activities with peers, a factor more common in vulnerable teens who lacked self-esteem.

The Adolescent Peer Group

Teenage peer groups have been the topic of much sociological study, in part because of the troublesome features of their subcultures, such as conformity and consumerism, peer pressure to abuse drugs or alcohol, exposure to adult sexual encounters, bullying, hazing, gangs, and school violence. Seltzer (1982) defines the adolescent peer group as one that functions as an escape from dependency on parents and offers support and acceptance to members while trying out new independent social roles and identities. Erikson (in Seltzer) notes that in the absence of truly important roles for adolescents in Western society, the peer group forms out of necessity as a substitute structure to ease the transition in social status from family (during childhood) to the workplace (in adulthood). He notes that teens are eager to be affirmed by peers and willingly conform to peer social norms out of fear of rejection. The peer group serves three functions according to Erikson: (1) to protect one another against apparent loss of identity; (2) to provide feedback through social interaction, within which the teen members project, identify, and reflect off one another; and (3) to form subgroups or "cliques" that provide emotional support while members learn more realistic views of themselves through the eyes of others (Seltzer, 1982).

Ausubel (1954) defined the adolescent transition period as an ongoing reorganization of personality structure, gradually moving away from the "derived status" based on parental values and position, to a "primary status" based on performance within a peer group membership. It is the peer group experience that provides adolescents opportunities to try out different social roles and to alter aspirations for what they might become in adulthood based on a broader social perspective. This resonates with Mahler's view as extended into adolescence by Blos (1979) that the primary tasks of adolescence are separation (from parents) and individuation (form a new self-identity).

A related area of study dubbed "youth cultures" by Burlingame (1970) looks at the social norms and trends of entire younger generations. Aspects of youth culture have incorporated advances in technology and rebellion against adult values and societal bureaucracies, which collectively become the target of corporate marketing practices. The grassroots of such youth cultures is the adolescent peer group, within which interaction and peer feedback serve as the route to social identity in maturity. Sociological studies continue to track the distinguishing features or "youth culture" of each subsequent generation. Burlingame found that the peak adherence to youth culture occurs differently for boys and girls. For boys, adherence peaks in the 10th grade, with a potential appeal of risk, action, and danger. For girls, adherence develops through middle and late middle school, motivated mostly by opportunities for social esteem (popularity and social belonging).

For therapists, teachers, and parents, the high importance for teens of belonging to an adolescent peer group cannot be underestimated. In both popular literature and the media, high school students have been portrayed as highly status conscious, continually ranking one another (and themselves) in terms of status and popularity. Developmental theory supports this view that the peer group provides the most important context for development of social competence. Knowing this, therapists and others need to facilitate social participation in peer groups that would encourage each teen's strengths, abilities, and special talents in ways that would likely shape identity in adulthood.

The structure of adolescent peer groups has a profound effect upon who gets to belong and who does not. Milner (2004) elaborates on the social structure of adolescent peer groups through the application of status relations theory, including four key concepts:

1. *Conformity*—To the norms of the group, which are created by members with the highest status, including modes of dress, communication, and activity choices.

2. *Association*—Exclusively with other members, including (for teens) dining partners, friendships, even sexual partners.

3. *Inalienation*—Status as a member of a specific group, once attained, tends to remain stable, despite deviant behaviors.

4. *Inexpansibility*—Membership is limited in order to preserve status or value.

Milner's retrospective study of high school years for his college students revealed that there was usually a hierarchy among student groups, the top level being "cool kids" and the bottom level "nerds, geeks, or dorks," usually easily distinguishable by "how they dress and how they interact" (2004, p. 30). He further observed that students had to choose one group with which to identify and did not associate between groups. While multiple groups usually existed, most students modeled themselves after the more popular groups. Status could be structured around prevailing norms regarding the following characteristics: beauty, athletic ability, clothes and style, speech, body language, collective memories, humor (inside jokes), rituals (secret handshakes), popular music, dancing and singing, space and territory, and athletic uniforms. Milner notes that once status in the group is established, associating with other groups becomes possible and might even be a sign of greater social maturity.

The need for belonging and acceptance by one's peers makes teens vulnerable to peer pressure and that can be both good and bad. As teenage sons and daughters distance themselves and join peer groups, parents have less and less influence over their social development. It is this transition that is most important to attend to, especially for a teen who may not fit in with the more positive types of peer groups. Middle school is particularly difficult for early teens who don't fit in (Lavoie, 2008). "Middle schoolers draw boxes. And if you don't fit inside that box, you're rejected" (Rosen, 2008, p. 90). Loners who may be odd in some way also become more likely targets for teasing or bullying, adding to the painful isolation they feel as they question their own abilities and self-worth.

Assisting the so-called "square pegs" to fit in during middle school can be a challenge for teachers, therapists, and parents. Kids in this situation need to find others their age with the same strengths, talents, or special interests so that they can develop a positive self-identity in spite of being rejected by the "in-crowd." Fortunately, with the help of the internet, finding other kids with specific interests is not as difficult as it has been in the past. For example, Jake, a sixth grader, "loves ancient Roman history, hates small talk, (and) reads restaurant guides," clearly isolating him from the mainstream (Rosen, 2008, p. 90). Rosen advises parents to encourage kids like Jake to find their strengths and then join groups of others with similar interests, even if that means starting up a new group at school. When teasing or bullying is an issue, professional help may be needed to help these kids cope, an effort made easier in groups. Interventions for adolescents facing social isolation will be discussed further in Chapter 13.

Adolescent Social Behaviors

Adolescents typically experiment with many new social behaviors as they develop socially. Through their peer groups, they create social norms that may or may not resemble those of their parents, communities, or larger society. Some behaviors within the broad range of normal for teens include following fads, incorporating gender stereotypes, cheating and stealing, and casual sexual relationships. They can also be easily persuaded by images in the media and can benefit from adult expectations of positive social behaviors.

Fad Followers

With the exuberant energy adolescents can have, when they win a game, it is not surprising that they whoop it up in celebration as is often seen at the Olympics (Tracy, 2008). For norms on appropriate adolescent behaviors, it is typical for adolescents to use social comparison as guidelines for self-evaluation. In fact, according to research, when their social comparison group changes, their behaviors are altered (Crabtree & Rutland, 2001). Most noticeably, social comparison is common among teens in choosing clothing that is trendy with their chosen in-group. Recalling popularity of footwear from flip flops to Crocs and Uggs, it is easy to see local, national, and international fads. Some trends last longer than others, into adulthood or semi-adulthood, becoming embedded in the wider culture. During adolescence, and for adults who do not readily graduate from adolescent styles, fitting in by wearing the uniform is de rigueur (Tuttle, 2008). Even lyrics of some well-publicized songs follow trends of scorn for school spirit, discounting teachers, demeaning women, and portraying macho swagger as essential.

Gender Stereotypes

Some stereotypes of adolescent social behavior or outlook even include subjects pursued in high school, such as the notion that girls are not as strong in math as boys are (Begley, 2008), at least in the United States. Teams of students from Russia, Germany, and Bulgaria participating in the mathematical Olympiad have included numbers of girls. The stereotypes of mathematical ability are dependent on social, cultural, and school environments according to research carried out by Hyde and Mertz (2009).

Cheating and Stealing

Another trend among high school students, which seems to be becoming more acceptable to them, is lying, cheating, and shoplifting (Josephson Institute,

2009). Thirty percent of high school students admit to shoplifting from a store, while 64% say that they have cheated on a test. Josephson, founder and president of the Josephson Institute, an ethics organization, asks what the social cost becomes for future society. It appears that these behaviors among adolescents may be due to norms socially condoned among them.

Sexual Relationships

Casual relationships among adolescents, frequently called *friends with benefits*, and other unprintable labels, refer to relationships of a physical and emotional nature, which may include sexual aspects without the expectations of a more romantic or formal relationship. The relationship can continue over time with commitment being voluntarily constricted and geared toward satisfying sexual needs, aside from romantic or emotional needs. Some of these relationships in addition include support, friendship, and social enjoyment. Negative aspects of these social interactions include pregnancy, sexually transmitted diseases, extension of psychological immaturity, sexual addiction, and the perspective of *technical virginity* as an aspect of oral sex.

Media Communications

Social messages in television programs and movies often present unrealistic romantic expectations to adolescents, indicating that relationships and sexual interactions are always perfect without communication between the couple. Many adolescents and young adults believe that their partners should know what they need without communicating it because of the romanticized and reductionist storylines presented in "chick flicks." Interactions unfortunately often do not portray what is involved in developing trust and commitment within a couple's social communications and, in fact, indicate that love exists from the moment people meet (Holmes, 2008). Dr. Holmes is collecting data online for further study of media and relationships.

In a study of Web usage of social sites by teens, Dr. Moreno (2009) organized a study comparing groups who were given a head's up about their profile's contents regarding sexual issues, drinking, smoking, and drugs with groups who were not given a warning. The warning indicated that it would be wise to revise their Web page to better protect their privacy for future social and business contacts. Three months after the warning, 42% of the teens had modified their social page, while, in a control group, only 29% of the group not contacted had done so. Dr. Moreno encourages parents to review their teens' social Web pages with them and advise the teens not to expose their less responsible behaviors for public consumption.

Positive Social Behaviors

While adolescents are often seduced into exciting, but dangerous, experimental behaviors by their peers, the greater majority find social support from their families, neighborhood pals, teammates, school friends, and religious groups. While teens have fewer meals with their families than middle schoolers, Eisenberg (2008) found that in families where adolescents had five or more family meals per week, girls reported less substance use—marijuana, cigarettes, and alcohol. Perhaps the support of family meals is perceived differently by boys.

As Levitt (2009) traveled around the United States photographing teenagers, she was struck by their confidence and pride in their accomplishments. The assurance of these teens shone through in their photographs. They danced, sang, and performed for her without embarrassment or nervousness. While many of them were unique as individuals, she was told that they found companionship and similar lifestyles from communicating with other teens on the Web who had similar interests. She entitled her book, *We Are Experienced.*

Multiple sources indicate how important it is for parents to talk to teens about sex, pregnancy, and responsibility for a child born without planning. However, general talking is also needed to develop conversational skills. Teens need dinner with their family as frequently as possible for day-to-day social interaction, which provides the bedrock of social participation.

Life Tasks of Adolescence

Simpson (2001) reviews more than 300 recent studies of the prevailing theories and research on adolescence and summarizes them in the following 10 developmental tasks of adolescence:

1. Adjust to sexually maturing bodies and feelings

2. Develop and apply abstract thinking skills

3. Develop and apply a more complex level of perspective taking

4. Develop and apply new coping skills in areas such as decision making, problem solving, and conflict resolution

5. Identify meaningful moral standards, values, and belief systems

6. Understand and express more complex emotional experiences

7. Form friendships that are mutually close and supportive

8. Establish key aspects of identity

9. Meet the demands of increasingly mature roles and responsibilities

10. Renegotiate relationships with adults in parenting roles

Adolescents work on these tasks within the context of their social roles and occupations. While the cognitive aspects may be accomplished in the classroom as part of the role of a student, those involving moral judgment and decision making often occur within friendships or peer relationships outside of school. In expressing more complex emotions and forming close relationships with peers, teens begin to participate in higher-level supportive cooperative groups. Within these groups, they learn how to express empathy for others and to give and receive social and emotional support (Donohue, 2008; Mosey, 1986). For the first time, friendships outside the adolescent's family become deep and meaningful and function as a basis for new areas of self-identity. This is one of the reasons many of the social ties made in high school seem to last for many years into adulthood and are the most highly-valued friendships throughout one's life.

Simpson's breakdown of adolescent life tasks can also serve as a guideline for therapists, educators, and community organizers when designing appropriate learning experiences for youth, as well as understanding and problem-solving dilemmas that arise with adolescent individuals or groups. For example, educators might present scenarios that evoke discussion about acceptance of cultural diversity among students in the classroom. Therapists may work with individual teens in ways that encourage creative problem-solving when addressing conflicts with peers or parents. Adolescence may, in fact, be the ideal age group for volunteer community projects that bring teens into contact with populations with special needs, such as the homeless, poor, elderly, or otherwise disadvantaged groups. Such experiences encourage broader, more complex perspective taking while at the same time addressing the needs of their communities. Community leaders working with such volunteer groups need to facilitate the development of empathy and social understanding through open group discussions of issues raised by participants. Research shows that in order to accomplish the goal of higher level thinking about complex social issues, participants need opportunities to interact with each other, compare viewpoints, and process the meaning of volunteer experiences involving diverse groups.

Adolescent Roles and Contexts

Teens in the United States take on many new social roles during their adolescence. In addition to continuing roles of family member, friend, and student, after-school activities can include sports teams, bands, chorus, dance or drama groups, and many other special interests. Religious youth groups, Boy or Girl Scouts, other community-based groups, and employment outside the home often round out the busy lives of today's teens. For those who can afford it, computers and cell phones add yet another dimension to adolescent social participation, as communication with others can potentially continue almost nonstop day or night.

From an occupational standpoint, social participation continues to occur at the three basic group levels: parallel, associative, and cooperative. Attending classes in middle and high school remains largely parallel for classes with 20 to 30+ students listening to one teacher. Students take notes, write down assignments, and may ask or answer questions related to the topic of the lecture or presentation. Associative group characteristics emerge in class discussions or when subgroups form, such as teacher-initiated group projects or student-initiated study groups. Characteristics of these groups include helping one another with learning tasks and sharing or exchanging roles in the context of a defined group outcome. Examples are study groups working on raising the school's average on a state exam or members of a school band putting on a concert. From these associative group experiences during school, cooperative groups naturally flow as students take on more leadership roles in and out of the classroom. Sports teams competing with other schools are good examples of cooperative groups. Team members work together in a give-and-take manner, spontaneously trading roles in order to score goals, points, or touchdowns. Groups outside of school may spontaneously form to raise money to buy sports equipment for the team or just to hang out (Figure 7-1).

Supportive cooperative groups emerge spontaneously in clusters of teens for whom social and emotional aspects of the group take on greater importance than any one task or goal. Team spirit forms as players bond with one another emotionally, and this social bond helps the team to work better together and to put forth greater effort so as not to let one another down. Schwartz (2007) notes that there is such a thing as *too much* team spirit, causing members to continue to play football even with

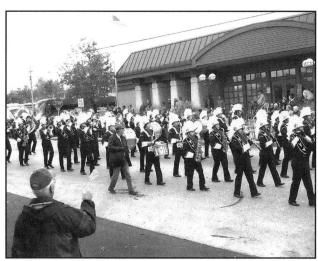

Figure 7-1. Teens can participate socially in their communities through activities such as marching in a Memorial Day Parade. High school marching band is an example of a basic cooperative group.

an injury. As one high school football player states: "It's not dangerous to play with a concussion. You've got to sacrifice for the sake of the team. The only way I come out is on a stretcher" (Schwartz, 2007, p. 1). Concern over fitting in and not letting friends down, or a macho mentality, may also explain why teens feel such extreme loyalty to neighborhood gangs or continue to participate in groups involved with drug or alcohol abuse, reckless driving, unsafe sex, or other risky behaviors. Support for teens facing difficult decisions, through guidance and open communication with parents and other responsible adults, can help to balance the need to fit in with the ability to exercise good judgment about when to participate and when to refrain from participating in specific social groups or situations (Simpson, 2001). The protective function of continued adult guidance and dialogue throughout adolescence will be further discussed in the section on barriers to social participation later in this chapter and in Chapter 13.

Teens in Families

Most academic disciplines would agree that the family serves as the primary context for social development of teenagers in the United States. However, in the 21st century, family must be broadly defined because of its many variations in today's culture. One in five children lives with just one biological parent, and many structures exist that affect adolescent socialization. For example, teens stay in school longer than previous generations and do not have parental supervision throughout most of the day. When both parents work out of economic necessity or choice, adolescents may receive goods

and technology instead of needed attention from parents (Milner, 2004). Ideally, as teens develop more mature social skills, they also raise their level of participation in family life, often taking on household tasks for working parents or caring for younger siblings. Parental expectations guide the extent to which teens take on more responsibility within the home. Still, there is a point during mid-adolescence that the peer group and the larger community surpass parents as the primary influence on social development.

An adolescent develops a higher degree of social competence when parental discipline is based upon support and affection, use of reasoning to control behavior, and emphasis on independence and achievement (Garberino, 1992). Social competence, the goal of socialization during adolescence, may be defined as a set of skills, attitudes, motives, and abilities needed to master the principal settings that an individual can reasonably expect to encounter in the social environment. Social competence maximizes one's sense of well-being as well as enhancing future development. Different social environments encourage different types of competence. For example, city-dwelling teens develop a "street smart" awareness that helps them survive a variety of dangers and pitfalls while participating in selected social groups. Adolescents growing up in rural communities may develop an expectation of friendliness, helpfulness, and mutual support that comes with the relative safety of living in a neighborhood where everyone knows and looks out for one another. Likewise, the context of peer groups and the norms within it also have a profound influence on the eventual identity and self-worth of emerging young adults.

Friendships in Adolescence

Friendships deepen with increased cognitive ability. Childhood friendships focus on external concrete aspects, such as playing ball or eating lunch together. In adolescence, friendship requires more abstract expectations, such as trust and loyalty, sharing secrets, and offering mutual support and empathy. Dunphy (1963) offers a five-step model for teen friendship development:

1. *Separate microsystems*—Groups that tend to "hang out" together

2. *Mesosystems*—Intergroup contact increases

3. Unisex groups break down as leaders enter heterosexual relationships

4. Groups of both genders are fully integrated

5. Couples sometimes replace individuals as the major format of social life

This progression varies in different cultures and circumstances (Figure 7-2).

Individually, teens mutually agree to become friends based on feelings of liking (affection) as well as how they treat one another (social behaviors). Ongoing friendships, often initially based on similarity or proximity, can adapt in various settings, and intimacy is quickly restored despite separations. Through friendships, teens learn to reflect on the self, taking a third-person perspective and making introspection and empathy possible (Selman, 1980).

Adolescent Volunteers in the Community

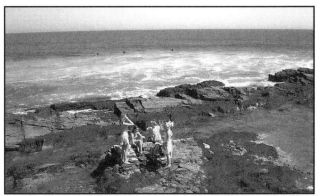

Figure 7-2. Teen girls "hang out" while their boyfriends ride the waves.

Service learning, a recent educational trend that links community outreach to educational objectives, currently occurs in 33% of schools in the United States (Hanc, 2008). This trend marks a change in the way teens are viewed in society, focusing on their energy and talents as assets for the community, rather than as liabilities and users of resources. For example, sixth graders in Arlington, Virginia participated in an "Earth Force" program as part of their science curriculum. This program includes six steps: (1) assessing their community's environmental issues, (2) selecting a problem, (3) examining the human role, both positive and negative, (4) deciding on a solution, (5) implementing an action plan, and (6) evaluating the results. The Arlington sixth graders found that a local stream served as a dumping ground for discarded computers, monitors, and TVs. Their investigation identified the lack of a recycling program for electronics, and their plan included creating one called, "We'll bring it to you," which provided curbside pickup of such items and arranging for their proper disposal. The sixth graders recruited volunteers from a local high school as well as parents and family members and collected more than 200 items in a single weekend. In 2007, their efforts earned them the President's Environmental Youth Award. According to their science teacher, "these kids feel so empowered, like they can change the world…and in their community they truly have" (Hanc, 2008, p. 82).

According to a survey conducted by the Higher Education Research Institute of UCLA (2005), 71% of high school seniors volunteer on a weekly basis. In a nationwide survey (Corporation for National and Community Service, 2005), 77% of middle and 83% of high schools reported offering community service opportunities for students. Participants in service learning experience a heightened sense of self-efficacy as well as an increase in personal and social responsibility, according to the Learn & Serve Clearinghouse Report (2007). Besides the obvious benefits of such programs for the community, participating teens learn valuable lessons in giving, especially when the volunteer project is one researched and designed by the teens themselves. Students practice reading and writing while researching potential community problems, they practice social interaction skills through group problem-solving and decision-making strategies, and they learn how to negotiate the workings of local political and social systems during the process of implementing their plans. Teens who volunteer often need the help of a teacher or other adult leader in order to process their experiences and to appreciate the impact of their project for both themselves and society. Table 7-2 lists some of the volunteer organizations in which teens can participate.

Teens taking on volunteer work in their communities report how much maturity they gained from seeing the span of life, realizing the value of what they had in their family, and gratification experienced in helping others. One teenager admitted that volunteering cured her of her own bullying of others as the responsibility empowered her, and she no longer needed to forcibly flaunt power over others.

In a positive participation program, teen athletes promote social interaction by volunteering in Lynbrook High School's Athletes Creating Excellence Club. High school athletes visit three middle schools to play a set of games designed to develop communication skills, sportsmanship, and teamwork. The adolescent athletes make a commitment to be drug- and alcohol-free. These values are discussed by the teens with the middle schoolers as they interact around sports games.

When the University of Essex in Britain indicated that a longitudinal study of high school seniors found that the more friends you have in high school, the higher your salary will be, then social skills appear in a new light (Daum, 2009). It is not surprising then that a teen is suing a social Web site and classmates for millions for suffering from ridicule, public hatred,

Table 7-2

EXAMPLES OF SERVICE LEARNING ORGANIZATIONS

ORGANIZATION/WEB SITE	DESCRIPTION
The League www.theleague.org	Uses sports league framework, with teachers as coaches, students as players, and class itself a "team." Scores based on dollars donated or items collected are posted on a web-based "scoreboard."
Giraffe Heroes Project www.giraffe.org	Refers to people who "stick their necks out" for good causes. Students choose, research, and implement solutions for community problems.
Earth Force www.earthforce.org	Focuses on environmental issues in communities, using a six-step process: assessing local environment, selecting a problem, examining the human role, deciding on a solution, implementing an action plan, and evaluating the results.
America Scores www.americascores.org	A multi-prong program combining soccer (teamwork and physical fitness), poetry (reading and self-expression), and developing service programs for their community.

Adapted from Hanc, J. (2008). Higher learning. *Family Circle*, September. Retrieved from www.familycircle.com/family-fun/volunteering/volunteering-through-school

and disgrace on the Web site (Epstein, 2009). We need to ask if the rate of sexually transmitted diseases is at a record high, is this a social indicator (Associated Press, 2009)? We also need to ask if health professionals and parents are teaching respect for members of the opposite gender and if learning politeness would take the fear from intergender relationships (Klass, 2009). Even newspapers are reminding teens to mind their manners and celebrate without intoxication during the prom experience when adolescents need to consider the social aspects of avoiding hurting feelings of others and drinking while driving (Pescatore, 2009). These issues lead into the next topic (Safe & Drug-Free Schools and Communities Act Program, 1994; Substance Abuse and Mental Health Service Administration [SAMHSA] & Office of National Drug Control Policy [ONDCP], 2009).

Formal and Informal Student Roles

The *International Classification of Function* (World Health Organization [WHO], 2001) specifies education as a major life area, including informal (noninstitutional), preschool (preparation), school, vocational training, and higher education. Formal student roles assume full-time attendance in a public or private educational institution. Informally, many teens take private lessons, participate in after-school learning activities, or attend camps and workshops during school breaks. These learning activities facilitate the resolution of Erikson's (1968) "industry versus inferiority" stage of psychosocial development,

building knowledge and skills needed for successful social participation in adulthood. When teens continue their educational pursuits after high school, enrolling in university or vocational education for several more years, Erikson's fourth developmental stage continues into the early 20s or longer.

Educational settings serve as the context for many formal and informal social relationships during adolescence, including relating with people of authority, equals (peers), and subordinates (younger age groups). Teachers, coaches, and religious or recreational activity group leaders often serve as surrogate parents in terms of their role in adolescent social learning. Simpson (2001) suggests that parents who cannot provide full-time supervision should direct their adolescent children toward other responsible adults in their communities to help fill their need for support and guidance. Through social participation in educational activities, teens learn many of the basics of complex interpersonal interactions, such as forming and terminating relationships, regulating emotions and behavior during interactions, interacting according to social rules, and maintaining culturally appropriate social distance (WHO, 2001) (Figure 7-3).

Teen Work Roles

Working for pay represents a part of the social ecology of adolescent life in the United States, and work experiences can provide positive guidance toward vocational development and career maturity

(Zimmer-Gembeck & Mortimer, 2006). By graduation from high school, an estimated 80% of adolescents will have worked part-time during their high school years. Boys begin earlier, sometimes starting to work for pay at age 12, and work more hours than girls (McDowell & Futris, 2001). The teens most likely to work are middle class, and the most common type of part-time work is in restaurants, fast food, or retail establishments; this work is often unrelated to future careers. Dollars earned at work most often are not saved but spent on materialistic pursuits, such as wardrobes, entertainment, drugs, and alcohol (Broderick & Blewitt, 2006; Steinberg & Cauffman, 1995).

The positive and negative effects of working while in middle and high school have been widely studied during the past 20 years. Some of the proposed benefits are learning how to find a job, exploring work preferences, and clarifying work values. Teens themselves report the perceived benefits of part-time work as becoming more responsible, managing time and money, establishing work ethics, and learning social skills (Mortimer, 2003). From a positive perspective, most working high school students successfully combined working and schooling, along with other typical teen activities such as socializing with friends, participating in extracurricular activities, and doing household chores, making employment just another component of a busy adolescent life (Shanahan & Flaherty, 2001).

According to some studies of attitude toward working in adolescence, parents and teachers tend to disagree. More than 85% of parents felt that early work experiences were beneficial and saw few problems with their sons and daughters working after school (Aronson, Mortimer, Zierman, & Hacker, 1996). Benefits such as responsibility, confidence, commitment to work, time management, interpersonal skills, and feelings of self-worth were viewed as markedly similar for parents and teens. Teachers, on the other hand, thought that students working should be discouraged because it detracts from what should be their main focus—attending and achieving in school (Greenberger & Steinberg, 1986). In fact, further evidence exists for both views, depending on the intensity of work (number of hours/week) and the quality of the work experience.

Negative consequences for employed teens, such as lower grades in school, school misconduct, theft, higher alcohol and drug use, and smoking, have been associated with longer hours of work (20+ hours/week) and disengagement from school (Largie, Field, Hernandez-Rief, Sanders, & Diego, 2001). Other researchers concur, finding that, in contrast, shorter hours and good work experiences

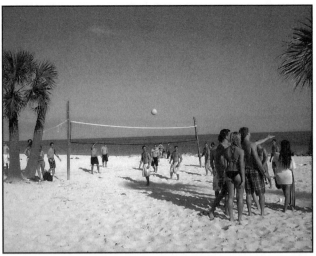

Figure 7-3. Spring breakers in Freeport, Bahamas, playing beach volleyball. Spring Break activity examples: "Insane Mardi Gras party in the square," all-day beach party, DJ spinning live, King and Queen of Spring Break contest, chugging contests, Bahamas Pong team tournament, glow party, "hot bod" contest, snorkeling trips, "booze cruise," rock climbing, water slide, dance contest "best of the Bahamas," and more. *What types of risky social behaviors might these activities encourage?*

are more likely to lead to feelings of self-efficacy and self-esteem. Other studies suggest that the negative consequences of longer work hours affect boys at risk for delinquency more than they do girls or low-risk boys (Wright, Cullen, & Williams, 1997). Conversely, negative attitudes, depressive affect, boredom, and life dissatisfaction among teens predicted subsequent unemployment after leaving school (O'Brien & Feather, 1990). Youth who lack the confidence, motivation, or resources for attending universities also tend to work longer hours during high school (Mortimer, 2003).

From a theoretical perspective, teens apply their work experiences to accomplish two important developmental tasks: (1) making career decisions that match one's talents and goals with available employment opportunities, including plans for acquiring the necessary education and training, and (2) developing a self-social-occupational identity, including autonomy and self-reliance. The right type of work experiences in adolescence can contribute to both of these goals, given certain optimal conditions for both workers and work contexts, which researchers are still attempting to identify. Some positive aspects of work environments that promote teen developmental goals include learning and using a variety of work skills, opportunities for social interactions that promote feelings of competence, and availability of role models and mentors in the adult worker role (Zimmer-Gembeck & Mortimer, 2006).

Several researchers recommend that schools take a more active role in facilitating students' transition to work (Stone & Mortimer, 1998). They could offer work internships that complement educational goals, making school more relevant to future work requirements. Teachers could include work experiences in class discussions, giving students opportunities to exchange information and/or to support one another. Teachers could help students to identify work goals and learn from their mistakes by asking them to reflect on, and write about, their experiences at work. More research is needed to fully understand the benefits and pitfalls of working in adolescence, to enhance teen work experiences, and guide students in selecting and shaping their workplace experiences to better facilitate the developmental tasks that will carry them from adolescence to adulthood.

Social Issues in Adolescence: Barriers to Social Participation

Much has been written regarding the problems facing teenagers today, including bullying, illegal drug and alcohol use, varying degrees of violence or criminal activity, and mental health issues such as depression and suicide. The high school years are the period when many major mental health conditions first appear, such as depression, schizophrenia, substance abuse, anxiety disorders, and eating disorders (Romer, 2004). A survey of mental health professionals in 2,000 public schools across the nation revealed that only 3% of schools practice some form of universal screening for mental health problems. Of those students identified as needing professional counseling, half or fewer actually received needed services. The lack of clear guidelines for identifying, referring, and providing appropriate treatment for middle and high school students with serious mental health issues is considered a serious crisis by Dr. Dwight Evans, Chair of the Department of Psychiatry at the University of Pennsylvania School of Medicine. An estimated 20% of adolescents have a diagnosable mental condition, 10% of whom have conditions that interfere with their daily functioning (Romer, 2004). The highest priority mental health problems identified in the Romer survey were depression, including suicide risk, anxiety disorders, illegal drug and alcohol use, truancy, and bullying.

Stress-Related Health Issues

Some evidence shows that the transition into "double digit" ages, often coinciding with entry into middle school, can trigger stress-related behavioral changes. In a study of more than 1,500 young teens, about 10% demonstrated the emergence of emotional health issues requiring medical attention (Schor, 1986). Schor found that psychological diagnoses for adolescents tend to correlate with predictable changes in social expectations that result from the onset of puberty, especially for girls. He calls for parents and teachers to identify signs of emotional difficulty earlier and to refer troubled preteens to health professionals who can help them cope with such stressful transitions.

Depression and Suicide

Suicide is the third leading cause of death among 10 to 24 year olds, and 16.9% of students in grades 9 to 12 have seriously considered suicide, according to a recent Centers for Disease Control (CDC) survey (2007). Emotional difficulties that underlie depression and suicide attempts frequently lead to recognizable negative consequences, including the following:

* Poor academic achievement
* Social isolation
* Failure to complete high school
* Self-medication with drugs or alcohol
* Promiscuity
* Involvement in the correctional system
* Lack of vocational success
* Inability to live independently
* Physical health problems

Suicide does not typically occur in isolation. Other factors are usually present, such as access to weapons, engaging in unprotected sex, clinical depression, bullying or ridicule by peers, tobacco use, or drug and alcohol use (Williamson, 2006). Some educational sources advocate teaching middle school students about the signs of depression, anxiety, and early signs of suicidal thinking as a part of school health education. Most kids do not have any conception of what depression is as an illness. They don't know the following subtle signs of depression:

* Criticizing yourself
* Feeling unwanted by others
* Cognitive difficulties
* Anxiety (performance, separation, or social in nature)

These early warning signs, left untreated, can lead to social isolation, depression, and ultimately, suicide (Williamson, 2006). Suggested strategies for suicide prevention are further discussed in Chapter 13.

Drug, Alcohol, Food Consumption, Reckless Driving

From a health perspective, taking drugs, drinking alcohol, and consuming sugary and fatty foods during the adolescent years all lead to compromised health as a teenager, leading to addiction, obesity, and diabetes. All three are also greatly influenced by the family and the social group with whom a teen associates. It is reported that teens are frequently overweight due to dropping out of physical activity when their peer group is no longer involved in sports or working out. In recent years, fortunately, there was a decline in teen pregnancy and smoking; however, driving at high speeds with other teens in the car is still the leading cause of death in this age group. About 50% of the deaths in adulthood are from health-related behaviors engaged in as adolescents, often promoted by teenage social groups (National Research Council and Institute of Medicine, 2009). Sad to say, about 10% to 20% of adolescents manifest a mental health problem without receiving care or intervention often because of the social stigma prevalent in high schoolers. Unfortunately, these experiences of mental illness can lead to teens dropping out of school before graduation (Taylor, 2006). Parents who want ideas about how to talk to their teens about drugs can go to the parent resource Web site www.drugfree.org. *Discuss the value of and privacy issues related to home, school, and athletic drug screens.*

Bullying and Victimization in High School

Bullying refers to negative physical or social actions that are repeated over time, by one or more people, toward a person who cannot easily defend him- or herself (Olweus, 1991). The problem begins before adolescence, with 10% to 20% of children identified as bullies in primary schools and 20% to 30% identified as victims (Smith et al., 1999). Both bullies and victims suffer psychosocial adjustment problems as well as internal psychological consequences (Hawker & Boulton, 2000). The relationship of bullying in school with consequent social adjustment has been studied by Scholte, Engeis, Overbeek, Kemp, and Haselager (2007). They found that children who bullied in both primary and secondary school (stable bullies) had a different outcome from those who engaged in bullying for only a short time (transient bullying). Stable bullies were more disliked, aggressive, and disruptive in adolescence. Stable victims have fewer friends and show overt signs of helplessness and distress (Hodges, Malone, & Perry, 1997; Perry, Willard, & Perry, 1990). This suggests that both bullying and victimization, when they are continuing patterns throughout the school years, are more likely to shape the identity of the adult personality in negative ways. Interventions by responsible adults will likely be necessary in order to reverse such socially negative outcomes. Yet, teachers and administrators, lacking in power to enforce any really effective consequences, do little to stop the "small cruelties" imposed by bullies that are common in school life, probably because their attempts to intervene do not stop the behaviors and often make matters worse (Milner, 2004).

Cliques, Gangs, and Youth Violence

Research shows that peer relationships form an essential part of teen social development, and members of the peer group offer each other needed social and emotional support in exploring different value systems and lifestyles that will become part of their adult identity. Thus, adolescent crowds and cliques can positively influence teens, surrounding them with others of similar social status and providing close friendships and potential dating partners. In this sense, membership in peer cliques and crowds forms a normal part of growing up (Bateman, 2009).

However, through middle and high school years, teens might also fall in with the "wrong crowd," which can subscribe to values and beliefs that are very different from those of adult society. When peer culture influences teens in negative ways, problem behaviors result, that can adversely affect adolescent social development. Parents, society, and the media have blamed peer pressure and negative peer cultures for any number of social problems, including alcohol and drug abuse, reckless or drunk driving, promiscuity, teen pregnancy, the spread of sexually transmitted diseases, drug trafficking, and at its extreme, gang-related violent crimes (Bateman, 2009).

A youth gang is commonly defined as a self-formed association of peers having the following characteristics:

- A gang name and recognizable symbols
- Identifiable leadership
- Geographic territory
- Regular meeting pattern
- Collective actions to carry out illegal activities (Howell, 1997)

An estimated 14% to 30% of adolescents join gangs at some point, and that trend, including both boys and girls, is increasing nationwide (Thornberry, Huizinga, & Loeber, 2004). Alarmingly, gang membership triples the likelihood of adolescents becoming involved in violent crimes when compared with nongang members. Furthermore, even when a teen member drops out, he or she continues the tendency toward violence learned as a gang member. Howell (1997) identifies cycles of violence between gangs, focusing on turf protection and expansion, member recruitment, and defending the honor of the gang. The increase in gang violence is exacerbated by increased availability of illegal drugs and firearms.

Why is it that youth gang members sustain much higher rates of delinquency and drug involvement? In a 2005 study (Gatti, Tremlay, Vitaro, & McDuff), three hypotheses were tested:

1. *Selection*—Those teens who tend toward aggressive behaviors seek out gang membership

2. *Facilitation*—Gang membership encourages increased involvement in violent crimes

3. *Enhancement*—Both selection and facilitation work together to increase violence

They found that gang membership facilitated increased delinquency for teens ages 14 to 16 years who remained in the gang for 1 year or less, while the enhancement hypothesis was supported for more stable members (remaining in the gang for all 3 years, ages 14 to 16). These researchers concluded that the best way to stop gang violence is prevention—taking steps to stop the formation and participation in gangs by providing other community alternatives or programs.

It has long been known that teens like their comfort zone group and use derogatory nicknames for teenagers in other groups. Because these trendy names change over time, they will not be mentioned as examples here; however, most readers will know examples from their adolescent years and locale. Some efforts to "mix it up" in some high schools have met with nonverbal responses, such as indifference, sarcastic eye rolls, shrugging sophistication, awkward silence, and nonparticipation in changing tables in the cafeteria (Teaching Tolerance, 2009). Verbal responses included, "This is stupid," "I don't want to sit with those people. They make fun of my accent, and call me names," "I miss my friends." Students labeled these responses as due to insecurity, shyness, and being scared. In this high school, the "Mix It Up at Lunch" day was planned by outside college students; it is preferable if the organization comes from the high school's own student government.

When planning was done by the high school students' own student council, one school had a mission of "celebrating diversity" among three major culturally-mixed racial groups. This philosophy encouraged the students to reach across social boundaries.

In this school, there was mixing of students in classes of various years, ethnicity, economic background, academic, artistic, and athletic focus, so that slang epithets such as nerd or jock stereotyping were not typical, and the "mix it up" day was successful. Students at this school had much to talk about. In other schools, handouts of topics and moderators at the lunch tables could be helpful (Teaching Tolerance, 2009). Other such programs will be discussed in Chapter 13.

Wayward Teens

If waywardness can be considered a separate role, many teens find themselves caught between the need to belong and the need to uphold parental values. Wayward teens may not fit the category of "troubled" but begin to show signs of breaking away from parents by engaging in what parents view as risky behaviors. Parents of the 1970s and 1980s have typically used a "tough love" approach, setting down the law and asking their wayward teen to conform to the rules or leave (Wyman, 1982). Parents of this millennium have learned a few things from the consequences of the tough love approach, and the pendulum seems to be swinging more toward a hands-on type of parenting, which offers attention and love rather than authoritative line drawing (Currie, 2004). Currie suggests a broader approach for schools and communities to offer guidance and support for potentially troubled teens, as described in Table 7-3. An example of one such teen who may be at risk engages in a family therapy session at the end of the next chapter, illustrating the need to view teen rebellion as a part of a family systems problem-solving approach.

Learning Activity: Role Playing

This activity works well with groups of 6 or 8 members. Each person chooses a partner with whom to spontaneously role play one of the scenarios. Members may draw numbers at random, or they may choose which scenario relates best to each of them. Alternatively, students can respond in writing, explaining why they chose certain responses, then share their reasoning process with the group and discuss the pros and cons of alternate responses.

Using the social skills and competencies discussed in Chapters 1 and 3, describe how you would respond to each of the following social dilemmas:

1. Your best friend in middle school invites you to a party on Saturday, and you know that your friend's parents are away. If you tell your parents this, they will not allow you to attend.

Table 7-3

RECOMMENDATIONS FOR CREATING A CULTURE OF INCLUSION AND SUPPORT FOR TROUBLED TEENS

1. *Places to go*—Alternative programs, places to hang out, places to spend the night

2. *Things to do*—Available activities that welcome teens, such as recreation centers and volunteer groups that discuss, organize, and provide needed community services

3. *Inclusionary schools*—Allowing for a wider range of social and recreational activities

4. *Community of shepherds*—Responsible adults that teens can turn to for guidance

5. *New kinds of counseling*—Mental health treatments

6. *Family-friendly policies*—Humane work policies

Adapted from Currie, E. (2004). *The road to whatever: Middle class culture and the crisis of adolescence.* New York, NY: Holt & Company.

2. As a high school senior, you have dated the same person for more than a year and would like the relationship to be exclusive. A friend has just told you that your steady was spotted around town with another partner.

3. A friend who used to be close withdraws from the relationship, seems preoccupied, and looks depressed. Today, you receive a long letter describing hopelessness about the future, expressing appreciation for your friendship, and basically saying goodbye.

4. As a college student, you have let yourself fall behind on reading and assignments in several classes and now face midterm exams next week. It is Sunday night before the first exam, and you have more than 200 pages to read as well as class notes to study. Your suitemate, who has the same class, offers you a copy of the exam, stolen from a fraternity file by another student.

5. In the same scenario as above (#4), a senior student sitting next to you in the library offers you a "wake up" pill for free, which is "guaranteed" to enhance alertness and memory for at least 12 hours. You have never used any illegal drugs before, but find this prospect a better alternative than failing your midterm.

6. As a new graduate, you have been searching for a job in your field of expertise for more than 6 months, while living at home with your parents. Although you can still earn some money babysitting for neighbors, it is not enough to pay the rent for your own apartment. Your boyfriend (or girlfriend) wants to get serious and asks you to move in with him (or her). You do not feel the same desire for intimacy but feel compelled to become independent from your demanding and impatient parents.

Script: Student Government Decision During Senior Prom Committee Meeting

Scenario Description

This scenario was chosen because there was a high school where this proposal caused an incredible controversy, leading to one student being expelled. In an after-school meeting, six student government officers of the senior class of a local high school discuss their plans for the senior prom. They compose the Senior Prom Committee for the year and are meeting in an empty classroom.

Seating Chart

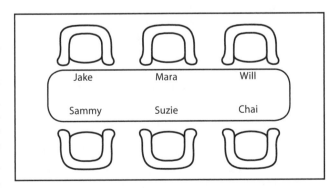

Action Begins Here

Jake: This is our meeting devoted to deciding what we want to do for the Senior Prom.

Mara: Let's do something different this year. Because our school is small, let's partner up with a neighboring school for the prom.

Will: Which school did you have in mind?

Mara: Zen High (*chief competitor school in football*).

Jake: I don't like those guys. They're our arch enemies! Another school might be okay.

Suzie: I think that Zen High School would be awesome. I know some of the kids over there.

Will: Do you think that it would be a good social mix?

Sammy: What do you mean by that?

Will: Well, they are of a different cultural background, but you might not think that's PC.

Chai: What's PC?

Will: Politically correct.

Chai: You know, having the prom with another school might cut into our school spirit and make it feel not so special for our class. The prom is the last time our class gets to be together before we graduate.

Suzie: You may be right. When we take pics, I would prefer it be just with our own class.

Will: Yeah, but having two high schools could lower the cost everyone has to pay. Maybe some of the merchants in both towns would subsidize the mixing when we talk to them about sponsoring us. That would help pay for the band.

Suzie: Are there some kids this year who can't afford to go to the prom? Or to pay for post-prom activities or trips?

Chai: Probably from Zen there would be.

Mara: I think that we should sound out some of the kids from Zen, and also we should talk to our principal about it. They could talk to their principal, too.

Jake: I'll talk to our principal about it.

Mara: I'll sound out some of the kids from Zen. Suzie, would you join me? I know where they hang out.

Suzie: Yeah. Okay.

Chai: I'm still not so sure if as many kids would come… Would having Zen kids there change what sometimes happens at post-prom parties and trips?

Will: Well, let's gather information and find out what other kids in the class think, too.

Mara: Yeah, let's not be Zen-o-phobic!

The End.

Discussion

1. What problems do you foresee in this prom suggestion?

2. What reasons are there for going with this idea?

3. What reasons are there for not doing so?

4. What is the purpose of a prom? What is it supposed to accomplish?

5. What economic aspects of a prom might divide a class socially?

6. What sometimes happens during post-prom parties and trips? What might be some social pressures to engage in risky social behaviors?

7. How does this scenario demonstrate social relationships with peers from different social groups?

8. How do committee members regard authority figures? What might be some reasons to involve the principal or other adults in the decision?

9. Which Kohlberg principles and levels of moral development does this discussion demonstrate? Why?

10. Considering Simpson's life tasks of adolescence, which tasks are evident in this discussion, and how might their accomplishment impact the outcome?

References

Aronson, P. J., Mortimer, J. T., Zierman, C., & Hacker, M. (1996). Adolescents, work, and family: An intergenerational developmental analysis. In J. Mortimer & M Finch (Eds.), *Understanding families* (Vol. 6, pp. 25-62). Thousand Oaks, CA: Sage.

Associated Press. (2009). Report: Tween, teen years crucial to health. *Newsday*, Jan. 6, A27.

Ausubel, D. (1954). *Theory and problems of adolescent development*. New York, NY: Grune & Stratton.

Bandura, A. (1964). The stormy decade: Fact or fiction? *Psychology in the Schools, 1,* 224-231.

Bateman, H. V. (2009). *Adolescent peer culture: Overview*. Retrieved January 20, 2009 from education.stateuniversity. com/pages/1738/Adolescent-Peer-Culture.html

Begley, S. (2008). Math is hard, Barbie said. *Newsweek, October, 27,* 57.

Blos, P. (1979). *On adolescence: A psychoanalytic interpretation*. New York, NY: Free Press.

Bowlby, J. (1969). *Attachment: Attachment and loss* (Vol. 2). New York, NY: Basic Books.

Broderick, P. C., & Blewitt, P. (2006). *The life span: Human development for the helping professions* (pp. 325-327). Retrieved September 30, 2009 from www.pearsonhighered.com/educator/academic/product/0,3110,0131706845,00.html

Burlingame, W. (1970). The youth culture. In E. Evans (Ed.), *Adolescents: Readings in behavior and development* (pp. 131-150). Hinsdale, IL: Dryden Press.

Corporation for National and Community Service. (2005). *Building active citizens: The role of social institutions in teen volunteering. Brief 1 in the Youth Helping America Series.* Washington, DC: Author.

Crabtree, J., & Rutland, A. (2001). Self-evaluation and social comparison amongst adolescents with learning difficulties. *Journal of Community and Applied Social Psychology, 11,* 347-359.

Currie, E. (2004). *The road to whatever: Middle class culture and the crisis of adolescence.* New York, NY: Holt & Company.

Daum, M. (2009). With friends like these, who needs strangers? *Newsday, March 12,* Retrieved from www.newsday.com

Donohue, M. (2008). *Social profile manual.* Unpublished manuscript.

Dumont, M., & Provost, M. (1999). Resilience in adolescents: Protective role of social support, coping strategies, self-esteem, and social activities on experience of stress and depression. *Journal of Youth and Adolescence, 28,* 343-363.

Dunphy, D. (1963). The social structure of urban adolescent peer groups. *Sociometry, 26,* 230-246.

Eisenberg, M. (2008). Family meals and substance use: Is there a long-term protective association? *Journal of Adolescent Health, 43,* 2.

Epstein, R. J. (2009). *Oceanside teen sues Facebook, ex-classmates for $3M.* Retrieved from www.newsday.com/long-island/nassau/oceanside-teen-sues-facebook-ex-classmates-for-3m-1.896009

Erikson, E. (1963). *Childhood and society.* New York, NY: Norton.

Erikson, E. (1968). *Identity: Youth and crisis.* New York, NY: Norton.

Garberino, J. (1992). *Children and families in the social environment* (2nd ed.). New York, NY: Aldine Transaction Publishing.

Gatti, U., Tremlay, R., Vitaro, F., & McDuff, P. (2005). Youth gangs, delinquency, and drug use: A test of the selection, facilitation, and enhancement hypotheses. *Journal of Adolescent Psychology and Psychiatry and Allied Disciplines, 46, 11,* 1178-1190.

Gesell, A. (1933). Maturation and patterning of behavior. In C. Murchison (Ed.), *A handbook of child psychology* (2nd ed. rev.). Worcester, MA: Clark University Press.

Gilligan, C. (1982). *In a different voice.* Cambridge, MA: Harvard University Press.

Greenberger, E., & Steinberg, I. (1986). *When teenagers work: The psychological & social costs of adolescent employment.* New York, NY: Basic Books.

Hanc, J. (2008). Higher learning. *Family Circle,* September. Retrieved from www.familycircle.com/family-fun/volunteering/volunteering-through-school

Hawker, D., & Boulton, M. (2000). Twenty years' research on peer victimization and psychosocial maladjustment: A meta-analytic review of cross-sectional studies. *Journal of Child Psychology and Psychiatry and Allied Disciplines, 41,* 441-455.

Higher Education Research Institute of UCLA. (2005). *Volunteering and community involvement declines after students leave college.* Retrieved October 22, 2009 from www.gseis.ucla.edu/heri/PDFs/Atlantic_PR.pdf

Hodges, E., Malone, M., & Perry, D. (1997). Individual risk and social risk as interacting determinants of victimization in the peer group. *Developmental Psychology, 33,* 1032-1039.

Hoffman, M. (1980). Moral development. In P. H. Mussen (Ed.), *Carmichael's handbook of child psychology* (Vol. 2). New York, NY: Wiley.

Holmes, B. (2008). Rom-coms 'spoil' your love life. *BBC News.* Retrieved from www.bbc.co.uk/2/hi/uk_news/scotland/edinburgh_and _east/.stm

Howell, J. (1997). *Youth gangs.* Office of Juvenile Justice and Delinquency Prevention Fact Sheet, #72: December 1997. Retrieved January 19, 2009 from www.ncjrs.org/ojjhome.htm.

Hyde, J. S., & Mertz, J. E. (2009). Gender, culture, and mathematics performance. *Proceedings National Academy of Science USA, 106,* 8801-8807.

Josephson Institute. (2009). *Making ethical decisions: The six pillars of character.* Retrieved October 22, 2009 from josephsoninstitute.org/MED/index.html

Klass, P. (2009). Another awkward sex talk: Respect and violence. Retrieved April 30, 2009 from www.nytimes.com/2009/04/14health/14klas.html

Kohlberg, L. (1970). Moral development and the education of adolescents. In E. Evans (Ed.), *Adolescents: Readings in behavior and development.* Hinsdale, IL: Dryden Press.

Largie, S., Field, T., Hernandez-Reif, M., Sanders, C. E., & Diego, M. (2001). Employment during adolescence is associated with depression, inferior relationships, lower grades, and smoking. *Adolescence, 36,* 395-401.

Lavoie, R. (2008). *It's so much work to be your friend.* New York, NY: Touchstone.

Learn and Serve Clearinghouse. (2007). *Experiences that Matter: Enhancing Student Learning and Success, Annual Report 2007.Institution.* Retrieved May 20, 2010 from www.nsse.iub.edu/NSSE_2007_Annual_Report/docs/withhold/NSSE_2007_Annual_Report.pdf

Levitt, D. (2009). Making overtures. *Psychology Today, January/February,* 11.

Marcia, J. (1980). Identity in adolescence. In J. Adelson (Ed.), *Handbook of adolescent psychology.* New York, NY: Wiley.

McDowell, U., & Futris, T. (2001). *Adolescent employment fact sheet FLM-FS-8-01.* Retrieved September 30, 2009 from ohioline.osu.edu/flm01/FS08.html

Milner, M. (2004). *Freaks, geeks, and cool kids: American teenagers, schools, and the culture of consumption.* New York, NY: Routledge.

Moreno, M. (2009). Teens get Web warning. *Newsday, January 6,* A5.

Mortimer, J. T. (2003). *Working and growing up in America.* Cambridge, MA: Harvard University Press.

Mosey, A. C. (1986). *Psychosocial components of occupational therapy.* New York, NY: Raven.

National Research Council and Institute of Medicine. (2009). Report: Tween, teen years crucial to health. *Newsday, January 6,* A27.

O'Brien, G. E., & Feather, N. T. (1990). The relative effects of unemployment and quality of employment on the affect, work values, and personal control of adolescents. *Journal of Occupational Psychology, 63,* 151-165.

Olweus, D. (1991). Bully/victim problems among school children: Basic facts and effects of a school based intervention program. In D. Pepler & K. Rubin (Eds.), *The development and treatment of childhood aggression* (pp. 411-448). Hillsdale, NJ: Erlbaum.

Perry, D., Willard, J., & Perry, L. (1990). Peers' perceptions of the consequences that victimized children provide aggressors. *Child Development, 61,* 1310-1325.

Pescatore, L. (2009). Mind your manners: Prom-time etiquette is crucial for no hurt feelings. *Herald Community Newspaper. April 23,* 15.

Piaget, J. (1972). Intellectual evolution from adolescence to adulthood. *Human Development, 14,* 1-12.

Romer, D. (2004). *National survey on adolescent mental health.* Annenberg Public Policy Center of the University of Pennsylvania. Retrieved July 21, 2004 from www.appcpenn.org

Rosen, P. (2008). Square pegs. *Family Circle,* September, 89-97.

Safe & Drug-Free Schools and Communities Act Program. (1994). Retrieved from www.ed.gov/offices/OESE/SDFS/publications.html

Scholte, R., Engeis, R., Overbeek, G., Kemp, R., & Haselager, G. (2007). Stability in bullying and victimization and its association with social adjustment in childhood and adolescence. *Journal of Abnormal Child Psychology, 35,* 217-228.

Schor, E. L. (1986). Use of health care services by children and diagnoses received during presumably stressful life transitions. *Pediatrics, 77,* 834-841.

Schwartz, A. (2007). In high school football, an injury no one sees. *New York Times.* Retrieved September 15, 2007 from www.nytimes.com/2007/9/15/sports/football/15concussions.html

Selman, R. L. (1980). *The growth of interpersonal understanding: Developmental and clinical analysis.* New York, NY: Academic Press.

Seltzer, V. (1982). *Adolescent social development: Dynamic functional interaction.* Lexington, MA: Lexington Books.

Shanahan, M. J., & Flaherty, B. P. (2001). Dynamic patterns of time use in adolescence. *Child Development, 72,* 385-401.

Simpson, A. R. (2001). *Raising teens: A synthesis of research and a foundation for action.* Boston, MA: Center for Health Communication, Harvard School of Public Health. Retrieved 9/18/08 from www.hsph.harvard.edu/chc/parenting

Smith, P. K., Morita, Y., Junger-Tas, J., Olweus, D., Catalano, R., & Slee, P. (1999). *The nature of school bullying: A cross-national perspective.* London, England: Routledge.

Steinberg, L., & Cauffman, E. (1995). The impact of employment on adolescent development. *Annals of Child Development, 11,* 131-166.

Stone, J. R., & Mortimer, J. T. (1998). The effect of adolescent employment on vocational development: Public & educational policy implications. *Journal of Vocational Behavior, 53,* 184-214.

Substance Abuse and Mental Health Service Administration & Office of National Drug Control Policy (2009). *Office of National Drug Control Policy. Drug Free Communities Act.* Retrieved from www.SAMHSA.gov

Taylor, D. (2006). *NAMI Letter.* National Association for the Mentally Ill, October 2006.

Teaching Tolerance. (2009). Retrieved April 30, 2010 from www.tolerance.org/teens/stories/article.jsp

Thornberry, T. P., Huizinga, D., & Loeber, R. (2004). The causes and correlates studies: Findings and policy implications, *Juvenile Justice, 10,* 3-19. Retrieved from www.ncjrs.org/pdf-files1/ojjdp/203555.pdf

Tracy, J. (2008). Whooping it up? It's only natural. *Newsday,* August 13, A27.

Tuttle, S. (2008). Make. It. Stop. *Newsweek, August 1,* 2.

White, R. (1959). Motivation reconsidered: The concept of competence. *Psychological Review, 5,* 297-333.

Williamson, S. (2006). Schools and suicide. *Advancing Suicide Prevention,* January, 16-26. Retrieved January 19, 2009 from www.advancingsp.org/ASP_Jan_2006.pdf

World Health Organization. (2001). *International classification of functioning, disability, and health.* Geneva: Author.

Wright, J. P., Cullen, F. T., & Williams, N. (1997). Working while in school and delinquent involvement: Implications for social policy. *Crime and Delinquency, 43,* 203-221.

Wyman, C. (1982). Toughlove is touted by weary parents. *The New Haven Register, April 4,* 11, 13.

Zimmer-Gembeck, M. J., & Mortimer, J. T. (2006). Adolescent work, vocational development, and education. *Review of Educational Research, 76,* 537-566.

Additional Resources

Bandura, A. (1993). Perceived self efficacy in cognitive development and functioning. *Educational Psychology, 28,* 117-148.

Bowlby, J. (1988). *A secure base.* New York, NY: Basic Books.

Burney, R. (2002). *Enabling & Rescuing vs. Tough Love.* Inner child/codependency recovery page. Retrieved February 18, 2009 from www.joy2meu.com/tough_love.htm

Centers for Disease Control. (2007). Teen suicide rate: Highest increase in 15 years. *Science Daily.* Retrieved January 1, 2009 from www.sciencedaily.com/releases/2007/09/070907221530.htm

Egley, A. & O'Donnell, C. (2007). Highlights of the 2007 National Youth Gang Survey, OJJDP Fact Sheet, April. Retrieved January 20, 2009 from www.ojp.usdoj.gov

Hardy, C., & Prior, K. (2001). Attachment theory. In L. Lougher (Ed.), *Occupational therapy for child and adolescent mental health* (pp. 48-66). London, England: Churchill Livingstone.

Main, M. (1996). Introduction to special section on attachment psychology: 2. Overview of the field of attachment. *Journal of Consulting and Clinical Psychology, 64,* 237-243.

Partnership for a Drug-Free America. (2009). Parent resource at www.drugfree.org.

Pownall, S. (2001). Aspects of child development. In L. Laugher (Ed.), *Occupational therapy for child and adolescent mental health* (pp. 48-66). London, England: Churchill Livingstone.

chapter 8

Adult Social Development
Theories, Roles, and Contexts

Marilyn B. Cole, MS, OTR/L, FAOTA

This chapter covers multiple adult ages from young adulthood through middle adulthood. While young adults have already acquired mature social and group skills, social development continues throughout life. Because the rate and sequence of adult social development varies widely, this chapter will be organized into two categories independent of age ranges, theories, roles, and contexts.

Theories of Adult Social Development

Older theories, such as Erikson's (1978) psychosocial development theory, Jung's (1914) spiritual stages theory, and Levinson's (1978) life transitions theory, divide adulthood into early, middle, and late life stages complete with age ranges. While both current research and the demographics of aging render the sequence and age ranges obsolete, the developmental stages and life tasks remain valid and relevant. Gilligan (1982) adds a female dimension, giving renewed importance to social relationships in the development of adult social maturity. Updates to Piaget's (1972) cognitive theory also impact social development and help explain some of the adult role changes in midlife and beyond. Atchley's (1999) continuity theory, and more recently, Commons' (Commons, Armon, Kohlberg, Grotzer, & Sinnott, 1990; Commons & Richards, 1999) theory of positive adult development and Baltes' (Baltes & Baltes,

1990) selection and optimization with compensation theory (SOC) contribute to our understanding of the changes in social participation throughout an ever-increasing lifespan.

Erikson's Adult Psychosocial Development

In Erikson's (1978) adolescent life stage, titled identity versus role confusion, a psychological conflict must be resolved in order to prepare the young adult to enter the world capable of commitment and fidelity (Goleman, 1988). Fidelity, as used here, means that the personality is stable and that the person can project a cohesive sense of self when entering into relationships with others. Intimacy versus isolation, the next stage proposed by Erikson, requires the adult to make social commitments in ongoing relationships. He states, "You have to live intimacy out over many years, with all the complications of a long range relationship (in order) to really understand it" (Goleman, 1988, p. 20). Intimacy can pertain to marriage and parenting, as well as close friendships and redefined adult relationships within one's family of origin. Love in early adulthood often begins with passion and its physical and mental expression. As love matures in marriages and partnerships, the values of tenderness, caring, loyalty, and unselfish friendship nurture the spiritual bond with significant others. Mature adults who successfully resolve the issues of intimacy versus isolation are able to participate fully in a

Cole, M.B., & Donohue, M.V. *Social Participation in Occupational Contexts: In Schools, Clinics, and Communities* (pp 127-148).
© 2011 SLACK Incorporated

Table 8-1

LEVINSON'S ADULT TRANSITIONS AND LIFE TASKS

YOUNG ADULT TRANSITION	YOUNG ADULTHOOD	MIDDLE ADULT "MIDLIFE" TRANSITION	MIDDLE ADULTHOOD	OLDER ADULT TRANSITION	OLDER ADULTHOOD
Ages 17 to 22	Ages 23 to 39	Ages 40 to 45	Ages 46 to 59	Ages 60 to 65	Ages 65+
Dream		Young/old		Mortality	
Mentor		Destruction/creation		Physical decline	
Occupation		Masculine/feminine		Loss of productive role	
Marriage		Attachment/separation			

Adapted from Levinson, D. (1996). *The seasons of a woman's life.* New York, NY: Ballantine Books.

variety of social roles. For example, they can balance the need to work alone without compromising marriage and family commitments and involvement in their communities.

Generativity versus stagnation, Erikson's (1978) middle adult stage, represents a continuation of the balance of life roles. Generativity includes caring, empathy, and concern for others, as well as imparting one's expertise and wisdom to future generations (McAdams, Hart, & Maruna, 1998). In a longitudinal study, Westermeyer (2004) adds evidence to support Erikson's generativity stage for men assessed at age 21 and again at age 53. He found that "generativity was significantly associated with successful marriage, work achievements, close friendships, altruistic behaviors, and overall mental health" (p. 29). Favorable social relationships in early adulthood stood out as a significant predictor of the resolution of Erikson's generativity versus stagnation conflict in midlife (Westermeyer, 2004).

McAdams and de St. Aubin (1992) devised an assessment scale for different components of generativity, and subsequently found, in those ranked highest for "generative identity," many positive health features that impact individual well-being, including the following:

× A positive attitude toward the self

× Trusting, satisfying, and warm relationships with others

× Independence and self-determination in resisting social pressures

× Competence in managing the environment and making use of opportunities

× Goals in life and a sense of direction

× A sense of continuing development with a growing and expanding self (McAdams, de St. Aubin, & Logan, 1993)

This research suggests that generative features of social roles in young and middle adulthood could provide important life patterns that contribute significantly to successful aging in later life.

Erikson's generativity stage, once thought to end around age 60, has been shown to have greater significance in later life as well. Research findings of Shmotkin, Blumstein, and Modan (2003) confirm the health benefits of extension of the generativity stage into older adulthood. They found that people ages 75 to 94 years who volunteered in their communities maintained a higher mental functioning and greatly reduced mortality risk when compared with similarly aged nonvolunteers. These findings emphasize the importance of establishing patterns of social participation through the performance of meaningful social roles and occupations throughout young and middle adulthood.

Levinson's Life Transitions

Levinson's (1978) life transitions theory continues to constitute probably the most delineated theoretical description of the main developmental issues concerning adulthood (Coleman & O'Hanlon, 2004). He divides adulthood into three transitional phases, which he called the young, middle, and older adult transitions, each with specific age ranges. This theory is grounded in a longitudinal study with retrospective interviews of 40- to 45-year-old men. The periods in between the transitions represent relatively stable stages within which the structure of life remains constant (Table 8-1).

Levinson integrates earlier theories of Jung and Erikson in organizing the life tasks of each transitional period, using the concept of balancing opposites (Jung, 1914) and suggesting problems to be resolved (Erikson, 1978). Levinson saw life transitions as periods of psychological and social turmoil during which people re-evaluate their life goals and priorities, often choosing opposing goals that necessitate drastic changes in the structure of their lives. For example, a man at midlife may decide he has spent too much time at work and needs to restructure his time to become more family oriented. Sometimes, a new appreciation for his own mortality sends him on radical dieting and fitness routines and other measures to preserve a young self-image. He may decide to divorce his wife, to change careers, or to move to another part of the country; he may embrace the symbols of youth such as driving fast sports cars or dating women much younger than himself. It was Daniel Levinson who first called attention to the term *midlife crisis*, now commonly known by such stereotypical behaviors as described above. Once the changes are made, the man's occupations are reorganized around newly formulated goals and are likely to remain stable until the next transition. Following earlier developmental theorists, Levinson places high importance on an individual's social relationships with significant others, such as a spouse, family members, and mentors (Thomas & Kuh, 1982).

Life tasks are defined by Levinson as crucial problematic issue(s) concerning oneself and the external world (1978). The young adult transition involves the following four life tasks:

1. *Forming a dream.* Children often begin this process through fantasy play. Adolescents prepare to enter the adult world by envisioning the possibilities for what they will be when they grow up. Age 17, the beginning of Levinson's young adult transition, often marks the end of formal schooling and decisions about what to do after graduation. Going on to higher education involves making choices from among the earlier possibilities. Finding ways to define and pursue the dream to make it real becomes the first life task of the young adult transition.

2. *Finding a mentor.* Mentors usually belong to an older generation and have developed expertise and mastery of the ways of the world. Teachers, supervisors, and coworkers are examples of likely mentors. A mentor's role is to guide the young adult through early career paths, helping him or her avoid the pitfalls and encourage continued growth in the occupations of the worker role. In a broader sense, motivation for taking on men-

tor roles might emerge from Erikson's midlife generativity stage. Young adults need a mentor to help facilitate the realization of their dream.

3. *Finding an occupation.* This task is necessary in order to truly separate from parents and achieve financial independence. Going away to college, getting vocational training, or doing internships and apprenticeships may help facilitate living away from home while delaying the young adults' ability to support themselves financially.

4. *Marriage and family.* Getting married and having children may have typically occurred before age 22 at the time of Levinson's study (the 1970s) but often happens much later in today's social environment. This trend points to the influence of the larger social system on an individual's social development.

The midlife transition asks the middle-aged adult to resolve the following opposites, or polarities, as a way to re-evaluate his or her life so far and to make changes in his or her goals and priorities for the second half of life:

1. *Young/old polarity.* Middle adults facing their mortality, often for the first time, need to contemplate the effects of aging on their bodies and their lifestyle. Maybe some have already experienced the early signs of chronic illness or have begun to worry about the long-term effects of life habits, such as smoking, drinking, sleep deprivation, or a sedentary lifestyle. Changes in self-image may need to realign with the reality of aging and its effects on appearance and physical abilities. The occupations of young adulthood, such as athletics, extreme sports, and some work roles, must be reconsidered in light of changes in fitness, endurance, or physical appearance. Coping strategies form the basis for new habits and routines, as well as altered criteria for making occupational choices.

2. *Destruction/creation polarity.* When renovating one's kitchen, the first step would be to demolish the outdated cabinets, appliances, flooring, and even tear down walls (destruction) to make room for the shiny new stainless steel appliances, hardwood floors, beautiful new cabinets, and granite countertops that make up the newly designed kitchen (creation). Symbolically, destruction can be seen when men in young adulthood act aggressively to get ahead in their careers, effectively eliminating anyone or anything who stands in their way. At midlife, an appreciation for traditional ways emerges, along with the need to balance history with progress, combining what is best about the old and the new to form a better, more

integrated present and future. The opposite could also be true—a young adult who has struggled to start a small business or succeed as an artist, actor, or musician may realize at midlife that a more mundane job with a regular paycheck and health care benefits outweighs the importance of expressing oneself creatively.

3. *Masculine/feminine polarity.* Regardless of gender, each person possesses qualities, talents, and skills that are associated with either men or women, and these vary widely from one culture to another. For example, women in American culture may "typically" react more emotionally or interpret social situations more intuitively, while men tend to hide their emotions and take social situations at face value. At midlife, according to Levinson's theory, men begin to explore their more "feminine" natures such as developing more nurturing relationships with their children or taking on more domestic pursuits. Women who have focused on childcare and relationships in younger adulthood may develop more assertive behaviors, enter the workforce, or take on community leadership roles. In general, whichever side of the self lay dormant during young adulthood begins to emerge during the midlife transition.

4. *Attachment/separateness polarity.* This polarity focuses on long-term relationships and assessing the need to redefine them. The process of individuation, or further defining the self as separate from others, continues through each life transition. At midlife, men take note of their career path and the extent to which their work roles have changed their social identity. A man may look at his wife differently and may need to reassess the extent to which his wife supports or detracts from his current social identity. Women at midlife may find themselves less involved with meeting needs of children, and may consider re-entering the workforce or seeking education and/or training for a new career.

In more current writings, Levinson's main concept of "life structure" provides a good perspective for analyzing "how the self is engaged in the world" (Coleman & O'Hanlon, 2004, p. 33). Engagement with others, involvement, and commitment form the central forces for continued development in adulthood. Three elements of life structure include (1) the sociocultural world and its impact on one's opportunities and obstacles; (2) the self, incorporating one's social identity, social roles, and personality; and (3) one's participation in the world through relationships and social participation in families, schools, communities, and the workplace.

The writings of Gould (1978) have confirmed some of Levinson's findings, elaborating on the need for change at midlife by defining four illusions that must be given up: (1) always being the child of one's parents, (2) parents always available to help, (3) the simplified (childlike) view of the world will always be correct, and (4) there is no real death or evil in the world (Gould, 1978). Disillusionment at midlife for women might take the form of a realization that parents cannot continue indefinitely to influence their children or protect them. Levinson later studied adult development for women, following approximately the same sequence of stages as men, but with widely varying life structures, and considering both traditional and antitraditional life roles (Levinson, 1996).

Gilligan's "A Different Voice"

Gilligan (1982) critiques previous developmental theorists as studying only the development of men in adulthood. She looks at attachment as a positive and selfless measure of maturity rather than focusing on separateness and individuation. She summarizes the place of relationships in lifespan development as follows:

> Attachment and separation anchor the cycle of human life, describing the biology of human reproduction and the psychology of human development. The concepts of attachment and separateness that depict the nature and sequence of infant development appear in adolescence as identity and intimacy, and then in adulthood as love and work. (1982, p. 151)

Women (and men) spend much of their lives in intimate and generative relationships, yet self-development has previously taken precedence over relationships. Taking on the viewpoint of the female gender, Gilligan points out that mothering, in many ways similar to Erikson's generativity stage, begins for women at a much younger age, often before the age of 20. *Could it be that women reach this advanced stage of social maturity much younger than men?* In fact, true caring, as depicted in the stage of generativity, may in fact be developed not through individuation at all, as Erikson and Levinson contend, but rather through "the progression of relationships toward a maturity of interdependence" (Gilligan, 1982, p. 153). Gilligan makes a compelling case for the central role of social participation in the development of social maturity in middle adulthood.

Kohlberg and Wilcox: Theories of Moral Development

Lawrence Kohlberg (1973, 1984) developed his theory of moral development by studying how people used concepts to make decisions about right and wrong. The theory is based on the philosophical concept of justice. Kohlberg's principles applying to childhood and adolescence were discussed in previous chapters. As the sequential stages move beyond postconventional cognitive development, their definition becomes more abstract. The adult stages of moral reasoning according to Kohlberg are as follows:

- *Universal ethical principle*—Based on one's moral principles or conscience, such as the greatest good for the greatest number, sometimes in spite of or contrary to the rules or laws; "Doing the right thing" or "the Golden Rule." Moral dilemmas at this level often require adults to look beyond their own social cultural traditions and constructs of reality and to consider more universal human principles such as social justice, fairness, and equality of human rights.

- *Ontological religious approach*—Involves the cosmic and contemplative experience (adapted from Lewis, 2003, p. 12). This level may require a higher level of cognition than most adults achieve because it often involves integration of conflicting ideas and concepts into unified paradigms, a type of postformal thinking described in the next section.

Kohlberg's stages are loosely tied to age, but more so with cognitive development, which may explain why these later stages may not be achieved by many adults (Commons, Richards, & Kuhn, 1982). Wilcox (1979) generally concurs with Kohlberg, but adds to it the dimension of a social and spiritual perspective. She considers the following social factors in her determination of a person's level of moral reasoning: law, value of human life, view of society and community, view of authority, empathetic role taking, and personal meaning. As the occupational therapy profession reconsiders the spiritual context of occupations and their importance in life situations, Wilcox's theory may be worth another look.

Piaget and Beyond in Adult Cognitive Development

Adults are generally believed to have achieved the highest level of Piaget's (1972) formal operations stage of cognitive development by the time they complete their transition from adolescence to young adulthood. According to Piaget's conceptualization, adults apply formal operations in order to adapt to changing life situations, through the subprocesses of assimilation (fitting new information into existing concepts) and accommodation (changing existing knowledge structures to account for new information), in order to maintain a balance between internal needs and the demands of the environment.

Attempts to expand Piaget's view of formal thought have resulted in several theories of adult cognition known as "postformal" thought (Sinnott, 1993). These new "postformal" stages, like Piaget's formal operations, apply equally to problem-solving and decision-making strategies within social, interpersonal, moral, political, and scientific domains (among others). Postformal stages were proposed by adult developmental theorists because they found that Piaget's construct of formal operations failed to explain some of the complex reasoning processes evident in adulthood (Birney & Sternberg, 2006). Theories of postformal thought contribute generally to the field of positive adult development (Commons & Richards, 1999), which examines the ways in which development continues in a positive direction throughout adulthood.

Commons and Richards (1999) proposed a model of hierarchical competency (MHC) to describe the ongoing cognitive development that combines intellectual abilities with motivation and life experience, demonstrating that development continues in a positive trajectory throughout adulthood and well into old age. Evidence for the existence of these stages takes the form of empirical as well as analytical studies and has also been supported by neurological brain research (Bialystok & Craik, 2006). Researchers in various domains agree that postformal reasoning involves at least some of the following: perceiving, reasoning, knowing, judging, caring, feeling, or communicating in ways that are more complex, more all-encompassing than Piaget's formal operations.

Commons and Richards (1999) determined four stages of postformal thought in adulthood by devising a series of tasks and subtasks that required increasing levels of complex reasoning to complete, including both horizontal (classical, factual information) and vertical (hierarchical, organizational, transformational, novel, and creative) complexity. The hierarchy of stages was measured using mathematical axioms, resulting in the following four stages:

1. *Systematic order*—Defining relationships between various parts of a system, including multivariate causes, building matrices or models to describe complex interrelationships that also recognize the unifying structures of the system. An estimated 20% of the population currently function at the systematic order level without support.

2. *Metasystematic order*—Conceptualize entire systems interacting with each other, and describe metasystematic actions that compare, contrast, transform, and synthesize systems and result in metasystems or supersystems. Professors at top research universities might function at the metasystematic level.

3. *Paradigmatic order*—Create new fields from multiple metasystems by comparing, combining, reorganizing, or coordinating very large and seemingly unrelated fields of knowledge. When findings of a research study are inconsistent with existing paradigms, paradigmatic thinkers can modify existing paradigms or create new ones to account for previously unexplained phenomena. Paradigmatic thinkers can best be drawn from the history of science, who have defied traditional theories in order to justify or validate newly defined theoretical systems or paradigms. Einstein (physics) and Euclid (mathematics) are examples.

4. *Cross-paradigmatic order*—Cross-paradigmatic actions integrate paradigms into new fields that profoundly transform some large area of knowledge. Interdisciplinary studies do not fall into this category, however (they are more likely at the paradigmatic order). Very few people have achieved this level of logical thought. One example given is Charles Darwin, who intertwined the fields of biology, paleontology, geology, and ecology to form the field of evolution, an entirely new relationship among paradigms.

The social significance of postformal stages benefits both individuals and society. While most adults never reach the highest orders, everyone has the potential to increase their intellectual ability through lifelong learning, adult educational opportunities, and enriching life experiences. The most salient features of postformal thought—comprehension of the relativistic nature of knowledge, the acceptance of contradiction, and the integration of contradiction into inclusive systems—represent expansions in the degree of complexity of logical thought that develops during adulthood. These advanced cognitive abilities increase the individual's potential for conflict resolution, creative problem solving, taking leadership roles to impact public policy in increasing social and occupational justice, and enacting positive social change.

In occupational therapy, examples of theories that address cognition include Claudia Allen (Allen, Earhart & Blue, 1992) and Joan Toglia (2005), neither of whom focused on the impact of cognition on social participation. However, these theorists do provide a framework for considering potentially higher levels of complexity in solving the more difficult life problems. Some cognitive disabilities only become apparent when clients face challenging problems such as those encountered during adult developmental transitions. Examples might be making decisions about career changes, financial planning, beginning and ending spousal relationships, moving to new locations, and planning ahead for retirement. These developmental tasks require adults to integrate lessons from all of their previous experiences, to reflect, to re-evaluate, and very often to move to higher levels of postformal thinking in order to plan and execute radical changes in their life structure to accommodate changing goals and priorities in their lives. A potential role for occupational therapists might be to assist clients who, in the face of physical or cognitive disability, find themselves unable to resolve these difficult life transitions.

Atchley's Theory of Continuity

Atchley's (1999) view counterbalances the earlier stage theories, proposing that as people age, many established patterns of thinking, activity profiles, living arrangements, and social relationships tend to remain stable over time. These patterns, derived from studies of adult adaptation in middle and older adulthood, become an integral part of the person's self-concept and social and occupational identity. Continuity theory is a feedback systems theory in which adults continue to evolve as they engage in life experiences and use them to evaluate, refine, and revise their behavior patterns, leading those most open to learning to achieve exceptional adaptive ability and resilience. The elements of continuity theory include the following:

- *Internal patterns*—Self-concept, worldview, personal goals, moral framework, beliefs, attitudes, temperament, knowledge, and coping style, which are primarily self-determined.

- *External patterns*—Social roles and relationships, activities, living environments, and lifestyle. "Continuity of relationships preserves the network of social support that is important for creating and maintaining solid concepts of self and lifestyle" (Atchley, 1999, p. 11).

- *Developmental goals*—In Atchley's view, these goals are not predetermined or chosen by the individual, although they are influenced by socialization and culture.

- *Adaptive capacity*—As they evolve, adults have increasingly clear ideas about how to make effective decisions and which developmental pathways most likely lead to life satisfaction for themselves. In adapting to change, adults seek continuity and use established patterns, both internal (optimism, spirituality) and external (family relationships, support networks), as a means of coping.

Continuity theory offers an optimistic view of adult development, proposing that, as people age, they continue to learn from their experiences, leading to ever-increasing intelligence and reasoning ability and building strong foundations for adaptation in later life.

Baltes' Selection and Optimization With Compensation

Paul Baltes began developing his selection and optimization with compensation theory (SOC) in the 1980s in an attempt to unify previous theories of development and aging (Baltes & Baltes, 1990; Baltes, Reese, & Lipsitt, 1980). He reviewed the age and stage theories and determined that they did not account for the impact of social contexts and historical circumstances. His view at that time was called *lifespan development*, which encompassed both ontological (normal development) and biocultural (evolutionary) changes. As a theory of aging, SOC begins at birth. Baltes argues that the infant develops biologically determined milestones within the context of selection of life tasks aimed at growth and development, and this selection continues until the child reaches reproductive maturity. Growth tasks are "selected," contexts "optimized," and tasks not relevant to the overall goal of reproduction set aside, or "compensated" for by others. Throughout life, the adult selects high-priority tasks, optimizes effort and energy toward prioritized goals, and finds ways to compensate for other necessary tasks of life. Young adults, for example, may put major effort and resources into establishing a career and may set aside other tasks such as recreation or volunteering.

Social relationships or attachments play an important role in the SOC balancing process. Division of labor in the home, for example, allows one parent to work while the other maintains the home, raises the children, and maintains social connections with family and friends. When both parents work, compensation might take the form of having children attend day care after school, bringing home take-out dinners, and hiring cleaning services. Priorities change for individuals throughout life, and the occupations they choose to meet their goals serve to refocus their energy. As physical energy declines, rebalancing to continue social participation in one's family and community, or in a valued work role, requires increasing amounts of compensation through the use of social capital and community services for caregiving, transportation, and home maintenance.

Social Roles and Contexts of Adulthood

A role may be defined as a proper or customary function in society, such as the mayor of a town or a father in the family. A psychological definition is the rights, obligations, and expected behavior patterns associated with a particular social status (Reed & Sanderson, 1999). Reilly (1969) introduced role theory in an occupational framework, suggesting that roles and their inherent occupations are learned in the process of socialization. Occupational roles are defined as "life roles that the individual holds in society," such as student, parent, homemaker, employee, volunteer, or retired worker (Pedretti, 1996, p. 3). Creek (2002) defined role as "the set of expectations placed on an individual in a particular social context that become part of his identity and influence his behavior. Each person plays a large number of roles, such as worker, parent, friend" (p. 588). Hagedorn (1997) distinguishes between occupational and social roles. Occupational roles identify the person as a "doer" of specific jobs or tasks, while social roles identify relationships. Thus, while roles and occupations are related concepts, there are some roles that do not necessarily relate to specific occupations.

Reed and Sanderson (1999) caution that roles and their expectations vary with different cultures and must therefore be defined and evaluated within specific social contexts. For example, the role of a lawyer in a business environment is different from one in a private practice setting because of the differences between corporate and community cultures. Culture, as used here, means the manner in which people in an organized group, society, or nation interact with their physical and social environments. Culture is more general than ethnic groups or nationalities. It relates to the many sets of rules, procedures, and customary methods of interaction within a group and is based on shared beliefs, meanings, values, and conventional ways of doing things. In this sense, every group and subgroup to which an individual belongs has its own unique culture and its own unique set of roles and social expectations.

Social and occupational roles serve as one way to organize the many elements of adult social participation. Oakley's Role Checklist (Oakley, Kielhofner, Barris, & Reichler, 1986) lists the following commonly recognized adult roles: student, worker, volunteer, caregiver, home maintainer, friend, family member, religious participant, hobbyist/amateur, participant in organizations, and other. Three categories of social participation are listed in the American Occupational Therapy Association's (AOTA) Framework domains:

(1) *community*, including work, school, neighborhood, and organizations; (2) *family*, including successful interaction in desired family roles; and (3) *peer/friend*, including levels of intimacy and sexual activity (AOTA, 2008). The following subsections sample some of the roles typically played by adults in society, along with suggested connections to the occupations or tasks that accompany them. By the order of presentation in this text, it should not be presumed that any specific role holds more importance than any other.

Social Participation in Work Environments: Worker Roles and Contexts

Most adults place a high priority on paid work roles and often connect work-related occupations with identity. Studies show that work norms, also called work ethic, probably due to social pressure, produce a powerful influence over most adults to continue to live off one's own income. In regions where the social norm to work is high, unemployment rates remain low, and people out of work return sooner, avoiding at all costs the need to accept welfare benefits (Stutzer & Lalive, 2004). People with internalized social norms to work have significantly lower life satisfaction when unemployed, rendering them less desirable companions and reducing their enjoyment of leisure activities, which tend to be mainly social (Frey & Stutzer, 2002).

Every work environment has its own unique culture. Within it, there is usually a power structure and organization that defines varying levels of authority and different roles or job titles. For example, a university has a president, several vice presidents, deans of different schools or subdivisions, department chairs of different academic programs, and faculty members. Each role has a job description, a list of educational and experiential requirements, and a set of duties and responsibilities. Status within the university is expressed through ranking systems such as instructor, assistant professor, associate professor, and full professor. Longevity in the university culture is valued and rewarded by the granting of tenure. However, other scholarly achievements also play a part in promotion and tenure, such as the performance of research and publication, evidence of excellence in teaching, and voluntary work on interdisciplinary committees or the community.

As such, occupations are linked to work roles, and collectively their performances become a part of the overall function of the organization. Therefore, occupational performance of an individual within the organization provides a basis for value and compensation and may allow the individual to rise in status based on meeting or exceeding social expectations of the work role.

The organization of a grocery store might look quite different from that of a university. In a retail store, a general manager presides over various subdivisions of the store: purchasing, sales, customer relations, human resources, maintenance, and security. Each subdivision probably has a department head or supervisor, and depending on the hours of operation, there may be separate divisions for different shifts. Again, each role has a job description, along with specific skill and experience requirements. Unlike a university, longevity may not be valued, and innovation and creativity may be discouraged rather than rewarded. Productivity, a euphemism for getting the most work from the fewest employees for the least cost, is highly valued by companies that have something to sell and that seek the highest profit possible.

Roles in any work environment may be broken down into three categories: bosses or supervisors, workers or employees, and customers or clients. Each of these roles has culture-specific social expectations. Some general expectations, occupations, or tasks of these work roles are summarized here.

What are some social expectations of a boss or supervisor?

- *Leading*—Giving guidance to workers with regard to the tasks and overall objectives
- *Setting limits*—Making sure rules and procedures are followed, and taking action to correct infractions through disciplinary action or termination of workers
- *Solving problems*—Settling differences when co-workers disagree or fail to cooperate
- *Expediting*—Planning time, materials, and manpower as needed to meet the overall goals
- *Providing incentives*—Setting up work environments that encourage employees to work to their full potential, team building, morale
- *Providing a safe environment*—Minimizing stress, preventing physical danger or liability of workers, adapting to special needs of employees
- Hiring and providing training for new workers as needed; firing and replacing workers who do not live up to expectations
- Avoiding abuse of power in leadership role

What are some social expectations of a worker?

- Arriving and leaving work site on time

- Performing occupations required in one's job description

- Applying skills in a productive and efficient manner

- Appropriately dressing and grooming for work role

- Following rules, procedures, and safety precautions set forth by supervisor/company

- Accepting feedback and guidance, and making positive changes when needed

- Keeping a positive attitude, treating others with courtesy and respect

- Being a team player, cooperating with coworkers, doing one's share of the workload

What are social expectations of customers or clients?

- Clearly communicate the goods or services they need

- Pay for goods or services as required

- Understand and accept the terms and conditions of transactions

- Respect the boundaries of the business relationship

All of these social expectations must be interpreted and adapted when applied in specific work situations. For example, when a client visits a doctor's office, expectations are different from those of a customer in a department store. Work settings come in all shapes and sizes, with varying levels of management and requirements for workers. Role competence for the purposes of designing and evaluating occupational therapy interventions is defined as "the ability to effectively meet the demand of roles in which the client engages" (AOTA, 2008, p. 651). Occupational therapists may need to assist clients in meeting the social expectations of many different work environments. Teachers may be concerned with the preparation and training of students for a wide variety of worker roles and contexts.

Social participation at work has also been addressed by the *International Classification of Functioning, Disability, and Health* (World Health Organizaton [WHO], 2001). It offers the following categories: apprenticeship or preparation, seeking and acquiring a job, maintaining and terminating employment, remuneration or earning a living, and volunteering.

Social Participation in the Home Environment: Roles and Contexts

Anyone can easily identify at least 10 roles that occur in the home environment. Some of them tend to be gender specific, such as wife, mother, daughter, sister, aunt, niece, grandmother, and conversely, husband, father, son, brother, uncle, nephew, grandfather. Obviously, home situations and contexts vary widely with culture. There may be blended families with stepparents and stepchildren, half-brothers or half-sisters. Well-to-do families may include household workers, such as housekeepers, gardeners, cooks, and butlers, or live-in caregivers such as nannies or health caregivers for the elderly. Inner-city families may include aunts, uncles, grandparents, and cousins as well as mothers, fathers, and children. Single-parent households have become commonplace at all income levels in the United States and abroad. The social expectations for each of these roles varies widely and should never be assumed or stereotyped by therapists or educators.

Some family roles have been studied more than others. The following roles are selected as perhaps the most universal and thus serve as examples. Even the norms listed here will vary with different cultures. *What might be some examples of this for a spouse? A mother? A father?* As a learning exercise, try filling in the blanks for other family roles in Table 8-2.

Intimate Partner

As couples who have been married for many years will attest, marriage takes work. Sustaining positive feelings of connection through hard times can be an uphill battle, but one definitely worth the struggle. Volumes have already been written about what makes a marriage or sexual partnership last, keeping romance alive, offering kindness, caring, and physical comfort, and many other attributes. One such book, titled *The Love Dare,* offers a 40-day spiritual prescription for reviving love relationships (Kendrick & Kendrick, 2008) and is now also a movie titled "Fireproof."

Ross (2009) recently wrote about her experiences as an occupational therapist in home care, during which she encountered both positive and negative relationships among disabled clients and their spousal caregivers. She writes,

> Quite often marital discord was the undercurrent of my home visits. It was like a pile of overlooked or hidden agendas, and it definitely hindered progress... Unlike the circumstances of (other clients) where the sweetness of family strength and support were evident... illness for these couples exacerbated an already unpleasant situation. (p. 90)

Table 8-2		
SOCIAL EXPECTATIONS FOR TRADITIONAL AND NONTRADITIONAL FAMILY ROLES		
ROLE TITLES	SOCIAL EXPECTATIONS FOR BEHAVIORS WITHIN YOUR CULTURE	GIVE A SPECIFIC EXAMPLE OF HOW A PERSON HOLDING THIS POSITION WITHIN YOUR FAMILY INTERACTS WITH YOU
Stepmother or stepfather		
Grandparent		
Aunt		
Uncle		
Brother		
Sister		
Cousin		

She laments, "I believed I was unqualified to explore or analyze those relationships. Nothing in my schooling and little in the literature related to an occupational therapist's role in such circumstances" (Ross, 2009, p. 90). This experience highlights the need to include social participation in the professional education of occupational therapists among others, so that at least basic communication skills such as active listening, expression of empathy, and conflict resolution strategies might be incorporated into the home care interventions for clients who need to repair troubled marital relationships that affect caregiving and recovery from illness.

In evaluating one's relationship, it may be helpful to review the basic expectations for one's mate, although this varies widely among cultures and even among couples from similar cultures. Couples participate in social activities together and share the responsibility for establishing a lifestyle that allows them to maintain financial independence.

What are some social expectations for a spouse?

- Treat each other with love, caring, and respect
- Meet one another's sexual needs and need for affection
- Share the responsibilities of maintaining a household

- Communicate openly and solve one another's problems together
- Maintain loyalty and refrain from participating in extra-marital sexual relationships

Intimate relationships are highly private, and there is a tendency among professionals to avoid discussing them without an invitation to do so. Yet, there is no doubt their quality has significant consequences for all others who interact with the couple, either together or separately.

Sexual Participation

Sexuality, as a form of intimacy in dyadic relationships, is associated with happiness and overall well-being. Researchers have even found frequency and enjoyment of sexual intercourse to be a significant predictor of longevity (Nusbaum & Hamilton, 2002). Particularly for clients with physical disabilities, sexual participation should be an important part of occupational therapy evaluation and intervention (Santoro, Sobocinski, & Klippel-Tancreti, 2008). Therapists need to become more comfortable with opening a discussion with clients who wish to engage in sexual expression within their loving relationships. A surprising number of health conditions affect a person's sexuality, including spinal cord injury, head injury, cancer, multiple sclerosis, heart

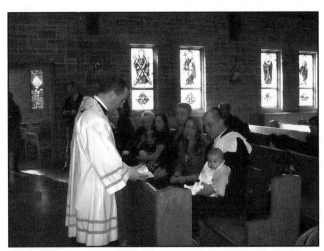

Figure 8-1. Family roles and contexts: Baptism marks a new beginning.

disease, stroke, and joint replacement. Educating clients about adaptive sexual positioning, as well as optimization and/or compensation for sensory, cognitive, fatigue, and pain issues can prevent injury and hasten recovery of this critical aspect of social participation and well-being (Vaughn, 2009).

Equally important to sexual participation is perceived body image, a concern that dramatically affects many aspects of social participation in dyadic relationships. Sexuality needs to be assessed by occupational therapists along with other activities of daily living (Vaughn, 2009). Intervention includes a dynamic problem-solving process with clients and their partners to overcome barriers, such as ways to conceal perceived disfigurements; experimenting with sexual positioning; and adapting contextual factors such as lighting, bedding, music, and timing, in order to enable more satisfying sexual participation.

Parenting Roles

As noted in the previous chapter on adolescence, parents (especially mothers) have been found to have a major influence upon their children's self-identity, values, and eventual social participation and leadership as adults in the larger social world (Ng, Ho, & Ho, 2008). While parenting is not a specific domain in the *Occupational Therapy Practice Framework*, "child rearing" is embedded in the description of instrumental activities of daily living (AOTA, 2008, p. 631). The ICF describes the parent-child relationship as

> Becoming and being a parent, both natural and adoptive, such as by having a child and relating to it as a parent or creating and maintaining a parental relationship with an adoptive child and providing physical, intellectual, and emotional nurture to one's natural or adoptive child. (WHO, 2001, p. 162)

For parents of young children, the occupational connection with this social role is clearest as the child needs physical caring—feeding, bathing, dressing, diaper changing, as well as engagement in play and learning activities with parents. However, emotional connection and social support for the child's growing needs can have even greater importance as the child learns to interact with others in the social world (Figure 8-1). Some guidance and discipline roles for parents have already been discussed in Chapter 1 in the section on family leadership.

As children move toward independence, parenting changes from one of total care toward a role of guidance and supervision. Simpson (2001) has summarized hundreds of research studies on the topic of parenting adolescents. She has posted a report on the Harvard School of Public Health Web site (www.hsph.harvard.edu/chc/parenting) to alert media, policy makers, and parents themselves about the role of parenting in addressing the many social and health risks teens face in our society, such as violence, abuse, mental illness, neglect, substance abuse, inadequate education, and sexually transmitted diseases. The bottom line is that parents who provide the following five specific types of guidance and supervision can play a major role in prevention for their teenagers.

1. *Love and connect*—Parents find ways to continue caring relationships and open communication with their teens while accommodating and affirming the teen's increasing maturity. Contrary to popular opinion, debate and conflict do not generally compromise underlying attachment. Parents are advised to support teens with warmth, interest, and respect while allowing differences of opinion and increased autonomy.

2. *Monitor and observe*—Parents remain aware of all teen activities including school performance, work, after-school activities, recreation, peer and adult relationships, and especially their internet relationships through direct communication and indirect observation. Involvement with other adults who interact with teens, such as teachers, coaches, recreation activity leaders, and other parents is a vital part of responsible parenting. Research shows that teens who communicate with their parents about their homework get better grades and exhibit fewer behavior problems in school (Garbarino, 1999; Miller, 1998; United States Department of Health and Human Services, 1997). Knowing after-school whereabouts is the best preventive strategy because the most common cause of mortality in teen years comes from the environment (accidents, violence). Parental communication about where teens spend time is

associated with lower rates of drug and alcohol use, teen pregnancy, delinquency, and reduced susceptibility to negative peer pressure.

3. *Guide and limit*—Teens need parents to uphold a clear but evolving set of boundaries, maintaining important family rules and values, but also encouraging increased competence and maturity. Parents continue to set moral and social rules and expectations for school, part-time work, chores at home, and other occupational areas (Gray & Steinberg, 1999). Research suggests avoiding forms of punishment that do physical or emotional harm (Eberly & Montemayor, 1999). Alternately, parents can use teaching through assignment of specific "punishment" experiences that fit the "crime" such as visiting a hospital where victims of drunk driving are treated if a teen has abused alcohol (or, better yet, volunteering there). It is often best to choose battles when it comes to punishment, letting minor infractions slide and focusing on the most important life lessons.

4. *Model and consult*—Parents provide ongoing information and support around decision making, values, skills, goals, and interpreting and navigating the larger world. Lessons learned by example have a more powerful impact; therefore, when safety is not a factor, parents should consider allowing teens to learn from their own mistakes or the mistakes of others known to them, always communicating and discussing the issues to encourage the reasoning process. Strategies for good decision making that are supported by research are further discussed in Chapter 14.

5. *Provide and advocate*—Parents continue to make available adequate nutrition, clothing, shelter, health care, and a supportive home environment with a network of caring adults. Simpson (2001) points out that barriers such as poverty, overwork, unemployment, and homelessness make this step more challenging. When unable to provide for basic necessities, teens need parents to provide "social capital"—that is, relationships within the community that supplement what the family can provide in the way of resources, guidance, training, and support. This function, also called advocacy, family management, sponsorship, or community bridging in the literature, has been observed in parenting across cultures and socioeconomic groups (Furstenberg, Cook, Eccles, Elder, & Smeroff, 1999; Myers-Walls, 1999; Smith, Cudaback, Goddard, & Meyers-Walls, 1994).

Couples new to parenting may find it helpful to review the social norms for the roles of mother and father that conform to their own culture. Examples of traditional social expectations are listed below.

What are some traditional social expectations for a mother?

- Meet the physical and emotional needs of children, including feeding them, keeping them clothed and clean, and responding to their need for comfort and love
- Taking care of health needs of children as needed
- Safeguarding the home environment to allow children limited freedom to move and play within defined spaces and under supervision
- Provide appropriate stimulation for children as they grow and develop, including toys, books, play and learning experiences with other children, and exposure to limited community and social situations
- Provide and maintain consistent routines for nutrition, cleanliness, maintenance of health, help with homework, social and solitary activity, periods of rest and sleep
- Apply appropriate discipline for children to help them learn the rules of life
- Shop, cook, do laundry, clean, and otherwise maintain a pleasant home environment

What are some traditional social expectations of a father?

- Supporting the family economically, paying the bills
- Supporting mother by participating in teaching and disciplining children as needed
- Maintaining order, discipline, and respect within the household
- Providing enrichment experiences for children, such as vacations, sports, or weekend entertainment activities
- Assisting with, encouraging, and checking on homework
- Involving children in maintenance of the home and yard as appropriate
- Making decisions, with input from family, to do what is best for all
- Protect children from inappropriate dangers, violence, sexuality, or other upsetting situations for which they are not emotionally prepared or mature enough to handle

In real life, perhaps there is no such thing as a "traditional" parent, as these roles vary widely by culture and individual. When working with clients who are parents, occupational therapists need to discuss their perceptions of what is expected of a parent and together make a list of preferred parental tasks so that interventions can focus on these specific abilities.

Facilitating the Transition to Adulthood

For many, parenting does not just stop when an adolescent graduates from high school. Parents may also need to help teens with their transition to adulthood. As they graduate from high school, teens' stress levels increase along with the need to make sometimes difficult choices about the next phase of their lives. While legal adulthood begins at age 18, few at that age in the United States are ready for financial independence. Some will go on to college or vocational school, while others continue their after-school jobs or find other low-paying jobs locally. Some teens get married, get their own living quarters, and begin families right after high school, but this move all but guarantees an uphill financial battle. More commonly, new graduates continue living with their parents while beginning their careers, continuing their studies, or just trying to figure out what to do next. Whether high school or college graduates, when postadolescents continue living with parents and "riding the gravy train," Asher (2008) suggests the following five-step plan:

- *Step 1:* Invest in the transition—Agree to pay for interview clothing and purchase or lend him or her a reliable car to drive to job sites; encourage the graduate to use available career services to develop a resumé and build job-seeking skills; find ways to make telephone and computer internet services available for searching and for communicating with potential employers.

- *Step 2:* Let him or her pursue real interests—Be open-minded about what kind of job your teen prefers, but also emphasize the need to support him- or herself at a reasonable level.

- *Step 3:* Require planning, activity, and reporting—In return for your financial help in Step 1, set some ground rules for daily tasks and structure. For example, your expectation is that he or she apply for five jobs each week. Even when unsuccessful in getting interviews, teens can participate in social networking activities, such as having lunch with friends who are employed or doing temporary jobs for friends and neighbors. Be sure to ask for a weekly progress report.

- *Step 4:* Volunteer—When the search goes on for more than 30 days, switch to volunteering 10 to 20 hours a week on a regular basis. The job search can continue while the teen gets some practice in "showing up on time and meeting the needs of others" (Asher, 2008, p. 45).

- *Step 5:* Set a deadline for the "end of the gravy train"—To prevent a full retreat from adult life, set a date after which you will require him or her to pay rent. A good guideline is 60 to 90 days. If a steady source of income is not found by the deadline, use a graduated payment schedule, such as $100 the first month, $200 the second, etc. That kind of money can easily be earned doing odd jobs, mowing lawns, etc.

Much has been written and studied about responsible parenting. Perhaps because norms vary widely with the many subcultures that exist in society, parenting skills are not taught in schools. It becomes the responsibility of parents to teach their children by example about how to be good parents. More about parenting skills training and approaches for problem behaviors will be covered in Chapter 14.

Extended Family Roles

The movie "The Godfather" and the television series "The Sopranos" serve as two examples of the extent to which families care and provide for each other. At the least, they celebrate together at holidays, birthdays, anniversaries, christenings, weddings, and wakes, often traveling for miles to attend these events (Figure 8-2). The helping hand sometimes extends to offering financial support to nieces, nephews, cousins, even distant relatives who

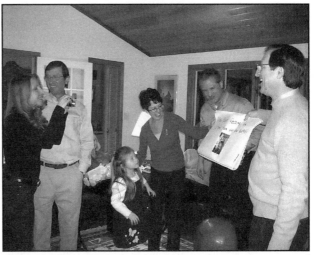

Figure 8-2. Birthday "roast" demonstrates how acceptance and belonging within the extended family group allows members to laugh at themselves and each other.

need a down payment for a home, tuition for a college education, or start-up money for a new business endeavor. Well-off members look first to relatives when hiring employees for their family business. Less fortunate parents look to well-connected relatives for help, such as getting sons and daughters accepted into choice educational institutions or finding them jobs when they graduate.

Families within many different cultures have similar interactions and expectations. Throughout adulthood, they provide each other with a sense of belonging, social support, and the security of knowing they can count on family in times of misfortune or adversity.

Genealogy, the study of one's ancestry, enjoys renewed popularity as the internet facilitates the search for lost relatives across the globe. New family Web sites appear daily, featuring family photo sharing, e-mail databases, and group calendaring—a listing of birthdays, anniversaries, and notices of family gatherings or reunions (Bhargava, 2007). An interesting variation is "zygotic social networking" (Wollan, 2007), in which family trees are formed online on the basis of a DNA test. For example, Genetree.com and Ancestry.com both begin with cheek swab DNA tests costing $100 to $200, followed by the opportunity to "build jumbo kinship networks" in cyberspace (Wollan, 2007, p. 1). Chung (2007) predicts that the internet is transforming the way families communicate, adding the visual dimension in which moving pictures would be dominant, moving the world one step closer to an "iconic society" (p. 2). This prediction applies to other social networks as well, citing the likely changes in social and cultural norms resulting from the explosion of online communities that enable people to meet each other in cyberspace, help and support one another, and build close relationships and restore common ties that bind people and strengthen human relationships (Chung, 2007).

Community Roles and Contexts

In addition to worker and student roles, other roles outside the home are that of friend, recreation/leisure participant, volunteer, advocate, and other community service roles. Each of these has its own set of social norms and expectations, as well as regional and cultural variations.

Friendship

Many adult friendships begin in childhood or adolescence, when peer relationships play a primary role in the development of social identity. Social identity refers to the way a person wishes to be viewed by others both inside and outside one's immediate social group. A person's primary social identity might relate to religion (a good Christian), ethnic group (Italian "piasano"), occupation (doctor, senator, soldier), social role (a good mother or friend), or other social group member (fraternity, democratic party, etc). Which of these is a priority for a given individual varies widely and may shift with maturity, changing circumstances, or advancing age. Friendships develop most easily between individuals who have a similar social identity, and "we become best friends with people who boost our self-esteem by affirming our identities as members of certain groups" (Weisz & Wood, 2005, in Karbo, 2008, p. 94).

What are some expectations of a friend?

- Crossing paths regularly and having things in common.

- Keeping up contact and communication.

- Emotional expressiveness and self-disclosure.

- Listening and unconditional support and acceptance.

- Loyalty and trust—Keeping promises and confidential information private.

- Reciprocity is key—Giving and taking, talking and listening, exchanging gifts or invitations, sharing burdens, and celebrating accomplishments with each other

According to Fehr (1995), "once a friendship is established through self-disclosure and reciprocity, the glue that holds it together is intimacy" (in Karbo, 2008, p. 93). In same-sex friendships, intimacy refers to a feeling of closeness and connection that comes from a history of responsiveness and an expectation of support and caring that can remain even over miles and years of separation. Overall contact (frequency of communication/interaction), closeness (extent of self-disclosure and emotional expression), and supportiveness (both honesty and being positive) predict whether a friendship is maintained (Karbo, 2008; Oswald, Clark, & Kelly, 2004) (Figures 8-3 and 8-4).

Groups of friends often function as social support groups for members with similar challenges and goals. For example, a group of five women coworkers with a desire to lose weight formed a "dieter's sisterhood" in their workplace, providing each other with low-calorie lunches, identifying junk-food-free work zones, exercising or walking together, and swapping other strategies to keep weight off. Together, they lost 100 pounds in 6 months (Eberlein, 2004). Another group formed online is "Raising Grandchildren," accessed by grandparents who found themselves "juggling preschool play dates and retirement planning," many

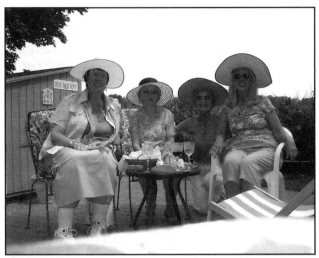

Figure 8-3. Friends gather for annual reunions each August for more than 25 years.

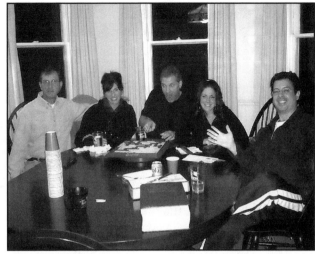

Figure 8-4. Fierce competition over a Scrabble game during an annual family retreat.

of whom met face-to-face at a campground in North Carolina (Eberlein, 2004, p. 65). With more than 6% of children under 18 in the United States living in grandparent-headed households, grandparents in this role often feel isolated from non-child-rearing peers and could use some help in connecting with one another in communities as well as online.

Social Participation in Leisure Occupations

Leisure occupations, defined by AOTA (2008) as nonobligatory activities that are intrinsically motivated, often involve some form of group interaction within community settings. For example, social participation in sports varies with the type and level of the sport, as well as the rules of the game. Playing golf, for example, can be a solitary occupation, but most golf courses require that players move together in groups of two, three, or four. If a solitary player shows up, he or she is matched up with a group before teeing off. Looking at a group of golfers as a social context, it is no surprise that the inexperienced members face high social pressure to keep pace, while the more skilled members need patience and self-discipline. For larger team sports, such as basketball, football, or soccer, it is not enough to possess good physical skills and knowledge of the rules of play. These recreational occupations require skills in team playing, cooperating with one another on the court or field for the benefit of the group as a whole. The metaphor of the team transfers to other aspects of life, such as community service, volunteer, and work settings where a similar form of cooperation is required for successful social participation.

Leisure activities provide many benefits for the adult social participant, including relief from stress, physical and mental exercise, and the freedom to

pursue one's interests and talents outside the context of work. For example, managers and their workers at an Exxon Mobil Oil Refinery are encouraged to participate in an annual city marathon, a pursuit that requires months of physical training. These employees spend many mornings and evenings running around their neighborhoods or working out in local gyms, preparing for the big event. Running provides needed physical exercise to otherwise sedentary workdays and facilitates camaraderie among coworkers at the water cooler, discussing the details of healthier diets and other fitness strategies.

Like other occupations in life, leisure pursuits become a part of each person's personal and social identity. Working can be boring or repetitive, but leisure activities are freely chosen because they provide pleasure, creative expression, and a sense of accomplishment to participants. Bundy (2001) proposed four factors present in any leisure experience: control by the individual, degree of motivation to take part, freedom from constraints of reality, and absorption in the task itself. As such, leisure activities rise above mere time use and become aligned with the person's spiritual dimension, the experience of meaning. Individuals can choose any task as a leisure activity—cooking, gardening, playing a musical instrument, collecting coins, learning to speak Japanese, or fixing up old cars—whatever motivates them or makes them happy. Some leisure activities are performed alone, while others occur within groups, classes, workshops, or other social contexts. Eventually, leisure activities pursued over time become a part of each person's identity and are acknowledged by others as important aspects of the person's social identity.

Volunteering and Civic Engagement

Volunteering is either formal (through community organizations) or informal (carpooling kids, exchanging caregiving) unpaid work. Contrary to popular beliefs, working adults volunteer more often than those who are retired. According to the US Bureau of Labor Statistics (2004), people ages 35 to 44 years are most likely (34.2%) to volunteer, followed closely by ages 45 to 54 (32.8%). In today's tight job market, some unemployed adults use volunteering as a way to acquire job skills, to enter business establishments that may potentially employ them, and to build social networks that may help them get hired. Professional or work-related organizations comprise another category of volunteering, such as joining a committee, taking a position on the board, or making a presentation at a conference. Participation in organizations related to one's work may be a requirement as well as an advantage for career advancement. Listing volunteer jobs can improve one's resumé and counts as experience on a job application.

Many young parents find themselves volunteering on behalf of their children, taking roles such as coaching peewee football or little league baseball, teaching children's religious classes, or leading a Boy Scout or Girl Scout troop.

Citizenship and Advocacy Roles

In the 2008 election, many United States citizens across the lifespan voted for the first time, a trend that will hopefully continue in the years to come. Participation in government varies widely among the nation's citizens and includes, at a minimum, reading about local politics, keeping informed and taking a stand on the issues affecting one's neighborhood and town, or at the opposite extreme, participating in state and national election campaigns or running for some level of public office oneself. Many adults become so absorbed in their own work and family life that they do not pay much attention to the multiple opportunities to participate in government at any level. It is not until people run up against legal or systems issues affecting them personally that they realize the importance of understanding the prevailing public policy and of making their voices heard.

Because of the current economic downturn, public policy with regard to housing, taxes, unemployment, disability income, medical insurance or coverage, investment, debt collection, and the availability of credit take on renewed importance. Additionally, there are many public services available to people facing economic or social difficulties, such as transportation, recreation, education, environmental protection, and public health. The following questions test your awareness of public policy in your own local area that relate to social participation and well-being:

- How can you learn about local candidates for your town's government in order to make a good decision when voting?

- What sources of income would be available to you if you lost your job?

- What steps can you take in your town to recycle unwanted electronics or batteries, cans, bottles, and paper and dispose of broken appliances or leftover building materials?

- What services does your town offer for trash collection and disposal of leaves, branches, and organic waste? What about toxic waste (batteries, petroleum products, old computers)?

- When caring for an older adult in your home, what health care services are available, and how much will they cost?

- If you have been involved in an auto accident and have received a ticket or fine that you believe is unfair, what recourses do you have to challenge an unfair accusation?

- If you find a stray dog living under your front porch, digging up your flowers and growling at your visitors, what can you do to find its owner or have it removed?

- If you have a good idea about how to solve a social problem, or if you have a complaint about being treated unfairly, what steps could you take to change existing policy? Which elected officials represent your interests, and how could you contact them?

- When state legislatures are in session they often hold public hearings in order to better understand the perspectives of consumers, and various stakeholders, with regard to a proposed law or amendment to existing policy. How can you learn about and participate in a public hearing in your state?

These questions barely begin to address the many ways in which public policy and government affect everyone. People who do not vote and do not take the time to become informed about public issues affecting them give up some of the fundamental rights they have as U.S. citizens.

Advocacy for ourselves and our families and friends will be an increasingly important adult role as government regulation becomes involved in many areas of our adult lives. For example, how do we present ourselves during medical and dental appointments? Advocacy means not blindly accepting what doctors and dentists offer, but also asking questions, requesting second opinions, and becoming informed about the state of current research, especially when facing serious health consequences. In being one's own advocate, professionals offer not only services, but advice and information based on their expertise. In today's society, many options need to be considered in safeguarding one's own health and well-being. For professionals such as occupational therapists, enabling clients to advocate for themselves and their loved ones might be the modern-day equivalent of the Chinese Proverb: "teaching them to fish" so they can "eat for a lifetime."

Learning Activity

All in a Day's Work

Do you believe that busy people get more done than others? Find out by interviewing the busiest adult you know. First, do a daily occupation analysis; ask the person to account for every hour during a busy day. Then, identify some categories—at least three—and color code them. For example, underline work tasks in blue, leisure activities in red, and self-care activities in green. Then, ask the person to consider the social aspects of daily activities. Circle all of the daily activities that involved another person.

Morning/Afternoon	*Evening/Night*
6 am	**6 pm**
7 am	**7 pm**
8 am	**8 pm**
9 am	**9 pm**
10 am	**10 pm**
11 am	**11 pm**
12 pm	**12 am**
1 pm	**1 am**
2 pm	**2 am**
3 pm	**3 am**
4 pm	**4 am**
5 pm	**5 am**

Discussion

1. What percentage of the person's time is spent in each of the categories identified?

2. What percentage of the person's time has a social component?

3. Consider how balanced this person's day is between work, leisure, self-care, and social versus isolated activities.

4. How does your interviewee feel about spending time this way? What changes would he or she wish to make? Why?

5. What can you learn from a busy person about how to use your time more effectively?

6. How does socialization, or interaction with others, facilitate or create barriers to meeting one's daily goals?

Script: Family Therapy Session With a Rebellious Teen

Seating Chart

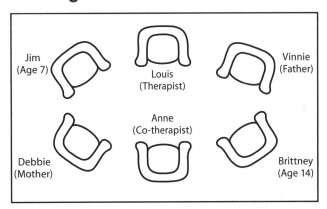

Characters and Situation Overview

This family has come together for marriage and family therapy because their daughter, Brittney, exhibits rebellious behavior and will not listen to her parents. Brittney's academic performance has declined since she began dating Mike (age 22) of whom both parents strongly disapprove. Jim, her younger brother, has twice tried to run away from home (once to a friend's house and once to his grandparents' house).

Brittney: (age 14) A high school freshman who has an older boyfriend, Mike, who works as an auto mechanic and drives a Harley Davidson motorcycle.

Vinnie: (age 45) An Italian Catholic, works as a college professor, married Debbie 8 years ago, and is the father of Jim (age 7) and Brett (age 4) and stepfather of Brittney. He loves Brittney like his own daughter and feels protective of her. It upsets him that Brittney no longer listens to him or obeys his rules.

Debbie: (age 43) Works part-time as a social worker. She comes from a strict Italian Catholic upbringing and wants to instill strong religious values in all of her children. She and Vinnie agree on these values but disagree about how to enforce them with Brittney. She worries that Brittney's rebellious behavior is having a negative influence on her younger brothers.

Jim: (age 7) A normally cheerful and obedient second grader who feels upset because of all the arguing at home; he has been neglected by his parents and abandoned by his older sister who has helped to care for him since birth.

Louis: (age 55) A psychologist specializing in marriage and family therapy in private practice.

Anne: (age 54) An occupational therapist with a master's degree in marriage and family therapy.

Two others not present at this meeting are Brett (age 4) and Roger (age 48), Debbie's ex-husband and Brittney's biological father, a stone mason by trade, who lives a carefree, single life and refuses to take on any responsibility for disciplining his daughter.

Action Begins Here

Louis: I'm impressed that you all got here with your busy schedules. That's a very positive sign.

Vinnie: Well, almost all. Debbie's mother is watching Brett, our toddler.

Anne: He is a bit young to sit through an hour session. Maybe we'll meet him another time.

Louis: What brings you to therapy today? *(pause, Debbie and Vinnie exchange looks)*

Debbie: I set up the appointment, so I'll start. We're having some issues with Brittney, and, as you said when we spoke over the phone, it would be helpful to hear from all the family members about how it's affecting our family.

Brittney: *(looking sullen)* How is this my problem? Jimmy ran away twice.

Louis: *(gently)* Hold on a minute, Brittney. You'll get a turn to talk in just a minute.

Debbie: *(continuing)* When I was Brittney's age, my father handled the discipline. When he grounded my sister and me, we stayed home. But when Vinnie tries to ground her, she argues back and disobeys him.

Vinnie: I love her like my own daughter. We used to be close, but when she turned 13, everything changed.

Brittney: You don't listen any more. You're too busy accusing me and calling my boyfriend names. He's not a "hell's angel" or a "grease monkey." You're not my real father, anyway. Why should I do what you say?

Debbie: Because he is the head of this family, and you live with us, not with Roger.

Louis: How often does Roger see Brittney?

Brittney: Not often enough. He treats me like a grown up. He lets me have fun. Not like you *(glares at Debbie).*

Debbie: About once a month, he'll take Brittney for a weekend, and they'll go to Six Flags or to a concert or a movie. It's true that he's the fun parent. He doesn't realize that a father isn't the same thing as a friend—discipline is part of being a parent, too.

Louis: Brittney, how do you see this problem?

Brittney: Mom and Dad don't realize I'm growing up. They still treat me like a little kid. But, I'm in high school. All my friends have boyfriends, and they go out on dates. Mom started dating my real dad when she was my age, and she got married right after high school. My dad was older than her. So why can't I have an older boyfriend? They don't even know Mike. He's really a great guy, and he makes me feel special. *(Vinnie shakes his head in desperation, and Debbie looks worried)* See, they won't listen.

Debbie: It's not that I won't listen, Brittney. I made a mistake to date an older boy in high school. I shouldn't have gotten married so young. It didn't work out very well, that's why Roger and I got divorced. I don't want to see you making the same mistakes I did.

Brittney: *(makes eye contact with Mom and appears to consider this idea)* Yeah, well....

Anne: Before we go on, let's give Jim a chance to speak. What do you think about what's going on at home?

Jim: Well, I don't like it when dad and my sister argue. They get really loud and slam doors, and then Brittney leaves on the motorcycle and doesn't come back until after I'm asleep.

Brittney: You're such a little tattle tale. What about when you went to Grandma's?

Jim: What do you care? You probably didn't even notice I was gone! *(wipes tears)*

Anne: Do you miss your sister when she leaves?

Jim: *(he nods, Debbie reaches over and rubs Jim's shoulder; he regains control)*

Anne: What happened that made you want to run away, Jimmy?

Jim: *(looks to Debbie for direction, she nods.)* Brittney wanted to leave right before dinner, and Daddy told her she had to stay and have dinner with the family. They were both shouting at each other, and I ran outside to tell them to stop...and *(sobs)...*

Louis: When and where did this happen?

Vinnie: Last weekend, Friday night, I think. Yes, because I had just pulled into the driveway, and Brittney comes out the door, all decked out in her skimpy top—I hate the way she dresses with her tummy bare....

Brittney: Everyone dresses like that. See, Mom, he doesn't listen.

Anne: Before we go there, let's hear Jim's side of the story. Jim, so your sister and your dad were arguing outside in the driveway, and you ran out. Then what happened?

Jim: I told them to stop, but they didn't. Brittney just told me to shut up *(more tears)*. And Daddy ordered me to get back into the house. Then I heard the motorcycle, and she went away again. Daddy's real mad, and he comes in still shouting. I figured he's mad at me, too. So I went into the garage, got on my bike, and rode to Grandma's.

Debbie: You see what I mean, Brittney? Jimmy sees you get away with it, and he thinks he can leave, too. But he's only 7.

Louis: How far away does Grandma live?

Vinnie: It's a 15-minute drive. I didn't think Jimmy even knew the way. It must have taken him an hour… and he didn't tell anyone where he was going. We called all his friends in the neighborhood, Billy Evans, the neighbor kid where he went last time.

Anne: He's done this before? Run away?

Debbie: A few months ago, he ran down the street to his friend's house and didn't tell us. But, Mrs. Evans suspected something and called us. We let him stay the night with Billy until everyone calmed down.

Vinnie: This time we got frantic, because we couldn't find him anywhere, and then we realized his bike was gone. So, we called the police. Jimmy gave us a real scare that time. It didn't occur to us he'd go that far.

Anne: Jimmy, what did you hope to accomplish by going to Grandma's? *(pause, no reply)* Did you want to give a message to your parents? What did you want from them?

Jim: I wanted everything back to normal—not everyone fighting. I wanted Daddy not to be mad at me.

Anne: That's really good, Jimmy. You're explaining how you feel very well. Did you tell Mommy and Daddy how you felt when you got back home?

Jim: *(shakes his head no)* Daddy yelled at me all the way home, and then he grounded me. Mommy told me she was glad I was with Grandma and I was okay. I ate some cookies and went right to bed. Then, Mommy and Daddy started yelling at each other.

Louis: I'm beginning to understand some of what's going on. Brittney's behavior may not be ideal, but she's right about one thing. When problems like this surface, it's rarely just one person's fault. The family is really a system, with each member's behavior affecting everyone else. Can you see that happening with you?

Debbie: Well, I can certainly see how the arguments between Brittney and Vinnie are hurting Jimmy. And they probably upset Brett, too.

Anne: And they affect your marriage as well. Didn't Jimmy say you argue with each other?

Vinnie: Only about how to discipline Brittney. If Brittney would just listen… Debbie's too soft on her, and then she expects me to be the bad guy.

Louis: Hold on just a minute, Vinnie. I'm not trying to blame you and Debbie for anything. It's understandable you are both concerned about your daughter. What you both need to ask yourselves, is what are you bringing to this problem that Brittney's behavior didn't cause? It's normal for her to want to go out on dates and to have fun. Don't you agree?

Vinnie and Debbie: *(both nod, yes)*

Louis: That's normal for her age. So what about this particular situation upsets you? Debbie's already admitted that she's worried about Brittney repeating her mistakes. This concern makes Brittney's behavior seem more troubling to you *(looking at Debbie)* than to your daughter. Because you know where it can lead, and you're projecting that onto her. Am I right?

Debbie: Yes, I see that, now.

Vinnie: You didn't tell me that before.

Debbie: I'm sorry, Vinnie. I guess I should have told you, too, Brittney.

Louis: What about you, Vinnie? What makes Brittney's behavior so upsetting for you, personally? Why do you choose to react the way you do?

Vinnie: Because I don't want to see her get hurt, and she's too smart for this guy. We hoped Brittney would go to college, get an education. This kid works on motors for a living. What kind of a future can he offer her?

Brittney: He's a mechanic, a good one, too. He has a steady job, and he makes good money. What's wrong with that?

Debbie: I'll tell you what's wrong with it. You're 14. He's what, 25?

Brittney: 22 *(with an exasperated sigh)*.

Debbie: You just started high school. That's a wonderful time in your life, when you should be making a lot of different friends and joining school activities, doing things other kids your age do. I never see you going out with girlfriends. Just Mike. Always Mike. I think you're missing out on a lot of fun you could be having in high school. You're growing up way too fast *(stops, teary eyed)*.

Vinnie: And what about academics? Brittney's grades took a nose-dive since she met Mike. I'm afraid she's throwing away her future. Before she even knows what she could have accomplished, she'll be barefoot, pregnant, and broke.

Brittney: I will not (*but she's suppressing a grin*).

Anne: And what about Jimmy? What's happening to him because of your preoccupation with Brittney?

Debbie: I guess we don't give him enough attention. All our emotional energy gets used up on Brittney. I'm so sorry, honey (*she leans over to give Jimmy a hug*).

Vinnie: Same with Brett. He's too young to understand, but he needs us, too. That's why we have to resolve this problem. So we can be a normal family again.

Louis: Well, I think we've all made an excellent start. What I'd like each of you to do for next time is to make a wish list. Write down the name of each person in your family and, next to it, one thing you love or admire about them and one thing you wish they would change or do differently. Don't talk about it ahead of time, but bring your list with you to the next session. Can you all agree to do that? (*all agree, but Jim looks confused*)

Louis: And Brittney, would you mind helping your brother with his list? I think it would be okay to talk about it with just your sister. Is that agreeable to both of you?

Brittney: Sure, bro. I can do that (*Jim grins at her*). I'm just glad I don't have to give up dating Mike.

Vinnie: Not yet! (*he frowns, then laughs*) Gotcha that time.

Anne: Anything else before we end?

(*silence, shaking heads no.*)

Anne: All right, then. We'll see you next week.

(*Vinnie pats Brittney on the back as they both stand to leave*)

The End.

Discussion

1. What was the intended goal of this session from the therapist's perspective?

2. How did it feel to be the character whose role you played?

3. How well did the two cotherapists work together? How did they divide up their leadership roles?

4. How well did the family members communicate with each other during the session? At what level (use Donohue's social profile levels from Chapter 3) of group interaction would you rate this session and why?

5. Identify and describe three conflicts between family members that were discussed.

6. How well did the therapists apply the conflict resolution methods described in Chapter 1?

7. What does typical social behavior look like for a 14-year-old girl such as Brittney? In what ways did her social behaviors deviate from the norm?

8. What type of discipline would you use in this home if you were Brittney's parent? Give an example of how your method would work.

9. In your opinion, what is the likely long-term outcome for this family? What are their strengths and shortcomings, and how likely are they to overcome current difficulties?

10. What was the purpose of the homework assignment given by the therapist, and how might the result be used in upcoming sessions?

11. Based on this discussion, what are the expectations of the mother and father for this family, and how do they compare with the traditional roles expressed in this chapter?

12. What life stages or transitions do you think these parents face, and how do they impact their family participation?

References

Allen, C. A., Earhart, C. A., & Blue, T. (1992). *Occupational therapy goals for the physically and cognitively disabled.* Bethesda, MD: American Occupational Therapy Association.

American Occupational Therapy Association. (2008). Occupational therapy practice framework: Domain and process (2nd ed.). *American Journal of Occupational Therapy, 62,* 625-683.

Asher, D. (2008). Lighting a fire. *US Airways Magazine, September,* 44-45.

Atchley, R. C. (1999). *Continuity and adaptation in aging: Creating positive experiences.* Baltimore, MD: The Johns Hopkins University Press.

Baltes, P. B., & Baltes, M. M. (Eds.). (1990). *Successful aging: Perspectives from the behavioral sciences.* New York, NY: Cambridge University Press.

Baltes, P., Reese, H., & Lipsitt, L. (1980). Life-span developmental psychology. *Annual Review of Psychology, 31,* 65-110.

Bhargava, R. (2007). *Features of the ideal family social network.* Retrieved September 5, 2008 from www.webpronews.com/blogtalk/2007/05/21/features-of-the-ideal-family-social-network

Bialystok, E., & Craik, F. I. M. (2006). *Lifespan cognition: Mechanisms of change.* New York, NY: Oxford University Press.

Birney, D., & Sternberg, R. (2006). Intelligence and cognitive abilities as competencies in development. In E. Bialystok & F. Craik (Eds.), *Lifespan cognition: Mechanisms of change* (pp. 315-330). New York, NY: Oxford University Press.

Bundy, A. (2001). Leisure. In B. Bonder & M. Wagner (Eds.), *Functional performance in older adults* (2nd ed., pp. 196-217). Philadelphia, PA: F. A. Davis.

Chung, I. (2007). *Roles and impacts of IT on new social norms, ethical values, and legal frameworks in shaping a future digital society.* National Science Foundation/OECD Workshop, Washington, January 31.

Coleman, P., & O'Hanlon, A. (2004). *Ageing and development.* London, England: Arnold/Oxford University Press.

Commons, M. L., Armon, C., Kohlberg, L., Grotzer, T., & Sinnott, J. D. (Eds.). (1990). *Adult development: Vol. 2. Models and methods in the study of adolescent and adult thought.* New York, NY: Praeger.

Commons, M. L., & Richards, F. A. (1999). Four postformal stages. In J. Demick (Ed.), *Handbook of adult development.* New York, NY: Plenum (Elsevier).

Commons, M. L., Richards, F. A., & Kuhn, D. (1982). Systematic and metasystematic reasoning: A case for levels of reasoning beyond Piaget's stage of formal operations. *Child Development, 53,* 1058-1068.

Creek, J. (Ed.). (2002). *Occupational therapy and mental health* (3rd ed.). London, England: Churchill Livingstone.

Eberlein, T. (2004). Lean on me: Sometimes a little support is the key to success. *Woman's Day,* Jan. 6, 62-65.

Eberly, M., & Montemayor, R. (1999). Chores. In C. A. Smith (Ed.), *The encyclopedia of parenting theory and research* (pp. 68-70). Westport, CT: Greenwood.

Erikson, E. H. (1978). *Adulthood.* New York, NY: Norton.

Fehr, B. (1995). *Friendship processes. Sage series on close relationships* (Vol. 12). New York, NY: Sage Publications.

Frey, B., & Stutzer, A. (2002). *Happiness and economics: How the economy and institutions affect human well-being.* Princeton, NJ: Princeton University Press.

Furstenberg, F., Cook, T., Eccles, J., Elder, G., & Smeroff, A. (1999). *Managing to make it: Urban families and adolescent success.* Chicago, IL: University of Chicago Press.

Garbarino, J. (1999). *Lost boys: Why our sons turn violent and how we can save them.* New York, NY: Free Press.

Gilligan, C. (1982). *In a different voice: Psychological theory and women's development.* Cambridge, MA: Harvard University Press.

Goleman, D. (1988). Erikson, in his own old age, expands his view of life. *The New York Times, June 14,* C1, C4.

Gould, R. L. (1978). *Transformations: Growth and change in adult life.* New York, NY: Simon & Schuster.

Gray, M., & Steinberg, L. (1999). Unpacking authoritative parenting: Reassessing a multidimensional construct. *Journal of Marriage and the Family, 61,* 574-587.

Hagedorn, R. (1997). Glossary. In R. Hagedorn (Ed.), *Foundations for practice in occupational therapy* (2nd ed., pp. 141-147). London, England: Churchill Livingstone.

Jung, C. G. (1914). *On psychological understanding. In Collected Works 3.* Princeton, NJ: Princeton University Press.

Karbo, K. (2008). Friendship: The laws of attraction. *Psychology Today,* Nov-Dec, 91-95.

Kendrick, S., & Kendrick, A. (2008). *The love dare.* Nashville, TN: B & H Publishing Group.

Kohlberg, L. (1973). Stages and aging in moral development: Some speculations. *Gerontologist, 1,* 497-502.

Kohlberg, L. (1984). *The psychology of moral development: Essays on moral development.* San Francisco, CA: Harper & Row.

Levinson, D. (1978). *The seasons of a man's life.* New York, NY: Ballantine Books.

Levinson, D. (1996). *The seasons of a woman's life.* New York, NY: Ballantine Books.

Lewis, S. C. (2003). *Elder care in occupational therapy* (2nd ed.). Thorofare, NJ: SLACK Incorporated.

McAdams, D. P., & de St. Aubin, E. (1992). A theory of generativity and its assessment through self-report, behavioral acts, and narrative themes in autobiography. *Journal of Personality and Social Psychology, 62,* 1003-1015.

McAdams, D. P., de St. Aubin, E., & Logan, R. (1993). Generativity among young, midlife, and older adults. *Psychology and Aging, 8,* 678-694.

McAdams, D. P., Hart, H. M., & Maruna, A. S. (1998). The anatomy of generativity. In D. P. McAdams, & E. de St. Aubin (Eds.), *Generativity and adult development* (pp. 7-43). Washington, DC: American Psychological Association.

Miller, B. C. (1998). *Families matter: A synthesis of family influences on adolescent pregnancy.* Washington, DC: National Campaign to Prevent Teen Pregnancy.

Myers-Walls, J. (1999). Advocacy. In C. A. Smith (Ed.), *The encyclopedia of parenting and research* (pp. 23-24). Westport, CT: Greenwood Press.

Ng, I., Ho, K. W., & Ho, K. C. (2008). *The role of families in shaping youth social participation: Evidence from Singapore.* Singapore: Nanyang Technological University.

Nusbaum, M. R., & Hamilton, C. D. (2002). The proactive sexual health history. *American Family Physician, 66,* 1705-1712.

Oakley, F., Kielhofner, G., Barris, R., & Reichler, R. K. (1986). The role checklist: Development and imperial assessment of reliability. *Occupational Therapy Journal of Research, 6,* 157-169.

Oswald, D., Clark, E., & Kelly, C. (2004). Friendship maintenance behaviors: An analysis of individual and dyad behaviors. *Journal of Social & Clinical Psychology, 23,* 413-441.

Pedretti, L. W. (1996). Occupational performance: A model for practice in physical dysfunction. In L. W. Pedretti (Ed.), *Occupational therapy: Practice skills for physical dysfunction.* St. Louis, MO: Mosby.

Piaget, J. (1972). Intellectual evolution from adolescence to adulthood. *Human Development, 16,* 346-370.

Reed, K., & Sanderson, S. (1999). *Concepts of occupational therapy* (4th ed.). Philadelphia, PA: Lippincott, Williams & Wilkins.

Reilly, M. (1969). The educational process. *American Journal of Occupational Therapy, 23,* 299-307.

Ross, M. (2009). *For the love of occupation.* Bethesda, MD: American Occupational Therapy Association.

Santoro, D., Sobocinski, S., & Klippel-Tancreti, C. (2008). Social participation. In C. Meriano & D. Latella (Eds.), *Occupational therapy interventions: Functions and occupations.* Thorofare, NJ: SLACK Incorporated.

Shmotkin, D., Blumstein, T., & Modan, B. (2003). Beyond keeping active: Concomitants of being a volunteer in old-old age. *Psychological Aging, 18,* 602-607.

Simpson, A. R. (2001). *Raising teens: A synthesis of research and a foundation for action.* Boston, MA: Center for Health Communication, Harvard School of Public Health. Retrieved October 5, 2008 from www.hsph.harvard.edu/chc/parenting.

Sinnott, J. D. (1993). Yes, it's worth the trouble! Unique contributions from everyday cognition studies. In J. M. Puckett & H. Reese (Eds.), *Mechanisms of everyday cognition* (pp. 73-95). Mahwah, NJ: Lawrence Erlbaum Association.

Smith, C. A., Cudaback, D., Goddard, H., & Meyers-Walls, J. (1994). *National extension parent education model of critical parenting practices.* Manhattan, KS: Kansas Cooperative Extension Service.

Stutzer, A., & Lalive, R. (2004). The role of social work norms in job searching and subjective well-being. *Journal of the European Economic Association, 2,* 696-719.

Thomas, M. L., & Kuh, G. D. (1982). Understanding development during the early adult years: A composite framework. *Personnel and Guidance Journal, 61,* Sept, 14-17.

Toglia, J. (2005). A dynamic interactional approach to cognitive rehabilitation. In N. Katz (Ed.), *Cognition and occupation across the life span* (2nd ed., pp. 29-72). Bethesda, MD: American Association of Occupational Therapy.

U.S. Department of Health and Human Services. (1997). *Understanding youth development: Promoting positive pathways of growth.* Washington, DC: Family and Youth Services Bureau.

Vaughn, D. (2009). The unspoken ADL: Helping patients regain their sex lives. *Today in OT, 2,* 24-25.

Westermeyer, J. F. (2004). Predictors and characteristics of Erikson's life cycle model among men: A 32 year longitudinal study. *International Journal of Aging and Human Development, 58,* 29-48.

Wilcox, M. (1979). *Developmental journey.* Nashville, TN: Abbington Press.

Wollan, M. (2007). Zygotic social networking. *The New York Times,* December 9. Retrieved December 9, 2007 from www.nytimes.com/2007/12/09/magazine/09zygotic.html?ref=magazine&pagewante

World Health Organization. (2001). *International classification of functioning, disability, and health.* Geneva, Switzerland: Author.

Additional Resources

Baltes, P. B. (1993). The aging mind: Potential and limits. *Gerontologist, 33,* 580-594.

Bandura, A. (1999). Social cognitive theory: An agentic perspective. *Asian Journal of Social Psychology, 2,* 21-41.

U.S. Bureau of Labor Statistics. (2004). *Volunteering in the United States, 2004.* Retrieved April 27, 2005 from www.bls.gov/news.release/volun.nr0.htm

Weisz, C., & Wood, L. (2005). Social identity support and friendship outcomes: A longitudinal study predicting who will be friends and best friends 4 years later. *Journal of Social and Personal Relationships, 22,* 416-432.

chapter 9

Social Development in Older Adulthood
Theories, Transitions, Roles, and Contexts

Marilyn B. Cole, MS, OTR/L, FAOTA

Theories of Social Development in Older Adults

As the older adult population increases each year, the *Occupational Outlook Handbook* predicts a higher-than-average increase in the need for occupational therapists along with other health and social service professionals in the area of gerontology (U.S. Bureau of Labor Statistics, 2009). Along with increases in numbers, other changes in the demographics for older adults include more years of good health, higher employment rates continuing after retirement age, and the trend toward aging in place. No longer can older adulthood be perceived as a series of losses and physical decline. Changes in the character of the older population have given birth to new and updated theories of older adult development, new research regarding the process of aging, and a greater understanding of the social factors that influence successful aging and prolong healthy life. This chapter includes a review of relevant psychosocial theories of aging and the roles and contexts within that older adults engage in occupations that facilitate continued social participation in their homes, neighborhoods, and communities.

Erikson's Late Life Developmental Stages

Erikson's sequential developmental conflicts to be resolved involve an ever-widening social radius across the lifespan (Erikson, 1978). Stage 7 (generativity versus self-absorption) and Stage 8 (integrity versus despair), Erikson's psychosocial stages affecting older adulthood, have also been validated and adapted through research to better explain the psychological and social issues that affect social participation through the older years. Vaillant (1993) noted that generativity went beyond mere parenthood to include active involvement in mentoring, teaching, coaching, or caring for the next generation or the wider community. In a longitudinal study, Westermeyer (2004) confirms the achievement of generativity in 53% of the sample and further notes that this advanced developmental stage was significantly associated with successful marriage, work achievements, close friendships, altruistic behaviors, and overall mental health. Additionally, this study identified good peer social adjustment and a warm family environment at midlife as significant predictors for the achievement of generativity. Erikson's generativity stage, once thought to predominate ages 50 to 60, can easily be conceived to continue well into the 80s and 90s for many older adults. This makes sense when one thinks of the number of people ages 60 to 65 who either actively volunteer or continue to work because their continued good health and vitality give them no reason not to do so. Those who are retired continue a busy and active lifestyle that includes many levels of social participation with families and communities. Generativity involves the desire to use one's knowledge and experience to guide the next generations, as well as to contribute to specific

Cole, M.B., & Donohue, M.V. *Social Participation in Occupational Contexts: In Schools, Clinics, and Communities* (pp 149-168).

professions or fields of expertise, to advocate for social causes, and to serve the needs of communities and of society. This focus synergizes with Laslett's Third Age mandate to use wisdom and experience of one's life to solve social problems and fulfill the unmet needs of society (Cole, 2008a, 2008b).

Erikson's eighth stage, integrity versus despair, addresses the need to reflect upon one's life and to evaluate its meaning as a whole. Integrity necessitates the resolution of psychological inconsistencies, such as repairing or renewing old relationships, finishing or finding closure for unresolved life problems, or reaffirming one's religious beliefs (Goleman, 1988). Reminiscing, writing one's memoirs, and participating in religious organizations and events are occupations that assist older adults with the resolution of Erikson's eighth stage. These introspective journeys have a spiritual quality, and their prevalence in later life resonates with the theories of gerotranscendence as well as Baltes' selection and optimization with compensation theory (SOC) and with Laslett's Fourth Age. Joan Erikson, Erikson's wife and frequent collaborator, at age 93, wrote about the need for solitude as a possible ninth stage, a "deliberate retreat from the usual engagements of daily activity... a paradoxical state that does seem to exhibit a transcendent quality" (Erikson & Erikson, 1997, p. 25).

Continuity Theory

Continuity theory (Atchley, 1989, 1999; Atchley & Barusch, 2004) suggests that, as they age, adults make adaptive choices that tend to preserve existing internal and external structures and strive to maintain their self-identity and existing perceptions of self and the world. Atchley (1989) defined retirement as a four-stage process: honeymoon, disenchantment, re-orientation, and termination.

1. *Honeymoon phase*—New retirees actively pursue projects previously precluded by employment, such as traveling or remodeling their homes.

2. *Disenchantment phase*—Realization that retirement has not worked out as they had hoped, requiring retirees to cope with the negative realities of retirement, such as loss of income.

3. *Re-orientation phase*—Re-evaluation of life leads to restructuring of one's lifestyle, including a search for meaningful occupations and establishing a new daily routine.

4. *Termination*—Advanced aging and the onset of disability necessitate dependence on others.

These phases illustrate the process of continuous adaptation in the face of newly emerging realities, which Atchley bases on feedback system theories (Atchley, 1999). He contends that people develop a large array of mental frameworks, such as self-identity, personal goals, belief systems, as well as external patterns, such as lifestyle, social networks, and activity patterns. These conceptions of and adaptations to the world around them allow older adults to make effective decisions leading to adaptive change. Continuity theory supports the positive adult development perspective that, as people grow older, they build on prior life experiences to improve their adaptive strategies, making them better able to cope with change in older adulthood. Atchley's theory, which has been validated in more recent studies (Reitzes & Mutran, 2004), paved the way for the current separation of young-old from old-old, as evidenced in Laslett's Third Age model.

Laslett's Third Age Model

Peter Laslett (1989, 1997) proposed a new developmental theory in consideration of the reality of increased health and longevity of older adults in the populations of most developed countries. He divides human life into four "ages" which are: (1) childhood and preparation for work; (2) employment and raising one's family; (3) beginning at retirement and ending with the onset of dependency; and (4) encompassing physical decline, dependence, and disengagement. Laslett's most important contribution is his definition of the third and fourth ages, previously thought of as a single developmental stage of older adulthood.

Any professional involved with program planning and serving older adults cannot ignore the global phenomenon of the Third Age model (Christiansen, 2008). People who retire in their 60s often have 25 to 30 more years of health and well-being, a significant amount of time. Far from the gradual decline of earlier theories of aging, Laslett's Third Age model gives a positive perspective to the "age of active retirement" (Laslett, 1989). Freed from economic responsibility, older adults in the Third Age focus on a whole new set of life tasks: self-fulfillment, lifelong learning, civic engagement, and making a contribution to society.

Yet, this view also diverges from the concept of retirement as a perpetual vacation or devoting each day exclusively to leisure pursuits. Laslett contends that while governments continue to give financial support to retirees, they have a responsibility to use their time, energy, and unique skills to fulfill the unmet needs of society. Add to this the expected surge of baby boomers—born between 1946 and 1964, who will very soon reach retirement age—many of whom have firsthand experience in the how-tos of producing social change. Retirees during the

Table 9-1

CHANGING INTEREST IN ACTIVITIES BETWEEN THIRD AND FOURTH AGES

GREATER INTEREST BEFORE AGE 85 (THIRD AGE)	GREATER INTEREST AFTER AGE 85 (FOURTH AGE)
• Making and creating things • Shopping and buying things • Making plans for the future • Keeping up with hobbies • Entertaining others in your own home • Social events with new people • Taking care of people and things • Meeting new people • Concern regarding others' opinions of yourself • Sharing opinions and advice • Visiting new restaurants/places	• Hearing from family and friends • Spiritual life/prayer • Pleasure in the small things • Visiting with family • Religious services • Reading, puzzles, using the computer • Getting together with old friends • Keeping up with current events • Worrying about friends/family's problems • Spending time alone • Being a good neighbor • Visiting with old friends/neighbors

Adapted from Adams, K. B. (2004). Changing investment in activities and interests in elders' lives: Theory and measurement. *International Journal of Aging and Human Development, 58,* 87-108.

next decade, given the right incentives, may be able to influence public policy in ways that truly embrace the concepts of social and occupational justice. With both free time and finances at their disposal, Third Agers have both the means and opportunity to help make the world a better place for everyone (Harvard School of Public Health, 2004).

Laslett's Fourth Age model encompasses some previously defined life tasks of old age, including those of adjusting to physical decline and coming to terms with death. Although Laslett does not set age ranges for any of his life stages, this last stage usually begins after age 80 and involves some aspects of disengagement, as conceptualized by Cumming and Henry (1961) half a century ago. A contemporary version of disengagement, recently validated by Carstensen (1992) involves the voluntary narrowing of one's social circle and the deepening of long-term relationships with old friends and family, a phenomenon known as socio-emotional selectivity. The Fourth Ager does this in order to conserve physical and emotional energy, choosing to spend more time on solitary and spiritual endeavors (Adams, 2004). This aspect of the Fourth Age was validated by Tornstam (1989, 1997, 2000) in a theory known

as gerotranscendence. Tornstam contends that the oldest-old attempt to construct a new reality within which past and present become one in a cosmic and transcendent worldview. The transition from health to dependence often requires a host of social and community supporters, as the aging individual moves to a place where both physical and social needs can be met in a way that protects autonomy and quality of life.

Adams (2004), in studying some of the activities that particularly interested older adults, was able to identify a distinct shift in interest occurring in the mid-80s. While her study was not specifically aligned with Laslett, the shift appears to reflect differences with regard to social perspective. In Table 9-1, the first column represents the interests of older adults in the Third Age, giving high importance to establishing new social relationships and engaging in social activities. The second column reflects narrowing one's social circle to family and close friends, increasing spiritual pursuits, and preferring more solitary occupations. These are more typical of Laslett's Fourth Age and are further evidenced in the contemporary theories of social emotional selectivity and gerotranscendence (Cole, 2008a).

Socio-Emotional Selectivity Theory

Carstensen (1992) recognized a voluntary narrowing of one's social circle in the over-80 age group. Long-term friendships and family relationships take on a deeper meaning, while more superficial relationships are dropped. This voluntary disengagement allows older adults to conserve emotional energy, pace themselves, and reduce worry about others (Adams, 2004). Another study supporting socio-emotional selectivity theory (SST) suggests that social supports provided by new acquaintances within retirement communities are not as meaningful and do not replace the support of long-term friendships (Potts, 1997). In SST, an older adult's time orientation changes to focus on the present, while future and past diminish. Therefore, "when boundaries on time are perceived, present-oriented goals related to emotional meaning are prioritized over future-oriented goals aimed at acquiring information or expanding horizons" (Lockenhoff & Carstensen, 2004, p. 395). Future becomes less relevant as death approaches, while the past fades away along with the loss of contemporaries who remember them when they were younger. Emotional intensity appears to diminish in elders who have come to terms with mortality, perhaps because they have nothing left to fear. Those over 85 spend more time sleeping and feel fairly comfortable with spending time alone (Larson, Csikszentmihalyi, & Graef, 1982).

Gerotranscendence

This contemporary outgrowth of disengagement theory focuses on the positive potential of cognitive changes that occur as the aging individual constructs a new reality, one that shifts from pragmatic and performance-oriented to a more cosmic and transcendent worldview. This internal, contemplative way of life, which trades in meaningless socialization for solitude, appears to be accompanied by an increase in life satisfaction (Tornstam, 1989, 1997, 2000). The cosmic dimension, which conceptually unites the past and present, may symbolize true wisdom for the older individual. This concept is reminiscent of the Jungian self-realization or Maslow's self-actualization (Boeree, 2006). In this state, the individual feels free to select only activities that are meaningful and to ignore the necessity for social reciprocation or convention. Both SST and gerotranscendence support the concept of Laslett's Fourth Age, which begins with physical dependence.

Social Support Theories

This group of theories has various titles, including social convoys (Rowe & Kahn, 1998), social exchange theory (Keyes, 2002), role theory (Kielhofner, 2002), social support banks (Antonucci & Jackson, 2002), and social capital (Stone, 2003; Veninga, 2006). Evidence shows that social relationships provide individuals with identity, social roles, and social support. The positive effects of social connections, including increased health, happiness, and longevity, are well documented (Stone, 2003). Role theory has influenced the way occupations are selected and organized (Spencer, 2003). In occupational therapy, the Person-Environment-Occupation-Performance model (PEOPM) (Baum & Christiansen, 2005) and the Model of Human Occupation (MOHO) (Kielhofner, 2002) are two occupation-based models that view roles as central ideas. Roles define the tasks or occupations that people do with or for one another, and the expectations and criteria for the performance of occupations may be socially and culturally determined. Because the absence of social support has been associated with significantly higher mortality for older adults (Lyyra & Heikkinen, 2006), the formal and informal social networks of the elderly have been studied extensively. Social support for older adults may provide emotional comfort, guidance, companionship, information, and physical assistance. Exchange theories emphasize the reciprocity of social and emotional support given. Keyes (2002) reports that the discrepancy between hours given and received becomes more balanced with age, but for the oldest adults in the study, unequal exchanges produced worse emotional well-being. The support bank theory (Antonucci & Jackson, 2002) uses a similar exchange concept, likening the hours of social support given to bank deposits and support received to bank withdrawals. The caregiving hours accrued in younger years can be "cashed in" in later life, making the receiving of care more acceptable. Such social exchange bank deposits and withdrawals may be used to explain intergenerational caring. Parents who cared well for their children do not have to worry about becoming a "burden" in their time of dependency.

Baltes' Selection and Optimization With Compensation Theory

This theory applies to the entire lifespan, as reviewed in Chapter 8, but has particular relevance for the transitions of older adulthood, where life goals and priorities change with both retirement (Laslett's Third Age) and the onset of dependency (Laslett's Fourth Age). The rebalancing of life priorities may be best accomplished with careful planning, as one plans for retirement by saving and investing money, but also in establishing and maintaining social networks, civic engagement, and leisure activities apart from paid work throughout the adult years. Baltes' theory suggests that as older adults experience declining energy levels, physical capacities, and other limitations, they will choose top-priority occupations (select) and focus remaining resources (optimize) more narrowly on the most important activities (Baltes, 1997, 2005). Social and community resources will then be called upon to compensate for those necessary occupations that the older person either cannot do (such as driving or managing finances) or elects not to do (such as cleaning house, grocery shopping, and other instrumental activities of daily living) (Baltes & Carstensen, 1996). Baltes' SOC theory provides useful guidelines for intervention with older adults who need assistance with the transitions of older adulthood, described in the next section.

Wisdom in Old Age

Recent theories of aging challenge the prevailing belief that intellectual ability declines with age. Looking at brain activity studies in the context of lifespan development, Buckner, Head, and Lustig (2006) suggest that "regional changes in gray matter in aging... reflect the continuation of development and lifelong learning processes that sculpt cortical structures in an adaptive manner" (2006, pp. 34-35). In other words, older brains may adapt by getting rid of unnecessary areas in order to allow existing pathways to operate more efficiently, a process similar to clearing one's computer of old programs in order to install updates that increase speed and efficiency. Sternberg (1985) proposes a theory of developing expertise based on a triarchic (three-part) theory of intelligence: components, contexts, and experience. Only the first part (component intelligence) can be measured using traditional IQ tests. It includes knowledge acquisition, performance, and metacognitive or executive functions (planning, execution, evaluation). Contextual intelligence allows the individual to apply acquired knowledge to adapt to environments or to adapt the environment to better suit individual needs. The experiential component of intelligence builds on previous life experiences and involves a higher level reasoning process to build connections between apparently unrelated situations in order to develop novel solutions. This experiential aspect, related to the concept of fluid intelligence, also considers automatic processing as a subconscious process that frees limited resources for other activities (Birney & Sternberg, 2006). Sternberg's conceptualization underlies the notion that intelligence increases with age. The five skills in developing expertise include (1) metacognition, (2) learning, (3) thinking, (4) knowledge (declarative and procedural), and (5) motivation. The inclusion of motivation links intelligence with the social aspects of adaptation and helps to explain the wide variations in functional and cognitive decline with aging.

Baltes also studied several positive aspects of the aging mind, including intelligence, wisdom, and advanced and exceptional levels of human performance (Baltes & Smith, 1990, 2001). The achievement of wisdom includes exceptional insights into human development, good judgment, advice about difficult life problems, and the "fundamental pragmatics of life." In contrast to a decline in the mechanics of cognition in older adulthood, the pragmatic features of wisdom include culturally acquired information and knowledge that is likely to increase with age, through ages 70 to 80 and beyond. Baltes and Smith (1990) identified five criteria for the achievement of wisdom: (1) rich factual knowledge, (2) rich procedural knowledge, (3) lifespan contextualism (knowledge about the contexts of life and developmental characteristics over time), (4) relativism (knowledge about differences in value, goals, and priorities), and (5) uncertainty (knowledge and acceptance of the unpredictable nature of human life). Researchers still struggle with how to define and measure wisdom, and how its presence affects health and well-being is largely unknown. However, from a social perspective, a better understanding of others can facilitate empathy, compassion, and a warmer temperament between people. Additionally, the potential of wisdom implies greater, more important roles for older adults in addressing some of the difficult social problems faced by families, communities, and nations.

Transitions of Older Adulthood

Some of the transitions of older adulthood identified by Knotts (2008) include retirement, changes in health status, relocation or place transitions, and transitions in social relationships. The two predictable transitions of older adulthood reviewed here exemplify the many adaptations older adults will face in the process of growing older. Because loving and working provide overarching themes throughout life, their eventual disruption toward the second half of life gives older adults a shared experience upon which to build relationships. Although theories of grief and loss are fairly well known, theories regarding retirement have only recently begun to address the complexity and variation in social and occupational transitions of older adults and to further define what is necessary to cope with adversity in later years. Studies such as "Reinventing Aging" (Harvard School of Public Health, 2004), which considers the social consequences of growth and continued health in the aging population as upcoming baby boomers begin their transitions to retirement, give some surprising insights about the future roles and impact of retired older Americans.

Transition to Retirement

Chuck Yeager, renowned U.S. Air Force fighter and test pilot who trained and mentored NASA astronauts in the 1960s and 1970s, writes this of his retirement:

> My first months out of the service, I felt kind of lost. For the first time that I could remember, there were absolutely no demands on my time. I could do anything I wanted to do, when I wanted to do it. Or, I could do nothing. It made no difference. So all that freedom looked kind of empty. Then, too, there was the feeling that I had been dumped off the merry-go-round and left behind. (Yeager, 1985, p. 421)

His experience is not uncommon. Kerr (1998) quoted a similar account of retirement from a letter published in the *Los Angeles Times*:

> My first few years of retirement were hit-and-miss, start-and-stop. … Early on, I just wanted to be free. Within months I tired of all the freedom and sought commitment and structure and duties. Later I wanted friends but couldn't find good ones because I didn't know what I wanted to have in common with them. Then I sought activities but grew frustrated that activities consumed time but didn't satisfy intellect. … As kids, we are often asked what we want to be when we grow up, but adults are never asked what we want to be when we retire. (p. 25)

For some retirees whose sense of worth, pleasure, and fulfillment centered around their employment, without work's purposeful activity and social connections, retirement can be a very lonely place (1998).

Several theories reinforce the importance of the transition to retirement. Levinson's late-life transition includes coping with loss of the worker role but does not elaborate on it. While we now recognize wider variation of ages for the older adult transition (originally 60 to 65), the 5-year timeline and the steps he uses to achieve a successful transition are useful for better understanding of what is involved in transitioning to retirement. The steps outlined in Table 9-2 are adapted from Levinson's life transition theory (Levinson, 1978).

A longitudinal study of the retirement process as an occupational transition (Jonsson, Josephsson, & Kielhofner, 2001) attempts to support continuity theory in its use of narratives to link past, present, and future for a group of older workers interviewed before, during, and after retirement. Narratives have been found useful for understanding the impact of change upon personal life stories and are

especially revealing in understanding motivation and meaning (Mattingly, 1998). Participants who had been interviewed before and during retirement were asked in this study to reflect upon the process as a whole. Three themes are identified in the result:

1. Transition involves the interaction between personal narrative and the living world, which can introduce an "unstable landscape of life events."

2. Retirement is full of surprising experiences, such as the inability to recreate satisfying life routines, the lack of extra time they had anticipated, changes in the meaning of occupations when work is subtracted from the picture, and the inability to continue or recreate social relationships apart from the context of the workplace.

3. Confirmation of the importance of "engaging occupations" in the achievement of life satisfaction in retirement. An engaging occupation is one infused with meaning, enjoyment, challenge, intensity, and a commitment or connection with others (the community). Participants who lacked truly engaging occupations had more difficulty with the transition to retirement.

These findings suggest that retirement is a complex process full of unanticipated realities that do not always continue one's life narratives as expected. When change interrupts one's personal story, some re-evaluation, introspection, and restructuring may be needed to figure out how this new episode (retirement) fits into the ongoing life "plot." Participants in the study by Jonsson and colleagues (2001) had been retired for a minimum of 5 years, possibly validating the 5-year transition period predicted by Levinson. The study adds an occupational perspective to the transition, citing engaging occupations that provide a context for building new social connections as a key feature in restructuring one's life for a successful retirement.

Coping With Loss

Most adults, by the time they reach age 60, have experienced the death of a relative or close friend and have participated in the traditions regarding death within their religion and culture. Some social norms might be wearing black and visiting a funeral home to view the body in a casket and to comfort the family. A religious or memorial service may include various family members and close friends sharing memories of their loved one or community members speaking of the person's contributions to their community. There may be a cemetery burial or a cremation after which the person's ashes are spread in a designated location that has special meaning for the individual. These are formalized social rituals that assist the living in coping with a significant loss.

Table 9-2

STEPS IN LIFE TRANSITIONS APPLIED TO RETIREMENT

STEPS INVOLVED IN LIFE TRANSITION	APPLICATIONS FOR TRANSITIONING TO RETIREMENT
Re-appraising the past: Evaluating one's life achievements to date, remembering the dreams of one's youth, and assessing one's real achievements and their meaning with regard to earlier life goals.	What career or work goals have been met? Has the dream been fulfilled? If not, what about it is still important to you? What social or family-related goals have been met? What social or family roles are most important to continue after retirement?
Setting new goals for the next life stage: Re-evaluating past goals and rebalancing priorities for the future. Consider the life tasks of the Third Age here: self-fulfillment, creativity, using time and energy to fulfill unmet needs for the community and society.	What lifelong dreams can still be accomplished during the retirement years? What roles and occupations are most important and meaningful for your new or continuing social identity? How will you pursue self-fulfillment? Creativity? How can your unique knowledge and skills be best used to serve your community or society?
Re-evaluating social relationships with regard to newly created goals.	Are your current relationships still meeting your social/emotional needs? How do you need to change them to make them more fulfilling? To what extent will they support your newly set goals? How can you replace the social networks left behind at work? What new social roles can be established to connect with others in meaningful ways for yourself and society?
Creating a new life structure for the next stable life stage.	How can daily occupations be re-organized to move you forward toward accomplishing new goals for the future? What healthy habits need to be established in order to maximize function, minimize health risks, and maintain well-being and life satisfaction?

Adapted from Levinson, D. (1978) *Seasons of a man's life.* New York, NY: Ballantine Books.

Loss of a spouse or long-time life partner can be particularly devastating for an older adult, holding the top score on Holmes' Scale of stressful life events (Holmes, 1978). For the surviving spouse, grief follows, sometimes complicated by the caregiver-dependent relationship in cases of chronic illness or slow decline in functioning. Also complicating the picture for the older adult survivor are lost roles, occupations, or activity patterns associated with the deceased, such as those related to caregiving, for example. Adjusting to living alone after death of a spouse or life partner (or after divorce) presents some unique challenges, such as safety and security issues, learning new roles once performed by one's partner, and making new connections with others as a single person. Support groups in one's church,

community, or online are a good way to cope with this traumatic loss in later life.

The stages of grieving, familiar to most since Kubler-Ross first defined them in 1969, provide an understanding of the expected process of a normal grief response. The stages are (1) denial, (2) anger, (3) bargaining, (4) depression, and (5) acceptance (Kubler-Ross & Kessler, 2005). The signs and symptoms of grief defined in the *Diagnostic and Statistical Manual of Mental Disorders* (American Psychiatric Association [APA], 2000) can easily be recognized: numbness, crying, weakness, loss of concentration, sleeping and eating disorders, restlessness, self-reproach, survivor guilt, helplessness and hopelessness, and sense of the deceased's presence. Together, these symptoms closely resemble

Table 9-3

GRIEF VERSUS DEPRESSION

	GRIEF	DEPRESSION
Intensity	Less	More
Duration of symptoms	Shorter	Longer
External influence	Reaction to loss	Internal
Suicide risk	Low	High
Medication	Seldom used	Almost always used
Precipitating event	Loss of significant other	May not be one
Presence of psychosis	Never	Frequently
Functional impairment	Short duration	Longer duration

depression, an abnormal mood disorder that can last for months or years when left untreated. The main differences between normal grief and clinical depression are duration and severity. Normal grieving usually requires no medical or psychological intervention, and the typical timeline is as follows:

- × Initial functioning returns within about 2 weeks, normal daily functioning resumes.

- × Most signs and symptoms subside after 1 to 2 months.

- × The entire process takes about a year, with experiences of all seasons and holidays.

Knowledge about possible abnormal responses is particularly important because the grieving widow or widower has a higher risk for depression, which is best treated with a combination of short-term counseling and antidepressant medication. Therapists and caregivers as well as family and friends need to be aware of the differences described in Table 9-3.

Some other social relationship transitions include taking on a caregiving role, accepting caregiving from family members or health professionals, and building new social networks after relocation (Knotts, 2008). Many older adults find that pets offer companionship, comfort, relief from stress, and a focus for daily activity that can help to bridge some of the more difficult transitions. Dogs can offer some level of safety for people living alone, and walking the dog also offers opportunities to connect with others and share interesting stories (Coppola, 2008).

Roles and Contexts of Older Adulthood

Family Roles

Family roles continue into later life, although they change with greater maturity or new circumstances.

Spouse or Intimate Partner

Spousal relationships following retirement often involve a reorganization of family roles such as household responsibilities, budgeting and handling finances, planning social activities, or entertaining others in one's home. A wife who continues to work may feel less positive than her husband after his retirement (Henrietta, O'Rand, & Chan, 1993). One study reported 71% higher satisfaction with marriage after retirement and identified spousal relationships as the most important single factor influencing adjustment of life patterns (Rosenkoetter & Garris, 1998).

A wide variety of living situations and relationships exist in older adulthood according to Womack (2008). In addition to married couples, 30% of older men and 45% of older women live as divorced, never married, or widowed. Cohabitation among this group had increased six times by 1990 over the previous three decades (Chevan, 1996), and the trend continues. The growing number of nonmarital intimate relationships requires an expanded definition of intimacy in older adulthood to include a broad range of behaviors (Womack, 2008).

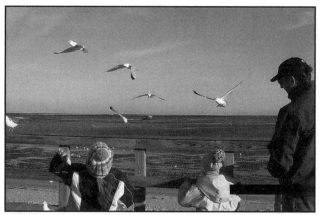

Figure 9-1. The grandparent role takes on added meaning when sharing activities such as feeding seagulls while on a winter walk to the beach.

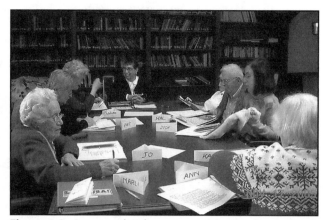

Figure 9-2. A mature level group; participating in a memoir writing group encourages members to share their collected wisdom with others.

Grandparent

Adults with grown children become grandparents at a broad range of ages and respond with a variety of grandparenting styles. Retirees with grandchildren may want to change their grandparenting style with retirement. Neugarten and Weinstein (1964) identified five patterns of grandparenting:

1. *Formal*—Limited contact with grandchildren with no parental responsibilities.

2. *Fun-seeking*—Frequent informal contact focused on sharing leisure activities (Figure 9-1).

3. *Surrogate*—Assuming parental responsibilities in the absence of parents who may be working or otherwise unavailable (usually grandmothers).

4. *Conveyer of family wisdom*—Special role of transmitting family history, culture or traditions, and of giving advice (usually grandfathers).

5. *Distant figures*—Contact limited to ritualistic events, such as birthdays and holidays.

Researchers have found that the fun-seeking and distant styles are more common for grandparents under 65 years, and both frequency of contact and role may change with retirement (Bonder & Hasselkus, 2003). Grandparents who are retired often take on parenting roles for their grandchildren, consisting of babysitting, caregiving, and offering financial support. Kornhaber (1996) found that children raised by grandparents tend to be more well-rounded, have greater respect for the past, are more likely to speak more than one language, perform better in school, and have a good sense of family and family values. When divorce threatens to cut off access to grandchildren, grandparents have fought for visiting rights in court (Bonder & Hasselkus, 2003).

Elder, Conveyer of Wisdom

The time may be right for a return to this ancient traditional role of elders once held in indigenous societies. Rather than limiting the conveying of wisdom to only grandparents, as noted by Neugarten and Weinstein (1964), communities and larger social groups might well benefit from the collective wisdom of older adults, given sufficient opportunity. Elders, cited by Enfield and Formichelli (2003) as "wisdom keepers" (p. 84), are more revered in Muslim, Hispanic, African, and Native American cultures than in mainstream America (Shalomi & Miller, 1995). The role of elder is mentioned here, not as a reality, but as an opportunity for therapists, agencies, and program planners to restore older adults to their rightful position of respect in society, "a challenging occupational developmental stage where people have the time and space to become more fully themselves, and to share with others the fruits and wisdom of their being" (do Rozario, 1998). Coming from the field of occupational science, this author suggests that society has much to learn from elders about the "art of being" as an occupational bridge to more fully understand the "art of living" (do Rozario, 1998, p. 125) (Figure 9-2).

Caregiver

More than 50 million people provide care for a disabled or aged family member or friend during any given year. Approximately 60% of family caregivers are women. The typical American caregiver is a 46-year-old married working woman caring for her widowed mother. Thirty percent of family caregivers are themselves ages 65 and older (American Association of Retired Persons [AARP], 2004). Some common caregiving tasks are listed in Table 9-4.

Caregivers who live with the disabled or aged person, such as a spouse, have a high risk for burnout

---

Table 9-4

COMMON CAREGIVING TASKS

- Administering medication, filling or refilling prescriptions
- Dealing with adverse effects of medication
- Providing help with activities of daily living—self-care
- Complying with medical follow-up (eg, changing wound dressing)
- Providing symptom management—vomiting, heat/cold, suctioning, positioning
- Following up with rehabilitation home programs, such as daily exercises
- Adapting the home to accommodate disability
- Notifying doctors, obtaining medical help
- Meal preparation and clean up
- Shopping/errands
- Attending to spiritual/religious needs
- Providing leisure activities/entertainment, companionship
- Managing finances
- Maintaining a clean and healthy environment

Table 9-5

SYMPTOMS OF CAREGIVER DISTRESS

- Feelings of sadness, depression, crying
- Anger, irritability, or hostility
- Guilt and self-blame
- Exhaustion due to caregiving burden
- Anxiety, fear, uncertainty
- Loneliness, isolation
- Strain on family and other sources of social support
- Neglect of own health and social/emotional needs

Adapted from Brintnall-Peterson, M. (2003). *Caregivers watch for warning signs of distress or depression.* Retrieved February 23, 2009 from www.uwex.edu/news/2003/6/caregivers-watch-for-warning-signs-of-distress-or-depression

---

or caregiver distress syndrome (Strawbridge, Wallhagen, Shema, & Kaplan, 1997). While this is not an official diagnosis, many research studies have identified some or all of these symptoms listed in Table 9-5. Studies show that certain circumstances carry a higher risk of distress, for example, caregivers of people with dementia are twice as likely to experience clinical depression (Brintnall-Peterson, 2003). Caring for people with behavioral abnormality, such as delusions; emotional or aggressive outbursts; or inability to focus, remember, and follow through on important tasks also carries a higher risk for symptoms of distress (Kreutzer, Gervasio, & Camplair, 1994; Riello, Geroldi, Zanetti, & Frisoni, 2002).

Interestingly, even though respite (relief from care-giving) was stated as a pressing need, most family care-givers in a rural setting did not use available respite services (Mast & Wakefield, 2003). Hoffman (2002), reporting on the Family Caregiver Self-Awareness and Empowerment Project, notes that many people who find themselves giving more and more care over time do not realize or acknowledge that this has become a major role in their lives. This lack of awareness makes caregivers less likely to seek help, support, or respite from others. Some of the caregiver needs identified in this report included the following:

- ⨯ Information, support, access to services, and resources

- ⨯ Understanding and cooperation from employers, family members, friends, and neighbors

- ⨯ Understanding and appreciation from physicians, health care providers, health plan administrators, and even strangers

- ⨯ Someone to talk to and share experiences with

- ⨯ New skills, including ways to communicate and solve interpersonal issues with clients, or medical management issues

- ⨯ Financial assistance to reimburse for the cost of home modifications, transportation, medical supplies, over-the-counter or prescription medications, and other incidentals related to the caregiving role

- ⨯ A place to go for a change of environment and a fresh perspective

As Hoffman reports, information provided to care-givers by health care organizations imparts facts and figures about the illness and its symptoms and statistics but fails to "delve into psychosocial issues" nor do these materials discuss self awareness, self-help, or sources of social or emotional support (2002). Caregiver distress self-report assessments may be found on several disability Web sites, including those of the Stroke and Alzheimer's Associations (www.strokeassociation.org; www.alz.org).

The incidence of family caregiving will likely continue to expand exponentially as the population of older adults increases and represents a significant societal trend as reported in the media (Hoffman, 2002). Given the expected increase of family caregiving for older adults with disabilities, it seems logical that the caregivers, and not the people with disabilities, would most likely seek out assistance from occupational therapists or others who have the expertise needed to simplify the caregiving role, such as modifying task environments to help people with cognitive deficits to continue to perform self-care tasks. Perhaps this population of caregivers represents an opportunity for occupational therapy

consultants to market their services within the umbrella of health care provided by community clinics and hospitals. However, reimbursement for such services may require changes in public or private medical insurance coverage (Bookwalter & Siskowski, 2009).

Community Roles

Civic Engagement/Volunteering

Like the ageisms of *elderly* or *senior citizen*, the term *volunteering* also connotes negative images of handing out flyers and ladling soup (Tanz & Spencer, 2000). Furthermore, volunteering has inconsistent meaning across economic and ethnic groups. For example, low-income communities may see volunteering and community service as a court-ordered punishment. Culturally, many immigrant and minority groups do not connect their own highly valued concepts of helping others with the word *volunteering*. Alternate terms, such as *civic engagement* or *community involvement*, expand the meaning of volunteering to include these additional sectors of society (Prisuta, 2003).

Today's Third Age active retirees prefer the term *civic engagement*. As a broader concept for serving one's community, civic engagement includes both paid and unpaid work, advocacy for social causes, participation in the democratic process, and lifelong learning (Cavanaugh, 2005). Along with the name change, the face of civic engagement in the hands of baby boomers is likely to take on a level of professionalism and respect that retirees once had during their careers. Civic engagement may also include paying a modest stipend for services of those in the lower economic subgroups, an incentive shown to be successful for informally engaging otherwise unavailable older volunteers (Kleyman, 2003).

The Statistics of Volunteering

Logically, one assumes that retired people have more time with which to serve as volunteers. However, in 2004, those over 65 years represented the lowest percentage (24.6%) for volunteering of any adult age group (U.S. Bureau of Labor Statistics, 2004). Younger adults 35 to 45 years old (34.2%) and 45 to 55 years old (32.8%), while still in the workforce, have a higher rate of volunteerism than those who are retired. With baby boomers reaching retirement, the situation is predicted to get much worse (Prisuta, 2003). An AARP survey (2003) of adults ages 50 to 59 years (primarily older baby boomers) found that half of this group who do volunteer do so mostly for "episodic special projects" (47%), and only 23% take on continuing volunteer roles. Himes (2001) found that "less than 30% of persons 65+ volunteer, and most of those do so for less than two hours a week" (Prisuta, 2003, p. 60).

Volunteering refers to unpaid work. The word implies that people participate in volunteer roles by choice and that these roles have some purpose or usefulness for others, the community, or society. According to the U.S. Bureau of Labor Statistics, in 2004, teenagers had a 29.4% volunteer rate (the highest increase over previous years), while those 65 and older averaged 24.6%, with this percentage declining as age increases. Those employed full- or part-time had a higher volunteer rate than those not in the workforce (2004).

According to Wyant and Brooks (1993), the concept of volunteering is becoming broader. In addition to the traditional volunteering for charity organizations, volunteering refers to community service learning, student internships, and court-ordered programs. These areas define the more formal volunteer roles. The more informal work activities people do without pay might include caregiving for children or aging relatives, home and yard maintenance, or providing occasional help to one's neighbors and friends. The domains of concern for occupational therapists outlined by the AOTA Framework are volunteer exploration and volunteer participation.

Volunteer exploration is defined as "determining community causes, organizations, or opportunities for unpaid work in relationship to personal skills, interests, location, and time availability" (AOTA, 2008, p. 632). In this aspect of volunteering, the tasks are similar to those required for seeking paid work. The older adult's knowledge, skills, and interests need to be evaluated and matched to available opportunities for local volunteer positions. Some older adults may need to take a closer look at the tasks and determine the activity demands required in the volunteer jobs being considered. AOTA (2008) defines activity demand as "the aspects of an activity, which include the objects, space, social demands, sequencing or timing, required actions, and required underlying body functions and body structure needed to carry out the activity" (p. 638). Most older adults with health limitations will need the help of an occupational therapist to correctly assess activity demands of a volunteer role. Retirees may need to look at their overall use of time to determine how much time would be optimal to devote to volunteering.

Volunteer participation is defined by AOTA (2008) as "performing unpaid work activities for the benefit of identified, selected causes, organizations, or facilities" (p. 632). Occupational therapists may assist clients in establishing needed skills, building or remediating required abilities for the tasks involved, and/or making the necessary adaptations to enable the client to participate in a volunteer experience safely.

Reasons for Volunteering

Giving back to the community; working for valued causes; making new friends; learning new skills; and finding expression for one's talents, skills, and creativity are some of the many reasons why people volunteer. Research has suggested volunteering as an enhancement for the transition to retirement (Dorfman & Moffett, 1987; Ellis, 1993; Rosenkoetter & Garris, 1998).

Because of the unavailability of younger volunteers, organizations have turned to retired older adults to fill the need. In 1987, 38% of people older than 65 served as volunteers in some capacity (Chambre, 1991). According to another source, 26% of older adults volunteer for organizations, 29% informally help the sick or disabled, and 33% help or care for their grandchildren (Caro & Morris, 2001). For many older adults, volunteering replaces the lost worker role, fills gaps in increased leisure time, and provides meaning or purpose in daily activities. However, Ewald (1999) points out that volunteering does not provide meaning if it is considered busy work. Good matches need to be made between a person's talents and a real need in the community for the elder "to mentor, educate, assist, and guide the next generation" (p. 325). Here again, occupational therapists need to develop knowledge of volunteer opportunities in order to use activity analysis and synthesis in matching volunteer roles with client abilities and priorities.

Benefits of Volunteering

While volunteering can have mutual benefits for people of any age, recent research tells us that those who benefit the most from volunteering are older adults. This age group has been widely studied, and the results demonstrate that volunteering prevents depression (Musick & Wilson, 2003), increases physical and psychological health (Backes, 1993; Greenfield & Marks, 2004), increases well-being (Morrow-Howell, Hinterlong, Rozario, & Tang, 2003; Wheeler, Gorey, & Greenblatt, 1998), and in many cases, prolongs life (Musick, Herzog, & House, 1999). For this reason, occupational therapy interventions with this population should include volunteer exploration, placement, and ongoing problem solving in the volunteer workplace.

The Healing Value of Volunteering

The enduring truth that helping others also helps yourself cannot be questioned. Many human interest stories in the media showcase the therapeutic value of victims and survivors helping others like themselves. Most self-help organizations have come into existence this way, including Alcoholics Anonymous, the Breast

Cancer Support Service, American Society of Pain Management, Compassionate Friends, and Weight Watchers. The timing of one's involvement in public sharing of one's experiences is critical and different for each individual. In the continuum of adaptation to chronic illness, early stages of shock, denial, and anger do not lend themselves well to any interventions, peer or otherwise. However, contacting a peer volunteer may overcome denial and increase one's readiness for therapy.

Civic Engagement Through Advisory Boards, Senior Centers, and Consumer Groups

Volunteering includes participation on appropriate advisory boards, community leadership groups, and advocacy groups. Sometimes, advisory board participation leads to continued employment opportunities. As older adults become more knowledgeable about public service opportunities, they will more easily find ways to become involved and to benefit from such connections.

Advocacy for Self and Others

Older adults may need to learn the role of advocacy for their own health and well-being. The skills of assertiveness discussed in Chapter 1 can find good usefulness in advocacy roles. Volunteering with school systems, community service organizations, and health agencies is a good way to learn how the system works and how to make it work for them, as well as finding helpful connections for enacting social change. Adults with acquired illness also identify *the system* of health service delivery to be a major obstacle to accessing services like occupational therapy, which would enable their continued participation in important life roles (Macdonald, 2000). Advocacy groups for other causes such as Defenders of Wildlife and the American Society for the Prevention of Cruelty to Animals (ASPCA) offer a variety of volunteer opportunities that can be easily found on their Web sites.

Religious, Ethnic, and Political Organizations

Statistics tell us that the lion's share of volunteering occurs through churches and religious organizations. This makes sense considering that, as people age, connections with their religious and cultural background take on deeper meaning. These organizations offer volunteer opportunities across the lifespan, and many older adults may already have established patterns of participation and service. As a social activity, volunteering may be a good way for older adults to keep in contact with others who share similar values and beliefs.

Lifelong Learner

Education in younger years had the prescribed purpose of preparing children and youth for adult life, including basic skills like reading, writing, mathematics, and training for specific careers. As adults, most workers have required educational updates in the form of continuing or in-service education or have opted to learn avocational skills through adult education. Lifelong learning has a different purpose entirely—to serve the educational needs of Third Agers in their unique life tasks of personal fulfillment, continued wellness and well-being, and preparation for civic engagement, a newly defined form of community service and advocacy.

Education "permanente," the French term that spawned the University of the Third Age (U3A) movement in the 1970s, epitomizes the lifelong learning concept in its broadest sense, as it encompasses formal, informal, incidental, accidental, and serendipitous learning (Hazzlewood, 2007). Thousands of U3As, a worldwide phenomenon that is least known in the United States, serve the lifelong learning needs of the healthy, actively retired population who are soon to become the majority of older adults as baby boomers enter the Third Age over the next 2 decades, and onset of the Fourth Age is further delayed by medical and cultural advancement. Public spending and government policy seems skewed disproportionately toward the minority Fourth Age while educational needs in the Third Age go unfunded and unmet (Jones, 2000).

Educational gerontology, a new academic discipline, focuses on the interface between adult education and social gerontology, the study for and about aging individuals (Withnall, 2002). It includes providing educational opportunities for older adults, educating the public about older adults, and educating professionals about working with older adults. Research in educational gerontology has much to offer occupational therapists, educators, and others who serve or create programs for older adults. Research has identified some of the motivations for older adults to seek educational opportunities:

- Keeping informed about health and wellness, creating and implementing healthy lifestyles

- Learning or training for service-related work serving humanity or community leadership

- Leisure occupations, learning new skills such as wine-making or Asian cooking, with subthemes of finding new friends and socializing

- Intergenerational interactions that allow learning from each other, such as computer training and gardening, or other combinations of interest to both generations (Tsao, 2004; Withnall, 2002)

The education of older adults also requires different methods than those designed for younger students. Traditional lectures and classroom procedures may be inadequate. Flexibility of instruction method and classroom arrangement are needed for adapting to a variety of special needs such as mobility issues, hearing and vision limitations, and method and speed of information processing. Small group seminar-style classes with opportunities for interaction and discussion are better suited to the learning needs of many older adults. Instructors who invite older learners to share their own related experiences and brainstorm about how new information may be applied create a richer, more enthusiastic learning experience for all involved.

Digital connection, using computers and the internet, stands out as an area of urgent need for older adult learners, not as an option but a necessity. As aptly noted by Prensky (2001), those who were educated during the last 2 decades of the 20th century have grown up with computers and technology as a way of life. Prensky dubs these youth and young adults, "digital natives," making the rest of us "digital immigrants" (2001, p. 1). Digital natives, because of their technological education and experience, have acquired not only different knowledge, but different patterns of thinking; in a sense, they have learned a different language. Soon to reach positions of authority, digital natives will no doubt reconfigure many of the ways of the world to their way of thinking, including some essential everyday activities such as making phone calls, banking, shopping, and traveling. For example, e-mail, online chats, and text messaging have already overtaken old-fashioned telephone calls for the younger set, forcing many grandparents to establish an e-mail account in order to communicate with their grandchildren. Bank tellers may disappear altogether as direct deposit replaces checks, people use ATM machines for cash, and receive and pay most of their bills online. Most major stores report ever-increasing sales from Web sites, as mall and Main Street shoppers continue to decline. Travel agents are another dying breed, as online Web sites offer bargain rates for flights, cruises, and hotels worldwide. *Is it any wonder today's older adults feel marginalized?*

Meanwhile, "digital immigrant" instructors and others struggle to keep up with the latest technology, but as Prensky observes, "a language learned later in life, scientists tell us, goes to a different part of the brain" (2001, p. 2). Anyone who has attempted to learn a new software program by reading the manual (whether in print or online) knows this to be true. The digital natives who wrote the manuals had no idea what digital immigrants did and did not already know

and could not fathom what features actually applied to their everyday life tasks.

Scott (1999) observes that older adults intent on learning new technology are neither technophobes nor passive dependents, but rather consumers needing to be informed. While knowledge of brain plasticity confirms the ongoing ability of older brains to learn new languages and many other things (Chui, 2001; Guttman, 2001; Prensky, 2001; Victoroff, 2001; Wolff, 2003), some older adults may find life more harmonious without cyber-learning. However, their apparent disinterest may also be due to a lack of opportunity (Withnall, 2006). A middle road might be offering cyber-learning at different levels for different needs. For example, "producing simple documents or greeting cards, playing games for fun while learning mouse skills, sending and receiving e-mail and accessing the internet for simple searching… may be enough for many older adults" (Hazzlewood, 2007).

Ironically, the best instructors for older adult learners are not digital natives, who tend to trivialize unfriendly software, blame problems on technophobia or inadequate hardware, and become impatient with the slower information processing or other adaptations on the part of the learner. When learning activities are congruent with the individual's learning style and are structured to motivate the learner, overall effectiveness is enhanced (Wakefield, 2001). Third Age lifelong learners who offer their skills as volunteers make more empathetic instructors of their peers and are increasingly becoming an integral part of the networks that make up learning communities. They point out the need for producers of technology to do away with planned obsolescence and unnecessary upgrades, which tend to outpace both the learning span and financial resources of many older adults (Hazzlewood, 2007).

Summary: What Is Successful Aging?

Along with increased numbers, significant changes in the dynamics of older adult roles in society seem likely. Already, the entry of baby boomers into the Third Age is challenging the negative stereotypes of aging and raising public consciousness about the lifestyle factors that influence wellness and longevity such as physical fitness and antioxidants in one's diet. Continued well-being, however, depends much more heavily on social connectedness (Figure 9-3).

A national profile of social connectedness, the results of a large-scale study funded by the National Institutes of Health (Cornwell, Laumann, & Schumm, 2008) find the following:

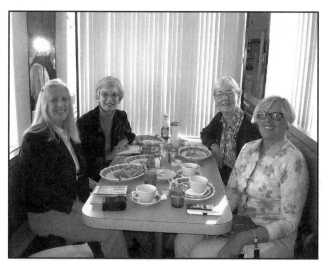

Figure 9-3. Third Age friends' continued social participation contributes to an ongoing sense of well-being after retirement.

- Age is negatively related to network size—As people grow older, social networks narrow and become limited mainly to primary group ties.

- Age is positively related to the frequency of association with neighbors, religious participation, and volunteering. Retirement and widowhood were found to increase connectedness with others in neighborhoods, religious groups, and the community.

- Age has a U-shaped relationship to volume of social connectedness—Contact volume declines through the young-old years, flattens through the old-old years, and increases again in the oldest-old age group. Life events, such as retirement, widowhood, and the onset of disability, are thought to influence this finding.

This comprehensive survey based on recent statistics (Cornwell et al., 2008) concludes that older Americans are well-connected. Results for young-old and old-old are consistent with social theories, such as Laslett's Third and Fourth Age models, and portray current older adults as resilient to potentially isolating events and motivated to continue social roles and activities through the transitions of older adulthood (Atchley, 1999; Baltes & Baltes, 1990; Cornwell et al., 2008). Social gerontologists view social integration as a key component of successful aging (Rowe & Kahn, 1998). Therapists and others serving the older adult population cannot ignore the importance of social participation for continued health and well-being. Interventions stressing wellness as well as rehabilitation strategies involving social reconnection for those with disability will be presented in Chapter 15.

Learning Activities

Developmental Interview With an Older Adult

Choose an older (over age 60) relative or friend who will trust you enough to answer your questions truthfully, and set up a time of about 2 hours for your interview. Include in identifying information, the person's age, current living arrangement, marital status, and current occupations.

Choose one theory of aging from those reviewed here. Write 10 open questions based on your chosen theory that will help you to understand how the older person has experienced a transition or resolved the life tasks that the theory outlines. Feel free to follow up any of these questions during the actual interview. Write the questions and summarize the answers in a 3- to 5-page paper. Tell why you chose the theory, whether or not your interview validated or refuted the theory, and why.

End your interview by asking what roles, contexts, and occupations might be included in this person's social identity? Ask the older person to show you or give you some specific examples of the most meaningful occupations in which he or she participates. End your paper with a brief description of your interviewee's social identity.

A Day in the Occupational Life of an Older Adult

With permission, spend a day with an older adult you met at a senior center or town library, and take photographs of the person while engaging in at least five different occupations or activities involving social participation. Before leaving, show the individual some of the pictures, and ask him or her to explain what is meaningful about each occupation or activity. Have the person sign a photo release explaining that his or her pictures will be used to make a photo diary as an assignment, and afterwards you will give him or her a copy of the diary to keep.

Make a digital photo album using at least five pictures of the person engaging in daily occupations with others. Along with each photo, write a short description of the occupation, where it took place, with whom (no last names, please), and what its meaning or significance was for the individual. Print the diary as an assignment. Be sure to follow up on your obligation to provide a copy of the occupational photo diary to the chosen individual.

Something to Live For

(Adapted from Leider, 2008)

Thinking about your own life experience and the beliefs, knowledge, skills, and wisdom you have acquired at this point in time, fill in the table below with at least five in each column: Gifts (talents and special abilities you possess), Values (beliefs, religious principals, or philosophical guidelines you live by), and Passions (causes, social issues, areas of knowledge or research, specific occupations, activities, or groups with which you feel strong emotional ties).

My Gifts	My Values	My Passions

Then, consider the list you have made and put a star next to the most important or top priority in each column. Following Leider's (2008) guidelines for finding your calling or what is most meaningful to you, take the top priorities of each column, and write them in the following blanks:

Using my special gift of _____ (top gift), and following my strong belief in _____ (top value), I will serve the cause of _____ (top passion) by taking the following actions:

1. _____

2. _____

3. _____

For example, one person nearing retirement might answer this way: *Using my special gift of leading therapeutic groups, and following my strong belief that each person has something unique to contribute to others, I will serve the cause of occupational justice by (1) connecting with my local senior center, (2) marketing and finding a pilot group of six to eight newly retired older adults, and (3) facilitating their ability to work as a team to identify the unmet needs in their community, choose one area to focus on, and create a plan for using volunteers to fill the need or to solve the identified problem.*

Script: Reminiscence Group

Seating Chart

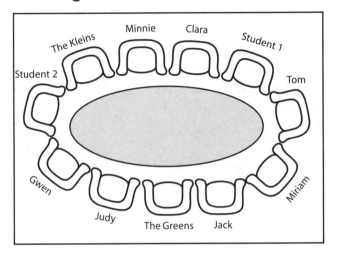

Setting and Participants

Eleven people ranging in age from 63 to 81 years old attend this group weekly. Membership is quite stable, although health issues and medical appointments sometimes keep these active older adults from coming to the group. The group meets in a somewhat affluent community center, with attendance permitted based on living in the neighborhood. There are two couples in the group. Two occupational therapy students are co-leading the group for 6 weeks. They had ascertained through an assessment that the group wished to have the opportunity to be in a reminiscence-oriented group during this time period. Activities range from discussion to a fashion show to sharing photos from the past.

Action Begins Here

Student 1: Today, we are going to carry out an activity you asked to do together—to share memories from the past that you can recall.

Student 2: So, everyone close your eyes a minute and think about what you might like to share with the group that is memorable for you.

Minnie: When I was married, my husband and I went on a honeymoon to Niagara Falls. I can still remember how beautiful it was, on the American and Canadian sides. When I want a moment of peace, I think about that gorgeous, natural flow of water...

Clara: When I was a child, my whole family traveled to Washington, DC, at the time when the cherry blossoms bloomed. We loved the monument, the White House, and the museums. When we left our home in upper Pennsylvania, spring was just starting, and as we drove south, more and more blossoms kept coming out until we arrived at the Capital where everything was in full bloom. I love the spring. It's my favorite time of year.

Mr. Green: On our honeymoon, we went to Maine. We drove in our old Chevy along the east coast through Connecticut and Massachusetts. Maine is rugged and foggy, another world.

Mrs. Green: We wanted to have seafood—shrimp, lobster, and clams—mouth-watering just to think about it.

Judy: My family was into seafood, too, but we fished ourselves for crabs, flounder, and bluefish. We had our own boat, which was great, so we could go out anytime. My father and brothers didn't mind that I would come along—even though I was a girl. Then, my mom would cook it all up for us. Delicious. We still like to sit around and eat a ton of crabs together.

Jack: Speaking of food, my family loved to go pick elderberries, and gather wild raspberries and strawberries out of the fields. Then, we'd make elderberry jelly. We lived near an old quarry where there were frogs. Believe it or not, I once caught a few frogs, and my mom cooked them up. They tasted good, like chicken.

Student 2: Lots of talk of food. What other memories do you recall?

Gwen: When I was getting married, my family was on a budget so I went to the fabric store to buy silk for my bridal dress. I loved sewing and was able to make it fit perfectly. That was a dream come true for me...

Tom: My dream come true was getting a train set for Christmas one year. I loved building a layout of hills and houses, tunnels and streams for my trains to ride around. Each year, my parents got me a few more cars to add to the train. My friends would come over to play with me with the train.

Student 1: We haven't heard from the Kleins yet. What memories would you like to share?

Mr. Klein: We don't want to spoil the atmosphere of these pleasant memories. We came from Europe in 1946, and so our memories are sad.

Judy: You can still share your recollections with us. That's why we have this group... we are your friends.

Mrs. Klein: We were in a concentration camp, which we were lucky to survive. We had little to eat, had to work hard, and were humiliated. David played the violin so that helped him to survive because our captors wanted him to play for them. I worked hard

making bricks. We never knew if we would get sick or be thrown into the "ovens."

Clara: How did you two meet?

Mrs. Klein: When the Americans came to the camp, we were given food, and Miriam was helping to dole out the food. I cried when I saw her. She was an old neighbor of mine, but now looked like a skeleton.

Miriam: The best day of our lives was the day we arrived in America. Seeing the Statue of Liberty moved us to tears. We had to work hard to rebuild our lives, but were so happy to be here.

Student 1: I'm so glad you shared your memories and experiences with us today. You brought the group closer together. Without that, we would not have really gotten to know you.

Student 2: If you still have flashbacks or issues on your mind from that time period, you could talk to the retired psychologist at this center. He would be very confidential about your details. We know that to survive, sometimes prisoners had to do things that were far outside what they wanted to do...

The End.

Discussion

1. Do you think that the students related well to the group members in this reminiscence group?

2. Did they end the group in an appropriate manner?

3. Should they discuss this group process in their supervision meeting with the social worker in the center? With their professor of the fieldwork course at school? With their fellow students in their seminar for this fieldwork?

4. Are the memories of the participants part of their adjustment to development of social participation at this stage of their lives?

5. Should the students ask the group if they would like to have another reminiscence discussion if there are only 2 weeks left? Or do they need to bring closure to their time with the group with another activity and leave further in-depth discussion to the social worker to carry on after they finish their fieldwork?

6. What other activities can assist Third and Fourth Age group members to transition well into this stage of human social development?

7. Should students also suggest that members of this group volunteer in their communities in order to expand their social development while retired?

8. Do the members of this group assume leadership roles?

9. What level of group participation does this group manifest?

References

Adams, K. B. (2004). Changing investment in activities and interests in elders' lives: Theory and measurement. *International Journal of Aging and Human Development, 58,* 87-108.

American Association of Retired Persons. (2003). *Managing in the middle: A survey of informal caregiving.* Washington, DC: Author.

American Association of Retired Persons. (2004). Caregiving in the US. National Alliance of Family Caregiving. Retrieved February 19, 2009 from www.thefamilycaregiver.org/who_are_family_caregivers/care-giving-statistics.cfm

American Occupational Therapy Association. (2008). The occupational therapy practice framework: Domain and process (2nd ed.). *American Journal of Occupational Therapy, 62,* 625-683.

American Psychiatric Association. (2000). *Diagnostic criteria from diagnostic and statistical manual–IV–TR.* Washington, DC: Author.

Antonucci, T. C., & Jackson, J. S. (2002). Environmental factors, life events and coping abilities. In J. Copeland, M. Abou-Saleh, & D. Blazer (Eds.), *Principles and practice of geriatric psychiatry* (2nd ed., pp. 379-380). New York, NY: Wiley.

Atchley, R. C. (1989). Continuity theory of normal aging. *Gerontologist, 29,* 183-191.

Atchley, R. C. (1999). *Continuity and adaptation in aging: Creating positive experiences.* Baltimore, MD: Johns Hopkins University Press.

Atchley, R. C., & Barusch, A. (2004). *Social forces and aging: An introduction to social gerontology* (10th ed.). New York, NY: Wadsworth.

Backes, G. M. (1993). Importance of social volunteering for elderly and aged women. *Z Gerontology, 26,* 349-354.

Baltes, P. B. (1997). On the incomplete architecture of human ontogeny: Selection, optimization, and compensation as foundation of developmental theory. *American Psychologist, 52,* 366-380.

Baltes, P. B. (2005). *A psychological model of successful aging.* Keynote Lecture, 2005 World Congress of Gerontology, Brazil. Retrieved November 5, 2006 from www.baltes-paul.de/SOC

Baltes, P. B., & Baltes, M. M. (Eds.). (1990). *Successful aging: Perspectives from the behavioral sciences.* New York, NY: Cambridge University Press.

Baltes, P. B., & Carstensen, L. L. (1996). The process of successful aging. *Aging and Society, 16,* 397-422.

Baltes, P., & Smith, J. (1990). The psychology of wisdom and its ontogenesis. In R. Sternberg (Ed.), *Wisdom: Its nature, origins, and development.* New York, NY: Cambridge University Press.

Baltes, P., & Smith, J. (2001). *New frontiers in the future of aging: From successful aging of the young old to the dilemmas of the Fourth Age.* Retrieved April 22, 2005 from www.valenciaforum.com/Keynotes/pb.html

Baum, C., & Christiansen, C. (2005). Person-environment-occupation-performance: An occupation-based framework for practice. In C. Christiansen, C. Baum, & J. Bass-Haugen (Eds.), *Occupational therapy: Performance, participation, and well-being* (3rd ed.). Thorofare, NJ: SLACK Incorporated.

Birney, D., & Sternberg, R. (2006). Intelligence and cognitive abilities as competencies in development. In E. Bialystok & F. Craik (Eds.), *Lifespan cognition* (pp. 315-330). New York, NY: Oxford University Press.

Boeree, C. G. (2006). *Personality theories.* Retrieved November 19, 2006 Retrieved from www.ship.edu/-cgboeree/Jung

Bonder, B., & Hasselkus, B. (2003). Families and professionals, therapeutic considerations. In B. Bonder & M. Wagner (Eds.), *Functional performance in older adults* (2nd ed., pp. 487-499). Philadelphia, PA: FA Davis.

Bookwalter, R., & Siskowski, C. (2009). Family caregivers: Doing double duty. *Today in OT, 2,* 28-32.

Brintnall-Peterson, M. (2003). *Caregivers watch for warning signs of distress or depression.* Retrieved February 23, 2009 from www.uwex.edu/news/print.cfm?release

Buckner, R. L., Head, D., & Lustig, C. (2006). Brain changes in aging: A lifespan perspective. In E. Bialystok & F. Craik (Eds.), *Lifespan cognition* (pp. 27-42). New York, NY: Oxford University Press.

Caro, F. G., & Morris, H. (2001). Maximizing the contributions of older people as volunteers. In S. Levekoff, Y. K. Chee, & S. Nugochi (Eds.), *Successful & Productive Aging.* New York, NY: Springer.

Carstensen, L. L. (1992). Social and emotional patterns in adulthood. *Psychology and Aging, 7,* 331-338.

Cavanaugh, G. (2005). Civic engagement: American Society of Aging helps lead new approach to retirement. *Aging Today, 26,* 16.

Chambre, S. M. (1991). Volunteerism by elders: Demographic & policy trends past & future. In *Resourceful Aging Today & Tomorrow Conference Proceedings, Vol. II, Volunteerism.* Washington, DC: AARP.

Chevan, A. (1996). As cheaply as one: Cohabitation in the older adult population. *Journal of Marriage & Family, 58,* 656-667.

Christiansen, C. (2008). Envisioning a key role for occupational therapy to support healthy aging in the 21st century. In S. Coppola, S. Elliott, & P. Toto (Eds.), *Strategies to advance gerontology excellence* (pp. 501-512). Bethesda, MD: American Occupational Therapy Association.

Chui, H. (2001). *Cognitive marauders.* Downey, CA: McCarron Clinical Research and Education Center.

Cole, M. (2008a). Theories of aging. In S. Coppola, S. Elliott, & P. Toto (Eds.), *Strategies to advance gerontology excellence* (pp. 135-162). Bethesda, MD: American Occupational Therapy Association.

Cole, M. (2008b). Retirement, volunteering, and end of life issues. In C. Meriano & D. Latella (Eds.), *Interventions in occupational therapy* (pp. 371-401). Thorofare, NJ: SLACK Incorporated.

Coppola, S. (2008). A transactional approach to understanding meanings and benefits of occupation in older adulthood. In S. Coppola, S. Elliott, & P. Toto (Eds.), *Strategies to advance gerontology excellence* (pp. 15-58). Bethesda, MD: American Occupational Therapy Association.

Cornwell, B., Laumann, E., & Schumm, P. (2008). The social connectedness of older adults: A national profile. *American Sociological Review, 73,* 185-203.

Cumming, E., & Henry, W. (1961). *Growing old: The process of disengagement.* New York, NY: Basic Books.

do Rozario, L. (1998). From age-ing to sage-ing: Eldering and the art of being as occupation. *Journal of Occupational Science, 5,* 119-126.

Dorfman, L., & Moffett, M. (1987). Retirement satisfaction in married and widowed rural women. *The Gerontologist, 27,* 215-221.

Ellis, J. (1993). Volunteerism as an enhancement to career development. *Journal of Employment Counseling, 30,* 127-132.

Enfield, S., & Formichelli, L. (2003). Lessons from Grandma: The wisdom of our elders may be the best life tool available to us. *Delicious Living, January,* 84-88.

Erikson, E. H. (1978). *Adulthood.* New York, NY: Norton.

Erikson, E. H., & Erikson, J. M. (1997). *The life cycle completed.* New York, NY: Norton.

Ewald, P. R. (1999). Future concerns in an aging society. In W. C. Chop & R. H. Robnett (Eds.), *Gerontology for the health care professional.* Philadelphia, PA: F. A. Davis.

Goleman, D. (1988, June 14). Erikson, in his own old age, expands his view of life. *The New York Times, C1,* C4.

Greenfield, E. A., & Marks, N. F. (2004). Formal volunteering as a protective factor for older adults' psychological well being. *Journal of Gerontology Series B: Psychological Sciences and Social Sciences, 59,* S258-S264.

Guttman, M. (2001). The aging brain. *USC Health Magazine,* Spring.

Harvard School of Public Health. (2004). *Reinventing aging: Baby boomers and civic engagement.* Report highlights. Retrieved March 28, 2006 from www.hsph.harvard.edu/chc/reinventingaging/report

Hazzlewood, J. (2007). *You're never too old to be a cyber opsimath.* ASCCA National Conference. Sydney, Australia.

Henrietta, J., O'Rand, A., & Chan, C. (1993). Gender differences in employment after spouse's retirement. *Research on Aging, 15,* 148-169.

Himes, C. L. (2001). Elderly Americans. *Population Bulletin, 56,* 3-40.

Hoffman, M. (2002). *Self-awareness in family caregiving: A report of the family caregiver self awareness and empowerment project.* Bethesda, MD: National Alliance for Caregiving. Retrieved February 23, 2004 from www.cargiving.org

Holmes, T. (1978). Life situations, emotions, and disease. *Psychosomatic Medicine, 9,* 747-754.

Jones, B. (2000). *Smoothing the pillow? Or revving up and plugging in? Seniors and information technology. Premier's Forum on Ageing* (pp. 22-31). Sydney, NSW: Department of Aging, Disability, and Home Care.

Jonsson, H., Josephsson, S., & Kielhofner, G. (2001). Narratives and experience in an occupational transition: A longitudinal study of the retirement process. *American Journal of Occupational Therapy, 55,* 424-432.

Kerr, T. (1998). Occupational performance in retirement. *Advance for Occupational Therapy Practitioners, July 27,* 25-26.

Keyes, C. L. (2002). The exchange of emotional support with age and its relationship with emotional well-being by age. *Journals of Gerontology Series B: Psychological and Social Sciences, 57,* P518-P525.

Kielhofner, G. (2002). *Model of human occupation* (3rd ed.). Baltimore, MD: Lippincott, Williams & Wilkins.

Kleyman, P. (2003). Study shows how older volunteer force in US could double. *Aging Today, 24,* 1. Retrieved March 28, 2006 from www.agingtoday.org/at-241/Study_Shows_How.cfm

Knotts, V. K. (2008). Transitions for older adults. In S. Coppola, S. Elliott, & P. Toto (Eds.), *Strategies to advance gerontology excellence* (pp. 109-130). Bethesda, MD: American Occupational Therapy Association.

Kornhaber, A. (1996). *Contemporary grandparenting.* Thousand Oaks, CA: Sage Publications.

Kreutzer, J. Gervasio, A. & Camplair, P. (1994). Patient correlates of caregivers' distress and family functioning after traumatic brain injury. *Brain Injury, 8,* 211-230.

Kubler-Ross, E., & Kessler, D. (2005). *On grief and grieving: Finding the meaning of grief through the five stages of loss.* New York, NY: Scribner.

Larson, R., Csikszentmihalyi, M., & Graef, R. (1982). Time alone in daily experience: Loneliness or renewal? In L. A. Peplau & D. Perlman (Eds.), *Loneliness: A sourcebook of current theory, research, and therapy.* New York, NY: Wiley-Interscience.

Laslett, P. (1989). *A fresh map of life: The emergence of the Third Age.* Cambridge, MA: Harvard University Press.

Laslett, P. (1997). Interpreting the demographic changes. *Philosophical Transactions of the Royal Society of London: Series B, Biological Sciences, 352,* 1805-1809.

Leider, R. (2008). *Something to live for: Finding your way in the second half of life.* New York, NY: Barrett-Koehler.

Levinson, D. (1978) *Seasons of a man's life.* New York, NY: Ballantine Books.

Lockenhoff, C. E., & Carstensen, L. L. (2004). Socioemotional selectivity theory: Aging and health: The increasingly delicate balance between regulating emotions and making tough choices. *Journal of Personality, 72,* 1395-1424.

Lyyra, T. M., & Heikkinen, R. I. (2006). Perceived social support and mortality in older people. *Journals of Gerontology: Series B, Psychological Sciences and Social Sciences, 61B,* S147-S152.

Macdonald, K. C. (2000). Experiences of five women adapting to physical disability. *The Israel Journal of Occupational Therapy, 9,* E39-E62.

Mast, M. & Wakefield, M. (2003). *Rural family caregivers' perceptions of facilitators and deterrents to the use of in-home respite.* Alzheimer's & related diseases research award fund: Final report. Retrieved February 23, 2004 from www.vcu.edu/vcoa/2003finalreport.html

Mattingly, C. (1998). *Healing dramas and clinical plots: The narrative structure of experience.* Cambridge, MA: Cambridge University Press.

Morrow-Howell, N., Hinterlong, J., Rozario, P., & Tang, F. (2003). Effects of volunteering on the well-being of older adults. *Journals of Gerontology: Series B, Psychological Sciences and Social Sciences, 58,* S137-S145.

Musick, M. A., Herzog, A. R., & House, J. S. (1999). Volunteering and mortality among older adults: findings from a national sample. *Journals of Gerontology: Series B, Psychological Sciences and Social Sciences, 54,* S173-180.

Musick, M. A., & Wilson, J. (2003). Volunteering and depression: The role of psychological and social resources in different age groups. *Soc Sci Med, 56,* 259-269.

Neugarten, B. L., & Weinstein, K. (1964). The changing American grandparent. *Journal of Marriage and the Family, 26,* 199-204.

Potts, M. K. (1997). Social support and depression among older adults living alone: The importance of friends within and outside of a retirement community. *Social Work, 42,* 348-362.

Prensky, M. (2001). *Digital natives, digital immigrants.* Retrieved April 15, 2010 from www.marcprensky.com/writing/Prensky%20-%20Digital%20Natives,%20Digital%20Immigrants%20-%20Part1.pdf

Prisuta, R. (2003). Enhancing volunteerism among aging boomers. In Harvard School of Public Health, *Report of conference on baby boomers and retirement: Impact on civic engagement.* Retrieved March 28, 2006 from www.hsph.harvard.edu/chc/reinventingaging/report

Reitzes, D. C., & Mutran, E. J. (2004). The transition to retirement: Stages and factors that influence retirement adjustment. *International Journal of Aging and Human Development, 59,* 63-84.

Riello, R., Geroldi, C., Zanetti, O., & Frisoni, G. (2002). Caregivers' distress is associated with delusions in Alzheimer's patients. *Behavioral Medicine.* Retrieved February 23, 2009 from www.findarticles.com

Rosenkoetter, M. M., & Garris, J. M. (1998). Psychosocial changes following retirement. *Journal of Advanced Nursing, 27,* 966-976.

Rowe, J., & Kahn, R. (1998). *Successful aging.* New York, NY: Pantheon.

Scott, H. (1999). Seniors in cyberspace: Older people and information. *Strategic Ageing: Australian Issues in Ageing, 8,* 1-37.

Shalomi, Z. S., & Miller, R. S. (1995). *From age-ing to sage-ing.* New York, NY: Warner Books.

Spencer, J. (2003). Evaluation of performance contexts. In E. Crepeau, E. Cohn, & B. Schell (Eds.), *Willard & Spackman's Occupational Therapy* (10th ed., pp. 427-449). Philadelphia, PA: Lippincott, Williams & Wilkins.

Sternberg, R. (1985). *Beyond IQ: A triarchic theory of human intelligence.* New York, NY: Cambridge University Press.

Stone, W. (2003). *Ageing, social capital and social support.* Australia Institute of Family Studies submission to the house of Representatives Committee on Ageing Inquiry. Retrieved November 20, 2008 from www.aifs.gov.au/institute/pubs/research

Strawbridge, W. J., Wallhagen, M., Shema, S. & Kaplan, G. (1997). New burdens or more of the same? Comparing grandparent, spouse, and adult-child caregivers. *The Gerontologist, 37,* 505-509.

Tanz, J., & Spencer, T. (2000). Candy striper my ass! *Fortune, 142*(4), 156-160.

Tornstam, L. (1989). Gerotranscendence: A reformulation of disengagement theory. *Aging, 1,* 55-63.

Tornstam, L. (1997). Gerotranscendence: The contemplative dimension of aging. *Journal of Aging Studies, 11,* 143-154.

Tornstam, L. (2000). Transcendence in later life. *Generations, 23*(4), 10-14.

Tsao, T-C. (2004). New models for future retirement: A study of college/university-linked retirement communities. *Dissertation Abstracts International Section A: Humanities & Social Sciences, 64* (10A), 3511.

U.S. Bureau of Labor Statistics. (2004). *Volunteering in the United States.* Retrieved April 3, 2006 from www.bls.gov/news.release/volun.nr0

U.S. Bureau of Labor Statistics. (2009). *Occupational outlook handbook.* Retrieved February 6, 2009 from www.bls.gov.oco.ocosf078

Vaillant, G. E. (1993). *Wisdom of the ego.* Cambridge, MA: Harvard University Press.

Veninga, J. (2006). *Social capital and health: Maximizing the benefits.* Health Canada Reports & Publications. Retrieved November 26, 2006 from www.hc-sc.gc.ca/sr-sr/hpr-rpms/bull/2006-capital-social

Victoroff, J. (2001). *Saving the brain.* Downey, CA: Keck School.

Wakefield, L. (2001). *Helping flexible learners to identify their learning styles and preferences.* Paper presented at the 10th NCVER National Conference, Geelong, Australia, July 10-13.

Westermeyer, J. (2004). Predictors and characteristics of Erikson's life cycle model among men: A 32 year longitudinal study. *International Journal of Aging and Human Development, 58,* 29-48.

Wheeler, J. A., Gorey, K. M., & Greenblatt, B. (1998). The beneficial effects of volunteering for older volunteers and the people they serve: a meta-analysis. *International Journal of Aging & Human Development, 47,* 69-79.

Withnall, A. (2002). Three decades of educational gerontology: Achievements and challenges. *Education and Aging, 17,* 87-102.

Withnall, A. (2006). Exploring influences on later life learning. *International Journal of Lifelong Education, 25,* 29-49.

Wolff, L. (2003). *Brain research, learning and technology.* Retrieved October 20, 2004 from www.techknowlogia.org

Womack, J. L. (2008). Occupations of older adults. In S. Coppola, S. Elliott, & P. Toto (Eds.), *Strategies to advance gerontology excellence* (pp. 59-89). Bethesda, MD: American Occupational Therapy Association.

Wyant, S., & Brooks, P. (1993). The changing role of volunteerism [Abstract]. *Pap Ser United Hosp Fund NY, 23,* 1-37. PMID:10183986 [PubMed-Medline].

Yeager, C. (1985). *Yeager, an autobiography.* New York, NY: Bantam Books.

Additional Resources

Buettner, D. (2008). Find purpose, live longer. *AARP,* Nov-Dec., 32-34.

Kubler-Ross, E. (1969). *On death and dying.* New York, NY: Macmillan.

Sternberg, R. J. (1999). Intelligence as developing expertise. *Contemporary Educational Psychology, 24,* 359-375.

Social Participation Assessment

chapter 10

Social Participation and Disability Research

Mary V. Donohue, PhD, OTL, FAOTA

This chapter will direct the reader's attention to questions people have had about such an abstract concept as social participation. Beginning with colloquial questions, this chapter will then review the scientific basis for the therapeutic effect of social participation, beginning 2 centuries ago, spanning the years 1897 to the present. The factors associated with social participation range from providing people with a comfort zone to sustaining life in terms of survival. Research questions about social participation related to suicide, general mortality, heart disease, stroke, cancer, diabetes, and dialysis will be reviewed. Studies focused on age groups, negative interaction, the internet, and social participation will also be presented.

Social Participation Research Questions in Daily Life

Dean Ornish begins his book on *Love and Survival* (1999) by asking these basic questions related to situations of everyday life: "What's love got to do with it?" "If you became ill, is there a friend who would drive you to the hospital or would you have to take a taxi or ambulance?" "If you were broke, is there a friend who would loan you money?" "If you were sick, is there a friend who would help take care of your children until you felt better?" (pp. 28, 30). The direction of this line of questioning and the impact of possible responses are obvious to many people; however, others are outright skeptics about

the importance of social participation. Still others believe in the importance of social participation but do not incorporate this belief into their everyday lives. In any case, evidence-based research is necessary to provide a foundation for the rationale of social participation as a premise for a rich life as well as a condition for survival itself.

Durkheim: What Is the Relationship Between Social Participation and Suicide?

In the 1880s, Emile Durkheim's famous study empirically examined the association between suicide and social integration and moral regulation (1951). His data were collected from the statistics of several European countries. He postulated that egoistic suicide was associated with too little social integration, whereas altruistic suicide was associated with too much social integration. Egoistic suicides were carried out by isolated people, while altruistic suicides were committed by people willing to sacrifice themselves for the benefit of a group. Suicides due to moral regulation he labeled as *acute* or *chronic economic anomie* and *acute* or *chronic domestic anomie*. Anomie can be defined as a lack of purpose, identity, or ethical values, leading to disorganization or rootlessness in society or in an individual. The suicidal categories he describes as related to moral regulation have a social element as

Cole, M.B., & Donohue, M.V. *Social Participation in Occupational Contexts: In Schools, Clinics, and Communities* (pp 171-184).
© 2011 SLACK Incorporated

well. Economic conditions brought on by disasters, financial collapse, and immigration movements of large populations can cause despair about carrying out social responsibilities and cause a change in social status, leading to suicide. Durkheim associated acute and chronic domestic anomie with social mores in societies where widowhood, physical abuse, and disgrace are perceived as worthy of self-immolation or annihilation. The domestic category overlaps with his fatalistic category of childless and rejected women, slaves, the imprisoned, and those diagnosed with fatal diseases.

Recently, Kushner and Sterk (2005) contradicted Durkheim's study results, stating that the relationship between social cohesion and suicide had its limits because suicide is often highest among people with high levels of social integration. They state that looking again at his data on female suicide and suicide in the military limits Durkheim's proclaimed association of healthier people's relationship to high social cohesion. *How would you refute this line of thinking?*

Carpiano and Kelly (2005) responded that Kushner and Sterk downplay the importance of altruistic and fatalistic suicide associated with excessive integration. They point out that Durkheim proposed that both the extreme of too little or too much integration can lead to the pathology of suicide. Carpiano and Kelly in their response also refer to Putnam's definitive construct of social capital, which incorporates elements of economic, cultural, and human forms of capital, indicating that Kushner and Sterk have blended the concepts of social capital and social cohesion.

Relationships Between Social Participation and Cardiac Mortality

Multiple studies around the world have asked whether there is a relationship between social participation and cardiac mortality. A famous early study of people living in Roseto, Pennsylvania, (an Italian-American community) and other nearby towns was undertaken when it was noticed that the Roseto men had half the cardiac death rate of the national average (Stout, Marrow, Brandt, & Wolf, 1964). The lifestyle in Roseto typically had three generations in a house. There were many festivals, social clubs, and meals together every evening. There was a great deal of cultural, job, and family stability from about 1935 up to the 1960s. Death certificates from 1935 to 1985 were examined. During

the 1960s, lifestyle began to change, bringing about less cohesive family arrangements and fewer community relationships. People began to have fenced-in yards, private swimming pools, large single-family houses, and they began to move into suburban surroundings of Roseto. With these changes came an increase in the cardiac mortality rate. The data indicated differences in cardiac mortality rates between Roseto and other neighboring communities during the earlier period of greater social cohesion and support in Roseto as well as differences in the early and later Roseto community itself (Egolf, Lasker, Wolf, & Potvin, 1992).

Another well-known longitudinal study of 35 years is the Harvard Mastery of Stress Study (Russek & Schwartz, 2004). What it is best known for is responses to the questionnaire inquiring about feelings of parental caring. Identifying feelings of warmth and closeness to parents appeared to protect participants from coronary artery disease in midlife. While those who perceived warm and close relationships with their mothers and fathers only had a 45% rate of diagnosis with diseases including cardiac illness, hypertension, duodenal ulcer, and alcoholism, their Harvard peers who did not perceive themselves as having a warm relationship with their parents had a 91% rate of diagnosis with these illnesses. Parental social support thus appears to have provided a biological insurance against midlife illness.

Social networks have also been studied in conjunction with women suspected to have coronary artery disease (Routledge et al., 2004). Using the Social Network Index, 500 women were measured for psychosocial factors during a 2-year period. They were also assessed for coronary artery disease with quantitative coronary angiography. Women who reported having a greater number of people in their social network showed a decreased pattern of coronary artery disease. High social network scores were associated with lower ratings for coronary artery disease according to their angiogram stenosis measurements. In follow-up, mortality rates for low scorers on the Social Network Index had twice the death rate of high scorers.

In 2001, Ziegelstein examined the risk factor of depression after myocardial infarction. He found that patients with depression had less social support than those without depression. In fact, he found that patients reporting depression after a myocardial infarct are less likely to be married or to have at least one friend. They are also more likely to live alone. This type of social isolation has been reported on in a number of studies summarized by Ziegelstein and is associated with more frequent subsequent fatal and nonfatal cardiac episodes. High levels of social support decrease the impact of depression on mortality after myocardial infarct. One study Ziegelstein included in his summary study found that patients with depression who perceived that they had high levels of social support did not have a higher rate of mortality after myocardial infarct than patients who were not depressed (2001).

Lett et al. (2005) also did a primary review of social support as a risk factor, finding that low levels of support are associated with 1.5 to 2 times the risk for coronary heart disease. They indicate that it is not clear which types of support are associated with negative heart disease outcomes. This is an invitation to carry out further studies on this topic in the future.

In an effort to obtain further information regarding risk of patients for chronic heart failure, Schiffer, Denoliet, Widdershoven, Hendriks, and Smith (2007) decided to study patients with type-D personality. These are people who have high social inhibition and negative affect who tend to delay medical intervention. Three instruments were used to gather data: type-D Personality Scale, Health Complaints Scale, and the European Heart Failure Self-Care Behavioral Scale. These scales indicated that type-D personalities have insufficient self-management skills as indicated by a lack of reporting of symptomatology. The cardiac prognosis of such patients is risky due to their low social communication abilities, which interferes with reporting symptoms to their cardiologist or nurse.

Relationships Between Social Participation and Mortality

Some studies have looked at mortality in general, both including and without cardiac elements. An early, well-known study carried out in Durham, North Carolina, by Blazer of Duke University was begun in 1972 and examined social support and mortality in an elderly community focused on a group of 331 people older than 65 years (Blazer, 1982). Included in social support by Blazer were roles and available attachments, perceived social support, and frequency of social interaction. The study was conducted for 30 months after the preliminary evaluation. He identified 10 possible confounding variables, including age, sex, race, economic status, physical health, self-care, depression, cognitive functioning, and stressful life events.

Blazer examined each of the three major independent variables separately, finding that relative risks for mortality were associated in a rough calculation with impaired roles and lack of attachment

associated at 1.96 times greater than for those with socially related roles and secure attachment; for impaired social support as perceived by the participant at 3.86 times as great; and for impaired frequency of social interaction at 2.72 times as great. These three parameters of social support significantly foreshadowed mortality at 30 months going forward from the initiation of the study. In estimates of relative morality included in the regression model, the risk was 2.04, 3.40, and 1.88, respectively, for the three major factors. These three factors appeared to be distinct in both statistical calculations.

In a similar study conducted earlier, examining social networks and mortality in Alameda County, California, Berkman and Syme (1979) used the Human Population Laboratory survey. A random sample of almost 7,000 adults studied with a 9-year follow-up indicated that those who lacked social networks were more likely to pass away during the follow-up period than those who had a greater number of community and social ties. The risk comparing those most isolated with those who had more contacts was 2.3 times greater in men and 2.8 times greater in women for mortality. Of interest is the fact that the relationship between social ties and mortality was independent of the participants' reports on their physical health, socioeconomic status, and health practices, such as smoking, drinking, obesity, physical activity, and use of preventive health interventions.

In an effort to replicate the Alameda study, Schoenbach, Kaplan, Fredman, and Kleinbaum (1986) studied more than 2,000 participants in Evans County, Georgia, from 1967 to 1980. Using a tool similar to that of Berkman's Social Network Index, the analysis of their data pointed toward marital status, church activities, and other social networks as associated with survival over these years. There was lower survival rate among senior subjects with few social ties. They cited this aspect as the most important feature of the data.

Brummett et al. (2001) reported on a study that examined psychosocial characteristics of people with higher mortality rates in the Durham, North Carolina area to narrow down the detailed aspects of socially isolated people. The participants in this Duke University study had coronary artery disease. They found that those with three or fewer people in their social network had a risk of 2.43 times greater mortality (p = 0.001) for cardiac mortality and 2.11 times greater risk (p = 0.001) for all causes of mortality. They controlled for age and disease severity in this study. Aspects of income, hostility, and smoking status did not lower the risk from social isolation. Isolated patients did not differ from nonisolated patients on demographic indicators, physical functioning, or psychological distress. However, isolated patients reported less social support and were not as pleased with how they related to network members, despite the fact that they did not report dissatisfaction with the amount of social contact received. Associated physical and psychosocial variables did not differ significantly between isolated and nonisolated patients. Patients with small networks still had an elevated risk of mortality despite these other factors.

Locations as far flung as Australia and Canada found similar results in their longitudinal studies. In a study of 10-year survival in very old Australians, Giles, Glonek, Luszcz, and Andrews (2005) examined whether social networks with children, relatives, friends, and confidantes predicted survival after controlling for a range of demographic, health, and lifestyle variables. They found that greater networks of friends and confidantes were protection against mortality. However, the effects of social networks with children and relatives were not significant in relationship to survival over the 10-year period. It may be wondered whether children and families of the very old people in this study lived nearby.

In Canada, the researchers posed their question in a more positive vein, asking if social support and thriving health were associated. Richmond, Ross, and Egeland in 2007 measured the factors of social support related to positive interaction, emotional support, tangible support, affection, and intimacy. Among 31,000+ Canadians reporting on their health status, women reporting high levels of positive interaction were significantly more likely to report thriving health. In men, emotional support was related to thriving health. This study controlled for educational achievement and work status. Multivariate logistic regression analyses were used to estimate the odds of reporting thriving health, as this was a study based on self-report. Social support was the major independent variable. *Similar studies have been carried out in Sweden and Japan. You can find them online.*

The Relationship Between Social Participation and Stroke

A 5-year study, the Northern Manhattan Stroke Study, studied social isolation and outcomes post stroke. For both men and women (17% White, 27% Black, 54% Hispanic), this research found no association between post stroke outcomes and hypertension, diabetes, education, sex, insurance, occupation, marital status, or primary care physician in this multiethnic group. However, social isolation was associated with further stroke events after the initial stroke at a rate of 1.4 times in contrast to those who were socially related to others. Boden-Albala, Litwak, Elkind, Rundek, and Sacco reported on these findings in 2005.

Incidence of stroke among women with suspected myocardial ischemia was examined in conjunction with social networks of the participants. Routledge and colleagues (2004) believed that while the association between heart disease and social networks has been well-established, the relationship of stroke events in at-risk cardiac patients is currently not clearly confirmed. The participants were followed over an average of 6 years to track the incidence of stroke. Participants were given the Social Network Index to assess the frequency of 12 types of common social relationships and were evaluated using the Beck Depression Inventory. Women with smaller social networks had more elevated scores of depression. More isolated women had stroke occurrences at greater than two times the rate of those with a larger social network.

Relationships Between Social Participation and Cancer

In the realm of cancer research, there have been two types of studies: one type examining survival rate in conjunction with group therapy and another type looking at survival rate as associated with social networks. First, the research question about efficacy of group therapy will be discussed in conjunction with an ongoing controversy.

In 1989, David Spiegel and colleagues of Stanford University reported in *The Lancet* that psychosocial treatment for survival patients with metastatic breast cancer was extending their lifespan (Spiegel, Bloom, & Gottheil, 1989). He used professionally led support groups in what he calls supportive-expressive group therapy where women could share their fears and anticipatory loss of not being alive for milestone events in their families. Initially, it was feared that women might become demoralized by being in groups with others who might die. It appears that the women preferred to face their fears as they knew that they were all at risk of dying.

Over the years, other studies revealed mixed results while trying to replicate Spiegel's findings. Publications of comparable research indicated in four studies that there were both psychological and survival benefits of group therapy, while six other studies indicated that quality of life was improved by group therapy but not survival rates. Spiegel undertook another study in 1991 with a treatment of group therapy, psychotherapy, or educational materials alone. The women were followed for 10 years, with reports of improved levels of distress, anxiety, and pain. In this study, however, there was not a reduced survival rate associated with therapy. Those receiving therapy survived an average of 31 months, and the group receiving educational materials only lived an average of 33 months. Dr. Spiegel and colleagues conjectured that this change in results may have been brought about by an improvement in medical treatments and in the emotional climate for breast cancer patients now compared to during the 1980s (Spiegel et al., 2007). One subgroup did find that psychotherapy assisted women who had an aggressive type of breast cancer with estrogen receptive-negative tumors. These women lived an average of 30 months, which was 21 months longer than those who only received educational materials. The overall results of this study indicate that support groups help people live better, but not necessarily longer.

In another study employing treatment intervention for patients with malignant melanoma, Fawzy, Canada, and Fawzy (2003) followed participants with stage 1 cancer for 10 years. Those receiving intervention were given structured group meetings of 1.5 hours for 6 weeks including health education, stress management, coping skills, and psychological support. After 10 years, patients who had participated in the intervention survived longer; however, the effect of the psychosocial interventions diminished over time. The rate of recurrence for the control group (n = 34) was 11 people who subsequently died. In the intervention group (n = 34), nine people had a recurrence and died. However, the length of survival in the intervention group was significantly different over time.

Comparing the treatment group studies with general social support studies for people with cancer reveals a stronger result for social support. In one study of 2,835 women with stage 1 to 4 breast cancer, carried out from 1992 to 2002, 107 participants died from the cancer. Kroenke, Kubzansky, Schernhammer, Holmes, and Kawachi (2006) used the Berkman-Syme Social Network Index in 1992, 1996, and 2000 to assess the presence and availability of a confidante. Women who were socially isolated before their diagnosis had a 66% greater risk of general mortality and a doubled risk for cancer-specific mortality compared with women who were socially integrated. Women with social networks received radiation and tamoxifen with treatment more frequently than women who were socially isolated. Social networks were considered

to include close relatives, friends, and children. It was postulated by the researchers that social isolation may serve to limit access to care, particularly caregiving from friends and family, thus influencing outcome results.

Close relationships and emotional processing were studied by Weihs, Enright, and Simmens (2008) to "predict" mortality in women with breast cancer. Ninety women with stage 2 or 3 breast cancer were included in an 8-year study. In 21 women, the cancer reoccurred, and 16 died of cancer. Two types of close relationships were found to be associated with decreased mortality—a confiding marriage and a number of dependable supportive people in the community. Acceptance of emotion was also associated with lower disease progression. The researchers recommend that a larger study be carried out. A response to this study was published online in *Psychosomatic Medicine,* with a reply by the authors.

Relationships Between Social Participation and Diabetes

Social support and mortality among older people with diabetes was studied by Zhang, Norris, Gregg, and Beckles (2007). These researchers wished to ask the question: What pathways provide social support affecting diabetes' progression?

People 70+ years of age (n = 1,431) over the years suffered 387 deaths. Social support was assessed by gathering information on relatives, friends, neighbors, social events, churches, and senior centers. A regression analysis was used to find the pathway, and data on survival were analyzed to ascertain the relationship between social support and mortality. People who had moderate levels of support had a 41% lower risk of death, and people with high levels of support had a 55% lower risk of mortality. The study also identified 8 of the 11 regression models as showing that the effect of social support on mortality was influenced by moderator variables, such as physical and mental health status.

In a qualitative study of diabetes and family interactions among Blacks with Type 2 diabetes, Jones et al. (2008) wished to study the impact of family and friends on the management of diabetes care. They also wished to study the impact of a culturally designed group intervention. Participants were assigned to an individual education group or to a culturally tailored intervention group. Family members attended invited group sessions to obtain information about diabetes and to provide support for the person with diabetes. The data indicated that family and friends did impact the treatment and progress of the person with diabetes, sometimes positively and other times negatively. The information in this study demonstrated how difficult it can be to manage and control diabetes. For some participants, taking medications and monitoring glucose levels can be very challenging. *Why and when are qualitative studies used to ask research questions?*

Relationships Between Social Participation and Dialysis

Social support and survival in dialysis patients was the focus of a study by Thong, Kaptein, Krediet, Boeschoten, and Dekker (2007). They examined the process of dialysis in 528 patients in the Netherlands from 1998 to 2002. Patients' self-report was recorded on the Social Support List. Two aspects of social support were studied: interaction and discrepancy. When patients perceived a discrepancy between the support they expected, such as companionship and daily emotional understanding, and what they received, there was an associated increase in mortality. The association was similar for incident hemodialysis and peritoneal dialysis. These findings indicate the association between psychosocial risk factors and mortality in patients on dialysis.

Relationships Between Social Participation and Job Stress

Schnall, Lansbergis, and Baker (1994) compiled a summation of a number of studies of job strain and workplace social support. The effect of low social support on cardiac and vascular disease showed a positive association. One study of 288 male factory workers in New York City with a supportive foreman and coworkers indicated lowered blood pressure. Another study followed 7,219 employed Swedish men for 9 years, where isolated, high-strain work was associated with blood pressure with risk of hypertension.

In a 6-year prospective study of a French cohort of national gas and electric workers, four researchers asked if psychosocial work factors and social relations exert an effect on sickness absence. Melchior, Niedhammer, Berkman, and Goldberg (2003) studied middle-aged employees including 9,631 men and 3,595 women through self-report. Psychosocial work characteristics included social networks, personal social support, and social relations satisfaction. The researchers studied the frequency of short (<7 days), intermediate (7 to 21 days), and long (>21 days) absences. Among both men and women, the levels of decision latitude and personal social support below

the median predicted 17% and 24% increases in absence rates for these two factors. Low satisfaction with social relations and low social support at work led to a 10% to 26% excess in sick leaves among men. Other international studies of associations between social support and job stress may be found on the Internet.

Relationships Between Social Participation, Emotion Processing, and Social Skills in People With Schizophrenia

People diagnosed with schizophrenia were examined in a study by Schneider, Koch, Amunts, Bilker, and Ute (2006) for an ability to discern faces with and without emotion. Fifty people diagnosed with schizophrenia and 50 healthy people were matched for age, gender, and parental education. These participants were tested for the ability to identify faces displaying happiness, sadness, anger, and fear. This assessment revealed that people with schizophrenia were impaired in discrimination of emotional aspects of facial expressions compared to nonemotional aspects and memory. This impairment may cause misunderstanding in social communication and may be the basis for difficulties in social adjustment and participation in people with schizophrenia.

The Social Skills Performance Assessment was used by Harvey, Patterson, Potter, Zhong, and Brecher (2006) to determine if Quetiapine or Risperidone might improve social competence and social cognition. As part of an efficacy and tolerability study of atypical antipsychotics, 673 patients with schizophrenia were randomly assigned to the two medications. Both treatments enabled the patients to significantly improve their level of social competence. These results also supported the use of a performance-based competency assessment as an outcome measure for clinical medication trials.

A social skills training clinical trial at the UCLA Clinical Research Unit consisted of 200 possible interpersonal situations that used role playing methods to problem solve how VA patients could interact with others in the hospital, community, and family. This training was carried out 5 days a week for 2 hours a day with three patients and two therapists in each group. Additionally, once a week, a 2-hour session was devoted to the three patients, their parents and family members, with three cotherapists. The evening groups emphasized information, communication of feelings, making requests of others, active listening, and giving positive feedback. The clinical trial included a comparison group that received equally intensive holistic health therapy of jogging, meditation, yoga, art therapy, and insight-oriented family therapy. There was a third group of patients receiving standard hospital treatment. Patients were assessed at the beginning, middle, and 2 years after the study. Multiple types of measures were used to evaluate participants. After 1 year, the relapse rates were 21% in the social skills training group, 50% in the holistic health group, and 56% in the standard hospital treatment group. After 2 years, the patients from the holistic health group spent a significantly larger number of days in the hospital in contrast to the social skills training group. The carryover of the problem-solving social skills training resulted in generalization of both social skills and problem solving for these patients and families, with sustained social participation keeping patients out of the hospital.

Because the patient groups and family groups were combined in this first study, a second study was designed with family therapy using problem-solving role playing versus individual therapy. Only 6% of the family-treatment group relapsed during the 9 months of treatment; however, 44% of those in individual therapy relapsed. Details of the treatment for problem solving and communication skills are presented in Chapter 5.

"The Street Will Drive You Crazy" was published in *The American Journal of Psychiatry* by Luhrmann (2008) to help explain the concept of "high-cost social signaling" as being a hindrance for homeless people in acknowledging the label of "mentally ill" as applicable to themselves when they accept services. This concept represents the nonverbal signals society sends about success and being strong, by the clothes worn, the cars driven, and the job performed. Some people equate the acknowledgement of having mental illness as a weakness and being thought of as crazy. An ethnographic method of qualitative research was used to come to this conclusion: although homeless people may seem isolated, they are still influenced by the perceptions of society in general, creating pervasive social stressors.

Relationships Between Social Participation and Social Risk in Children

Burchinal, Roberts, Zeisel, and Rowley (2008) were curious about social risk and protective factors for Black children's academic achievement and adjustment during the transition to middle school.

Among the protective factors that these researchers found were good language skills and supportive parenting. Helping the children to anticipate less racial discrimination in the middle school was also supportive of a positive transition, especially in those previously exposed to adversity.

In a 2005 national poll sponsored by "America Speaks Out," 1,278 young people, ages 10 to 17, indicated that in urban, suburban, and rural neighborhoods they have serious concerns about their personal safety. Forty-four percent said that they needed to watch out for bullies.

- 4 in 10 said kids in their community fight too much.
- 3 in 10 said too many kids in their community have guns/knives/weapons.
- 3 in 10 stated that they do not feel safe walking alone in their community.
- 1 in 4 said that they do not have enough caring adults such as parents, coaches, and teachers in their lives.
- 45% wished that they had more adults they could turn to for help.

In a study of the "Steps to Respect" program, six investigators asked whether this intervention could reduce playground bullying. Frey et al. (2005) organized this study to randomly assign six schools of children in grades 3 to 6 (n = 1,023) to a bullying intervention program or a control condition. Pre- and post-test surveys of behaviors and beliefs about bullying were completed by the children. Observers also coded playground behavior, and teachers rated their classes. Analysis of changes in playground behavior demonstrated reduction in bullying and argumentative behavior among the intervention group children in contrast to the control group children. They reported increases in positive interactions and a reduction of destructive bystander behavior. Bystanders were taking more responsibility, and playground adult monitors were more responsive and less accepting of bullying/aggression than those in the control group.

Cyberbullying has also been studied recently in international venues. A survey by Beer (2006) states that research reveals cyberbullying to be a problem: flaming, online harassment, denigration, masquerading, and exclusion from an online group are common forms of cyberbullying. Online harassment and exclusion are the two most common occurrences. The internet is perceived as having a major role in teenage culture and has created a new locale for social interaction.

In a Research Brief, Smith, Mahdavi, Carvalho, and Tippett (2006) described their investigation into cyberbullying, published through United Kingdom government research reports. They identified seven categories of bullying: text messaging, video clip, cell phones, e-mail, chat room, Web sites, and blogs. About 20% of students polled said that they experienced cyberbullying at least once. About 6% had been cyberbullied for a few months. Phone calls, text messages, and e-mail were most commonly used in this British study. Chat room bullying was least common. About one-third of students had not told anyone about the incidents. Girls were more likely to be cyberbullied than boys. Students were asked how they perceived the impact of cyberbullying. Video or photo clips were perceived to have greater impact than traditional forms of bullying; however, Web site and text message bullying were considered about equal in impact to traditional bullying.

Cyberbullying among Turkish adolescents was also studied by Aricak et al. (2007), indicating that in a secondary school about 35% of the students had engaged in cyberbullying and about 23% had been bullying victims. Solutions for blocking the harasser were found by about 30% of the students.

For a PowerPoint presentation on cyberbullying, refer to www.pewinternet.org, NECC Internet Safety Town Hall (June 30, 2008) by Amanda Lenhart. The presentation is called, "Teens Online Stranger Contact and Cyberbullying. What the Research is Telling Us…" and is sponsored by PEW/Internet and American Life Project.

Look to another site, www.cyberbullying.us, for research with graphs and blog opportunities.

Relationships Between Aggression in Children and Intervention

Stauffacher and DeHart (2006) were curious about the transfer of aggressive behaviors in preschool children from home to school. In a longitudinal study of 46 children videotaped in free play situations at age 4 with siblings and at age 8 with peers, sibling aggression was displayed at a higher rate than with peers. Over time, there was a shift with relational aggression among siblings declining and aggression among peers increasing. The researchers conclude that it is important for early intervention in childhood so that the aggressive behaviors do not transfer to school.

In a study of mothers' responses to preschoolers' aggression, Werner, Senich, and Przepyszny (2006) examined mothers' affective and behavioral responses to their children's relational and physical aggression. The researchers used hypothetical stories for the mothers to read and questions to ask them about their responses in relational and physical situations of aggressive behaviors in children. Mothers reported their feelings, indicating that they would more readily intervene with physical aggression and less so for relational aggression in their children. The lack of intervention for relational aggression could impact children's future social competence.

Relationships Between Social Participation and Post-Traumatic Stress Disorder in Children

Kjorstad, O'Hare, Soseman, Spellman, and Thomas (2005) studied the effects of post-traumatic stress disorder (PTSD) on children's social skills. The *Social Behavior and Activity Observation Guide* included factors of tasks, structured games, interaction with adults, interaction with peers, and social behaviors. While PTSD had a negative effect on the social behaviors of children, this condition did not interfere with their participation in structured games. The scores for social behaviors including expressing emotions appropriately, controlling temper, and tolerating frustration were lower than anticipated; however, as this was a pilot study for the instrument used, it is not possible to make a clear comparison.

Relationships Between Social Participation, Shyness, and Sensory Processing

Two recent studies of shyness and sensory processing disorders in children relate to social participation in their designs. Shyness and the benefits of organized sports participation were examined in 355 elementary children averaging 10 years of age in Canada. The children filled out self-report assessments of their shyness and aggression, sport participation, and psychosocial adjustment. Parents also evaluated their children. The results after 1 year of study indicated that sport participation was positively related to positive adjustment of social skills. There was some evidence to suggest that sport participation can produce a protective role by reducing anxiety. The article titled, "Come Out and Play" by Findlay and Coplan (2008), discusses the role of sports as a social context that can amplify children's peer relations.

The study examining sensory processing asks how children's ability to participate in social activities is affected by this limitation. Two groups of children were compared, typically developing children and children with sensory processing difficulties (SPDs), by parents, teachers, and the children themselves. Social skills, problem behaviors, use of free time, activity preferences, and task competence were assessed. The findings indicated that children with SPD tended to have more problem behaviors and weaker social skills than their peers without SPD. Both groups of children had similar preferences for activities, but the children with SPD had fewer people in their social networks.

Look on the Internet for this dissertation study to be published in print.

Relationships Between Authenticity, Self-Esteem, and Aggression in Adolescents' and College Students' Participation

Impett, Sorsoli, Schooler, Henson, and Tolman (2008) wished to research the relationship of girls' authenticity in relationships and their self-esteem during adolescence. They used latent growth curve modeling to assess the association between relationship authenticity and self-esteem across 5 years with 183 girls. Girls in eighth grade who had high scores in relationship authenticity experienced greater increases in self-esteem over the course of adolescence. Girls whose scores in relationship authenticity increased also improved their self-esteem scores.

Adolescent inpatient aggression was examined in a study by Stafford and Cornell (2003) looking at characteristics of psychopathy. Psychopathy is described as disregard for social norms and values, habitual dishonesty, irresponsibility, shallowness, and lack of remorse. The Psychopathy Checklist was used to measure 72 adolescent inpatients' reactive and basic aggressive behaviors. Scores of higher psychopathy were related to greater manifestations of aggression. The authors remark that they hold open the possibility of change in adolescents. Nonetheless, the social dimensions of participation, such as attachment to others, feelings of empathy, and style of manipulation, appear to be related to inpatient adolescents' manifestation of aggression.

The relationship of anger and social skills to psychological symptoms in college students was studied by Conger, Conger, Edmondson, Tescher, and Smolin (2003). Seven hundred students were examined using the Brief Symptom Inventory, the State-Trait Anger Expression Inventory, and the Anger Inventory. Social skills were measured by the Social Skills Inventory and the Social Problem Solving Inventory. As far as social variables were concerned, problem orientation had the highest weights of any predictor variable. Problem orientation was associated with social sensitivity. Other results indicated that both anger and social factors were related to scores of psychological symptoms. Problem orientation appears to support appropriate social behaviors because it enables control and moderation of emotions. The results also suggest that usually high-anger individuals in college do not have strong negative immediate impact due to a lack of social knowledge; however, they do not implement the social skills that they have. The authors suggest therapy for controlling anger arousal. *What other explanation do you have for this discrepancy between knowledge and skill application?*

Relationships Between Social Participation and Internet Use

Shklovski, Kraut, and Rainie (2004) began researching the social consequences of using the internet, collecting data as early as 2000 with follow-up in 2001. Participants were asked about their social activities on the previous day, activities such as visiting, e-mailing, and calling friends and family. The results show a moderate relationship among these three types of social activities. The trend was that the more a person used the phone to contact a family member, the more often they also e-mailed and visited. Respondents communicated more in all three modalities with those they felt close to. The results of this study show that use of the internet reduces some social interaction, such as visiting. Among respondents who were heaviest users of the internet, the probability of visiting dropped from 70% to 49%. The authors treat the results as tentative, as patterns with internet use may have changed since 2001.

Young people's presentations of themselves and their relationships on a Swedish internet community were studied by Elm (2007). The meeting place online used for the study was Lunastorm, which was visited weekly at the time of this study by 500 Swedish young people ages 15 to 20. Girls tended to emphasize their general relationships, describing them with strong feelings. In the area of romantic relationships, however, both boys and girls used strong feelings to discuss the relationship and their partners.

A study in the Netherlands carried out by Van den Eijnden, Meerkerk, Vermulst, Spijkerman, and Engels (2008) looked at online communication, compulsive internet use, and psychological well-being among both male and female adolescents. In a longitudinal study of 6 months with 663 students, questionnaires were administered in a classroom setting. The results demonstrated that instant messenger use and chat room use were positively related to compulsive internet use 6 months later. High rates of instant messenger use were positively associated with depression 6 months later; however, it was negatively related to loneliness. This apparent contradiction in the results may raise questions about the perception of "loneliness" on the part of study participants.

Relationships Between Social Participation and Participatory Action Research

Participatory action research (PAR) has been lauded for its authenticity and empowerment of clients. This process of research includes planning of intervention programs and protocols with clients, patients, students, or community participants; follow-up study of interventions with involvement by participants; and planning of changes to the program in accordance with research findings and suggestions of participants. After implementation of the new program, examination of these interventions through further PAR methods is again carried out. It can be seen that this is a collaborative method to test intervention ideas and the use of new strategies in education, health, and community programs. This method employs professionals with expertise in teaching, therapy, medication, and activities, side by side with experienced students, clients, patients, and community participants who have been immersed in the protocol or program. PAR employs a sequence of cycles identifying the issues, illness, concerns, and problems as it proceeds. Reflection on learning from the actions is integral to this type of thoughtful and interactive intervention, instruction, and research. Everyone is involved as a participant. There are no passive recipients of instruction or intervention (Fals-Borda, 1955).

As an example of PAR, Taylor, Braveman, and Hammel (2004) worked together to present concepts and strategies of PAR for community social groups in two cases: examples of people with chronic fatigue syndrome and with autoimmune deficiency syndrome (AIDS). They provide a critical analysis of this approach in research and in practice situations.

Authentic participation in research includes personal and social decision making with consumer groups' goals, such as having a self-help organization, a center for independent living, and employment. There is discussion of how to involve participants with low energy levels and a state of deprivation in participatory research. Some adaptations were made to the usual procedures by the researchers for practical reasons based on the social and contextual environment of the participants.

While PAR sets out to empower students, clients, patients, and community group members, some critics (Cooke & Kothari, 2001) contend that it can be a political process designed by an "outsider" to achieve change in protocols and programs. Their work addresses the process of community and economic development through PAR. On the international scene, some critics of PAR consider it a way for international organizations to bypass local national institutions. However, such a bypass does not fit the original model of PAR. Kern has been leading a study (Kern, Kornblau, Roberts, & Mather, 2009) using PAR for people with heart disease by developing a health promotion education program for them. The study is focusing on self-management and health-promoting occupations for the participants.

Script: Student Research Dilemma

Setting and Participants

Three students are presented in several sessions of meetings to plan their masters' research project together. These students wish to carry out a qualitative study. They are meeting in an empty classroom in their academic department (Figures 10-1, 10-2, and 10-3).

Seating Chart

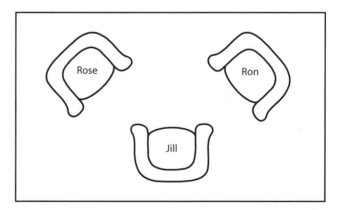

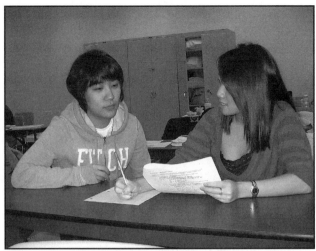

Figure 10-1. Qualitative research interview on social participation (Stony Brook University, Program in Occupational Therapy).

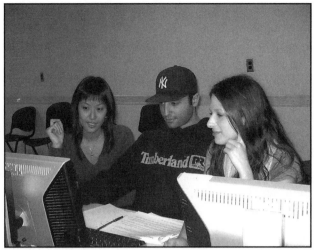

Figure 10-2. Analysis of group participation with computerized data entry (Stony Brook University, Program in Occupational Therapy).

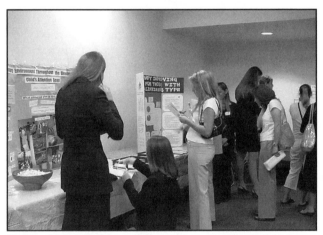

Figure 10-3. Students share their research projects at a conference for students and faculty at Quinnipiac University.

Action Begins Here

Rose: You both said that you'd like to do qualitative research. Do you have a question in mind?

Ron: Yes, I'd like to interview returning veterans from Iraq and Afghanistan.

Jill: That's a topic that would interest me, too. Our professor said we better find a topic that we are devoted to in order to maintain our commitment when the going gets rough.

Rose: What would our question be?

Ron: There were two that I had in mind: How do current support services help vets to re-adjust to past roles, especially if they are experiencing depression, post-traumatic stress disorder, or head trauma? I also was curious to hear from the vets as to how a holistic approach of occupational therapy could assist in complimenting re-adjustment services.

Jill: Maybe we could each do one interview, so we would have three veterans for our sample.

Rose: How can we contact them?

Ron: Let's go on the web and look at the VA Web site.

Jill: OK, let's all do that. How shall we handle the IRB form?

Rose: I'll get a copy of the form from the university Web site for Human Subjects, and we can fill it in together next week.

One month later.

Jill: I'm very discouraged. We received a letter from the IRB saying that, as first-year students, they don't think that we have the experience to interview returning veterans on such sensitive subjects as post-traumatic stress disorder and depression.

Rose: I talked to our professor, and she said that we can redesign our study.

Ron: Maybe we could interview therapists who work with the returning veterans and ask them our research questions. Let's divide up the VA Web sites we found and contact them again.

One week later.

Rose: Were you able to find any therapists working with these psychosocial aspects of returning veterans' adjustment? I could only find occupational therapists working with vets with physical disabilities.

Jill: That was my experience, too.

Ron: I found one occupational therapist who works at a VA hospital with veterans from earlier wars like Vietnam and Korea. He recommended that we contact an underground vets group that meet by themselves and pay their own professionals outside the VA system. We could interview those professionals.

Jill: Maybe we could do phone interviews.

Rose: Good idea. According to the IRB office, we need to draw up a Therapist's Consent Form/Letter and have those professionals sign it before we do the interviews by phone.

Jill: This study has become so far removed from our original plan.

Rose: OK, so this week we'll call people from the list we received on the Web site of the underground vets group.

One week later.

Jill: I found one therapist who is willing to do the interview by phone.

Ron: The two I contacted did not want to participate, so I'll have to keep looking. How did you do Rose?

Rose: I contacted one who wants to look over the Consent Form first before agreeing to be in the study. So, I sent him a consent letter 2 days ago.

Ron: This process is very slow, but our professor said that in our Power Point presentation we can report on our design, research questions, review of the literature, and the process with the obstacles we encountered.

Two weeks later.

Ron: I found an army occupational therapist working in a small community hospital in St. Louis who was willing to be interviewed.

Rose: My interview was with a psychologist re-adjustment counselor at a community Vet Center in Queens, New York.

Jill: I was finally able to interview a social worker readjustment therapist at the Vet Center in the local VA in Lower Manhattan.

Rose: Now, we can put together our presentation. I'm amazed that we accomplished this.

Jill: There were moments when I had my doubts about our topic and finishing it up.

Ron: It was frustrating, but I'm glad that we were able to do it!

The End.

Discussion

1. Did the three students carry out mutual group leadership? Did they all "pull their weight?"

2. Have you had similar types of frustrations in studies you are working on?

3. What other ways could they have changed their study design?

4. Did they indicate that they had prepared a script of questions to ask in the interview? Would you recommend that as a good idea? Is it also appropriate to deviate from the script when it seems warranted by the individual being interviewed?

5. Do you agree with the IRB decision that approaching veterans directly would have been too sensitive a subject for these students to handle? Could such discussion cause flashbacks?

References

Aricak, T., Siyahhan, S., Uzunhasanoglu, A., Saribeyoglu, S., Cipiak, S., Yilmaz, N., & Memmedov, C. (2007). Cyberbullying among Turkish adolescents. *CyberPsychology & Behavior, 11,* 253-261.

Beer, S. (2006). Magazine's research reveals cyberbullying problem. *IT NEWS Energy,* ITWire Technology Feature. Retrieved from www.itwire.com/content/view/4013/53

Berkman, L. F., & Syme, S. L. (1979). Social networks, host resistance, and mortality: A nine-year follow-up study of Alameda County residents. *American Journal of Epidemiology, 109,* 186-204.

Blazer, D. G. (1982). Social support and mortality in an elderly community population. *American Journal of Epidemiology, 115,* 684-694.

Boden-Albala, B., Litwak, E., Elkind, M. S. V., Rundek, T., & Sacco, R. L. (2005). Social isolation and outcomes post stroke. *Neurology, 64,* 1888-1892.

Brummett, B. H., Barefoot, J. C., Siegler, I. C., Clapp-Channing, N. E., Bytle, B. L., Bosworth, H. B., ... & Mark, D. B. (2001). Characteristics of socially isolated patients with coronary artery disease who are at elevated risk for mortality. *Psychosomatic Medicine, 63,* 267-272.

Burchinal, M. R., Roberts, J. E., Zeisel, S. A., & Rowley, S. J. (2008). Social risk and protective factors for African American children's academic achievement and adjustment during the transition to middle school. *Developmental Psychology, 44,* 286-292.

Carpiano, R. M., & Kelly, B. C. (2005). What would Durkheim do? A comment on Kushner and Sterk. *American Journal of Public Health, 95,* 2120-2121.

Conger, J. D., Conger, A. J., Edmondson, C., Tescher, B., & Smolin, J. (2003). The relationship of anger and social skills to psychological symptoms. *Assessment, 10,* 248-258.

Cooke, B., & Kothari, U. (Eds.). (2001). *Participation: The new tyranny?* London, England: Zed.

Durkheim, E. (1951). *Suicide.* Glencoe, IL: The Free Press.

Egolf, B., Lasker, J., Wolf, S., & Potvin, L. (1992). The Roseto effect: A 50-year comparison of mortality rates. *American Journal of Public Health, 82,* 1089-1092.

Elm, M. S. (2007). Young people's presentation of relationships in a Swedish internet community. *Young, 15,* 145-167.

Fals-Borda, O. (1955). *Action and knowledge: Breaking the monopoly with participatory action research.* Gainesville, FL: University of Florida Press.

Fawzy, F. I., Canada, A. L., & Fawzy, N. W. (2003). Malignant melanoma. Effects of a brief, structured psychiatric intervention on survival and recurrence at 10-year followup. *Archives of General Psychiatry, 60,* 100-103.

Findlay, L. C., & Coplan, R. J. (2008). Come out and play: Shyness in childhood and the benefits of organized sports participation. *Canadian Journal of Behavioural Science, 40,* 153-161.

Frey, K. S., Hirschstein, M. K., Snell, J. L., Edstrom, L. V. S., Mackenzie, E. P., & Broderick, C. J. (2005). Reducing playground bullying and supporting beliefs: An experimental trial to the Steps to Respect Program. *Developmental Psychology, 41,* 479-490.

Giles, L. C., Glonek, G. F. V., Luszcz, M. A., & Andrews, G. R. (2005). Effect of social networks on 19 year survival in very old Australians: The Australian longitudinal study of aging. *Journal of Epidemiology and Community Health, 59,* 574-579.

Harvey, P. D., Patterson, T. L., Potter, L. S., Zhong, K., & Brecher, M. (2006). Improvement in social competence with short-term atypical antipsychotic treatment. *The American Journal of Psychiatry, 163,* 1918-1925.

Impett, E. A., Sorsoli, L., Schooler, D., Henson, J. M., & Tolman, D. L. (2008). Girls' relationship authenticity and self-esteem across adolescence. *Developmental Psychology, 44,* 722-733.

Jones, R. A., Utz, S. W., Williams, I. C., Hinton, I., Alexander, G., Moore, C., ... & Oliver, N. (2008). Family interactions among African Americans diagnosed with type 2 diabetes. *The Diabetes Educator, 34,* 318-326.

Kern, S., Kornblau, B., Roberts, E., & Mather, P. (2009). *Using participatory action research to develop a health promotion education program for individuals with heart failure.* Panel conducted at the American Occupational Therapy Association 2009 Annual Conference, Houston, Texas.

Kjorstad, M., O'Hare, S., Soseman, K., Spellman, C., & Thomas, P. (2005). The effects of post-traumatic stress disorder on children's social skills and occupation of play. *Occupational Therapy in Mental Health, 21,* 39-56.

Kroenke, C. H., Kubzansky, L. D., Schernhammer, E. S., Holmes, M. D., & Kawachi, I. (2006). Social networks, social support, and survival after breast cancer diagnosis. *Journal of Clinical Oncology, 24,* 1105-1111.

Kushner, H. I., & Sterk, C. E. (2005). The limits of social capital: Durkheim, suicide, and social cohesion. *American Journal of Public Health, 95,* 1139-1143.

Lett, H. S., Blumenthal, J. A., Babyak, M. A., Strauman, T. J., Robins, D., & Sherwood, A. (2005). Social support and coronary heart disease: Epidemiologic evidence and implications for treatment. *Psychosomatic Medicine, 67,* 869-878.

Luhrmann, R. M. (2008). The street will drive you crazy: Why homeless psychotic women in the institutional circuit in the United States often say no to offers of help. *American Journal of Psychiatry, 165,* 15-20.

Melchior, M., Niedhammer, I., Berkman, L., & Goldberg, M. (2003). Do psychosocial work factors and social relations exert independent effects on sickness absence? A six year prospective study of the GAZEL cohort. *Journal of Epidemiology and Community Health, 57,* 285-293.

Ornish, D. (1999). *Love and survival.* New York, NY: Harper Perennial.

Richmond, C. A. M., Ross, N. A., & Egeland, G. M. (2007). Social support and thriving health: A new approach to understanding the health of indigenous Canadians. *American Journal of Public Health, 97,* 1827-1833.

Routledge, T., Reis, S. E., Olson, M., Owens, J., Kelsey, S. F., Pepine, C. J., ... & Matthews, K. A. (2004). Social networks are associated with lower mortality rates among women with suspected coronary disease: The National Heart, Lung, and Blood Institute-Sponsored Women's Ischemia Syndrome Evaluation Study. *Psychosomatic Medicine, 66,* 882-888.

Russek, L. G., & Schwartz, G. E. (2004). Feeling of parental caring predict health status in midlife: A 35-year follow-up of the Harvard Mastery of Stress Study. *Journal of Behavioral Medicine, 20,* 1-13.

Schiffer, A. A., Denoliet, J., Widdershoven, J. W., Hendriks, E. H., & Smith, O. R. F. (2007). Failure to consult for symptoms of heart failure in patients with type-D personality. *Heart, 93,* 814-818.

Schnall, P. L., Lansbergis, P. A., & Baker, D. (1994). Job strain and cardiovascular disease. *Annual Review of Public Health, 15,* 381-411.

Schneider, F., Koch, K., Amunts, K., Bilker, W., & Ute, H. (2006). Impairment in the specificity of emotion processing in schizophrenia. *American Journal of Psychiatry, 163,* 442-447.

Schoenbach, V. J., Kaplan, B. H., Fredman, L., & Kleinbaum, D. G. (1986). Social ties and mortality in Evans County, Georgia. *American Journal of Epidemiology, 123,* 577-591.

Shklovski, I., Kraut, R., & Rainie, L. (2004). The internet and social participation: Contrasting cross-sectional and longitudinal analyses. *Journal of Computer-Mediated Communication, 10,* 1-32.

Smith, P., Mahdavi, J., Carvalho, M., & Tippett, N. (2006). *An investigation into cyberbullying: Its forms, awareness and impact, and the relationship between age and gender in cyberbullying.* Research Brief, RBX03-06, July. Retrieved from www.dfes.gov.uk/research

Spiegel, D., Bloom, J. R., & Gottheil, E. (1989). Effects of psychosocial treatment on survival patients with metastatic breast cancer. *The Lancet, 2,* 888-891.

Spiegel, D., Butler, L., Giese-Davis, J., Copan, C., Miller, E., Domicile, S., ... & Kraemer, H. C. (2007). Effects of supportive-expressive group therapy on survival of patients with metastatic breast cancer: A randomized prospective trial. *CANCER,* September, 1.

Stafford, E., & Cornell, D. G. (2003). Psychopathy scores predict adolescent inpatient aggression. *Assessment, 10,* 102-112.

Stauffacher, K., & DeHart, G. B. (2006). Crossing social contexts: Relational aggression between siblings and friends during early and middle childhood. *Journal of Applied Developmental Psychology, 27,* 228-240.

Stout, C., Marrow, J., Brandt, E. N., Jr., & Wolf, S. (1964). Unusually low incidence of death from myocardial infarction. Study of an Italian-American community in Pennsylvania. *Journal of the American Medical Association, 8,* 1493-1506.

Taylor, R. R., Braveman, B., & Hammel, J. (2004). Developing and evaluating community-based services through participatory action research: Two case examples. *The American Journal of Occupational Therapy, 59,* 73-82.

Thong, M. S. Y., Kaptein, A. A., Krediet, R. T., Boeschoten, E. W., & Dekker, F. W. (2007). Social support predicts survival in dialysis patients. *Nephrology Dialysis Transplantation, 22,* 845-850.

Van den Eijnden, R. J. J. M., Meerkerk, G. J., Vermulst, A. A., Spijkerman, R., & Engels, R. C. M. E. (2008). Online communication, compulsive internet use, and psychosocial well-being among adolescents: A longitudinal study. *Developmental Psychology, 44,* 655-665.

Weihs, K. L., Enright, T. M., & Simmens, S. J. (2008). Close relationships and emotional processing predict decreased mortality in women with breast cancer: Preliminary evidence. *Psychosomatic Medicine, 70,* 117-124.

Werner, N. E., Senich, S., & Przepyszny, K. A. (2006). Mothers' responses to preschoolers' relational and physical aggression. *Journal of Applied Developmental Psychology, 27,* 193-208.

Zhang, X., Norris, S. L., Gregg, E. W., & Beckles, G. (2007). Social support and mortality among older persons with diabetes. *The Diabetes Educator, 33,* 273-281.

Ziegelstein, R. C. (2001). Depression after myocardial infarction. *Cardiology in Review, 9,* 1.

chapter 11

Social Participation Tools in Activity Settings

Mary V. Donohue, PhD, OTL, FAOTA

This chapter on social participation tools that can be used in activity settings is based on major studies in Chapter 8, whose tools have been used repeatedly in the past. It will also introduce other measures related to social participation, social networks, social roles, and social skills that appear to be most relevant and practical for assessment of these concepts. Calibration of these social factors is challenging to the authors of social measurement instruments and begins with defining these constructs and concepts. Briefly, social participation consists of interaction in activities with a social dimension, while social networks are made up of a linkage of people and groups that individuals are involved with at home, at work, or at leisure. Social roles are functional or official positions filled or fulfilled in human relationships, including familial, friendship, occupational, and group member or officer positions. Social skills are behaviors enabling interaction with other individuals or groups, which includes the ability to select and modify behaviors according to the specific relationship and setting. In discussing the tools in this chapter, their titles, authors, factors, format, and a description will be provided. For further information on these tools, the works of Hemphill-Pearson (1999) and Ascher (2007) present annotated details of purpose, population, timing, settings, materials, and sources. Web search engines are also valuable sources for exploration focused on any additional purposes of the individual reader.

Social Participation Measures

Parten's Participation and Mosey's Interaction Ordinal Scales

While not tools in the narrow sense of the term, Parten's sequence of descriptors for observation of activity group involvement are designated in three levels of play—parallel activity, associative play, and cooperative play—thus, creating an ordinal scaling of social participation. This continuum of social participation and interaction can be considered ordinal in nature as it places types of social involvement in a sequential order of natural growth and development (Figure 11-1).

In her description of parallel play, "The child plays independently, but the activity... brings him among other children. He plays with toys as he sees fit and does not try to influence or modify the activity of the children near him. He plays beside rather than with other children" (Parten, 1932, p. 250). In associative play,

The child plays with other children. The conversation concerns the common activity; there is a borrowing and loaning of play material... There is no division of labor and no organization of the activity... By his conversation... one can tell that his interest is primarily in his associations, not in his activity... merely doing whatever happens to draw the attention of any of them. (Parten, 1932, p. 251)

Cole, M.B., & Donohue, M.V. *Social Participation in Occupational Contexts: In Schools, Clinics, and Communities* (pp 185-198). © 2011 SLACK Incorporated

In cooperative play, "The child plays in a group that is organized for the purpose of making some material product, or of striving to attain some competitive goal, or of dramatizing situations of adult and group life, or of playing formal games." There is a division of labor, a taking on of different roles, and organization of the activity (Parten, 1932, p. 251). As an example, Parten uses the illustration of how activity at a sandbox could be done at all three levels. *Can you give examples to distinguish the behaviors of these levels?*

In her calibrated use of these levels, Parten used weighted scoring to differentiate the developmental social abilities and to attain a summated score for each child. She also used repeated measures, observing each child 60 times, in order to strengthen the statistical analysis and to obtain a broad picture of a child's performance. She considered changes in social participation part of the developmental process of socialization (Parten, 1932).

Mosey added to the scale of social participation of Parten by dividing the cooperative level into basic cooperative and advanced cooperative levels and adding a mature level of group interaction, thus, creating a five-level scale (1986; see Chapter 2). However, Mosey's work was not calibrated or analyzed empirically.

Knox Preschool Play Scale

Knox's Preschool Play Scale, revised in 1982, has four dimensions organized as subscales, with one subscale devoted to participation. All of the subscales are ordinal in nature, as they span the developmental periods of 0 to 72 months of age (0 to 6 years). Within 9 growth periods, Knox describes participation in great detail across four factors: type of interaction, cooperation, humor, and language. The text of this tool is rich in detail, providing good indicators of social behaviors considered typical in preschool children, and has been reported on in a book on play (Knox, 1997).

Social Participation Scale

A Social Participation Scale was developed by House, Robbins, and Metzner in 1982 and was used in a number of studies stretching from 1994 to 2008. This tool was also used to assess the level of participation in 10 social activities related to 8 clothing purchase decisions of rehabilitation clients (MacDonald, Bua-Iam, & Majunder, 1994). In 2002, a study in Ann Arbor, Michigan researched the effect of widowhood on social participation using the Social Participation Scale. Utz, Carr, Nesse, and Wortman (2002) were studying multidimensional aspects of both formal

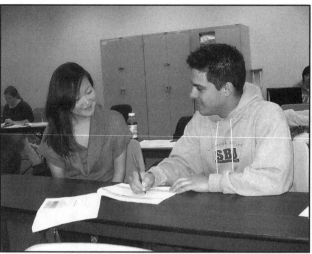

Figure 11-1. Reviewing social participation concepts of Parten's and Mosey's ordinal scale (Stony Brook University, Program in Occupational Therapy).

and informal social roles, which included meeting attendance, religious participation, and volunteer activities as formal aspects of social participation and phone calls and social contacts with friends as informal social participation. They found that both social strategies and resources influenced social participation. In a study carried out in Amsterdam, the Social Participation Scale was used to assess the relationship between societal participation, sociocultural activities, and word learning in older adults (Smits Maria, van Rijsselt, Jonker, & Hardy Deeg, 2004). This tool assisted these researchers in discovering that no one aspect of social participation independently predicted cognitive functioning; however, it revealed that organizational setting was an important influence.

Maier and Klumb (2005) used the Social Participation Scale to carry out a study in Berlin comparing time spent in social activities with direct interaction with others and time spent in social contexts while others are present with survival in older ages. Their findings imply that time spent conversing with friends has a stronger survival effect than time spent in activities with a social component; however, they recommend further research studying these two variables. Avlund, Lund, Holstein, and Due (2004) employed the Social Participation Scale in Denmark to evaluate social relations as a determinant of occurrence of disability in aging. They found that a large diversity in social relations and high scores of social participation were associated with prevention of disability risk.

In a study published in 2008, Dalemans, de Witte, Lemmens, van den Heuvel, and Wade employed the Social Participation Scale, along with 10 other

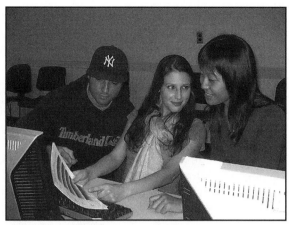

Figure 11-2. Using the social profile assessment tool to graph participation in an activity group (Stony Brook University, Program in Occupational Therapy).

instruments, as a measure for rating social participation of people with aphasia.

This group of researchers believed that the Community Integration Questionnaire was much closer to the concept of participation than nine other assessments evaluated. It is of interest that, despite its use in multiple studies in this country and abroad, the Social Participation Scale has not been reviewed by Buros' *Mental Measurement Yearbook.*

The RAND Social Health Battery

In 1984, Donald and Ware published an article about the RAND Social Health Battery used to measure social functioning in family, friendship, social, and community life. It consists of 11 items describing social connections in the format of a self-report questionnaire originally designed as part of RAND's Health Insurance Experiment. The frequency of going out, visiting another's home, telephone conversations, and volunteering in the community are included in this scale. Its validity was based on interviews with more than 4,000 people. Reliability of subscales of Social Contacts was 0.72, and 0.84 for Group Participation. The total score is a measure of social functioning as distinct from social support or role functioning.

The Social Profile

The Social Profile (Donohue, 2009) is a measure of social participation in activity groups that range from the family, to schools, clinics, clubs, and cultural, sports, or community groups. It is designed as a developmental sequence of interactive abilities in groups. Based on the work of Parten (1932) and Mosey (1986), the concepts of the five levels used in the Profile consist of *parallel, associative, basic*

cooperative, supportive cooperative, and *mature* levels of social function. The Social Profile's purpose reflects the principles of the World Health Organization's *International Classification of Functioning, Disability and Health* (2001), Chapters 7 and 9, emphasizing interpersonal interaction, relationships, and community, social, and civic life as essential to health (Figure 11-2).

The Social Profile has 40 items, divided into three topics of *activity participation, social interaction,* and *group membership/roles.* There are two versions of the Social Profile—the Children's Version and the Full Life Version. The first three levels of the Full Life Version make up the Children's Version. Studies of reliability, validity, and sensitivity have been carried out (Donohue, 2003, 2005, 2007).

Because groups and individuals may display and incorporate a number of levels in carrying out an activity, the instrument has been described as a profile, which can indicate the percentage of time spent at several levels during a session or across a longer period of time within a given activity. Adults participate at a parallel level in an exercise class despite their ability to interact at a mature level during other activities. Activities at times determine the level of group interaction of the individuals in the group. A highly structured AA meeting may only operate at a basic cooperative level, whereas a support group, focused on loss, may interact at supportive cooperative and mature levels. While this tool has not yet been published, it is described in Ascher's annotated index, *Occupational Therapy Assessment Tools* (2007, pp. 483-484). Additional information is provided on the Web site www.social-profile.com and online journals for the articles cited in this chapter (Donohue, 2009). Currently, Sok Mui Lim, an occupational therapist, is using the Children's Version of the Social Profile to study the social participation of children in Singapore as part of her doctoral research.

Social Network Instruments

Berkman's Social Network Index and Questionnaire

The Social Network Index was developed by Berkman (Berkman & Syme, 1979) to focus on the number of social ties an individual has and their relative importance. Using four network categories with various weighted scores, close contacts are given greater emphasis than acquaintances, as type and extent of social contact is calibrated in this index. The indicators of married partners, close friends and relatives, church membership, and informal and formal group associations, with the numbers of times encountered during a month, are specified. Employing this tool and the Human Population Laboratory Survey, Berkman and Syme (1979) participated in a ground-breaking study of Alameda county residents. In this study, they examined social networks, host resistance in physical health, and mortality. This work has been replicated in many studies mentioned in Chapter 7 (Berkman, 2007). A number of them have used the Social Network Index.

Mendes de Leon, Glass, and Berkman (2003) used the Social Network Index/Questionnaire to measure social engagement and disability in a community of older adults in New Haven, Connecticut. Strong social engagement in networks was associated with less disability.

Zunzunegui, Kone, Johri, Beland, Wolfson, and Bergman (2004) used variables of the Social Network Index in two French-Canadian communities to measure social networks and social integration. Health ratings were highly associated with a large level of social networks. Berkman's variables were used by Barnes, Mendes de Leon, Wilson, Bienias, and Evans (2004) during the Chicago Health and Aging Project in studying social networks and the levels of social engagement, finding positive correlations with cognitive function. Berkman's Social Network Index was also used by Kroenke, Kubzansky, Schernhammer, Holmes, and Kawachi (2006) to study social networks, social support, and survival after breast cancer diagnosis. Women who were socially integrated before diagnosis had lower levels of mortality than those with fewer social ties.

Social Network List

Hirsch (1979) developed a Social Network List with 13 network structure variables, including the size of the network, the number of confidantes, the dominance of relatives, and the density of the network. A premise of this list states that system and interactional variables help illustrate psychological strengths and weaknesses. Stokes (2007) studied satisfaction with social support by examining social network structure using Hirsch's list. The importance of the number of confidantes in the network emerged as paramount. Kazak (1987) studied stress and social networks in 1987 using Hirsch's Social Network List to study families with disabled children. The list revealed that mothers of disabled children had higher-density networks.

Lubben Social Network Scale

Lubben developed his Social Network Scale in 1988 to measure size, closeness, and frequency of a respondent's social network using 10 equally weighted items. This measure focused on the perceived support received from family, friends, and neighbors. There is a short version for clinicians and a longer version for social and health science research purposes, translated also into Spanish, Chinese, Korean, and Japanese. The scale has been used primarily with older adults. Low scores on this scale have been correlated with mortality, depression, and hospitalization for all causes. Lubben and Gironda (2003, 2004) have measured the benefits of social networks and the centrality of social ties to health status and the well-being of older adults.

Cohen's Social Network Index

Cohen developed a Social Network Index in 1991 to evaluate social participation in 12 kinds of social relationships, including those with an individual's partner, parents, in-laws, children, neighbors, friends, fellow workers, school friends, social, and sport, professional, civic, and religious group members. These relationships are assessed for contacts by phone or in person in 2-week periods and for the number of contacts they network with. This study is available online at www.psy.cmu.edu/~scohen/SNI.html. Using this tool, Cohen and colleagues have studied stress (Cohen & Wills, 1985), social support (Cohen, 1988), coping (Cohen, 1991), smoking and alcohol consumption (Cohen, Tyrrell, Russell, Jarvis, & Smith, 1993), and susceptibility to the common cold (Cohen, Doyle, Skoner, Rabin, & Gwaltney, 1997) as they relate to an individual's social network. This last study was rigorously designed with quarantine periods measuring the number of cold symptoms, viral cultures, and antibody response.

These objective illness criteria, with a decrease in the rate of colds, have an inverse association within increased social network diversity. The risk of colds increases among those with the fewest types of relationships. Data indicated that the number of relationships was not as important as having multiple types of relationships (Cohen et al., 1997).

Community Integration Questionnaire

Willer, with a group of professionals and consumers, developed the Community Integration Questionnaire (Community Integration Questionnaire [CIQ], 1998) as a tool to measure recovery from traumatic brain injury. Fifteen items related to home integration, social community integration, and productive activities are included. Scores are based on frequency of performing activities or roles, with secondary weight placed on activities done with assistance or jointly with others. The CIQ may be administered by phone or by the person with the traumatic brain injury. While formal training is not required to use the CIQ, it is recommended that new users contact Willer at the Centre for Research on Community Integration at the Ontario Brain Injury Association. Studies have provided evidence regarding reliability, validity, sensitivity, and other psychometric properties. The current version may be downloaded from www.tbims. org/combi/ciq/index.html. A new form, the CIQ-2, is being worked on through a NIDRR grant by Dijkers at Mt. Sinai School of Medicine in New York City.

Social Role Instruments

Adolescent Role Assessment

In 1976, Black developed a semistructured interview with a rating system of examining past and present roles, including 21 topics such as childhood play and current socialization in the family, at school, with peers, and in activities. The interview is a guide to having an investigational conversation with an adolescent. Content validity is based on developmental theories. Test-retest reliability for a small sample was 0.91. This tool has qualitative, narrative, and quantitative aspects.

Role Checklist

In 1982, Oakley began development of the Role Checklist as a self-administered questionnaire and rating form outlining the individual's perspective on participation in various life roles (Oakley, Kielhofner, Barris, & Reichler, 1986). The roles examined include student, worker, volunteer, caregiver, home maintenance, friend, family, religious, hobbyist, and organization participant (Dickerson, 1999). Reliability in test-retest averaged at 0.88. Concurrent validity with the activity configuration of Cynkin and Robinson averaged 0.78. The Role Checklist has been used in studies of community-living well adults and psychiatric and physical disability patients (Hemphill-Pearson, 1999). This study can be obtained from Frances Oakley of the Occupational Therapy Service of the National Institutes of Health (NIH). The Role Checklist was revised in 1988.

Role Activity Performance Scale

Good-Ellis developed the Role Activity Performance Scale (RAPS) in 1987 with colleagues working with psychiatric patients needing psychosocial intervention (Good-Ellis, 1999). It is a semistructured interview and rating scale using open-ended questions in 12 domains: work, education, home management, family, mate, parent, social relationships, leisure, self-management, health, hygiene and appearance, and treatment participation. These subscales are scored on a rating scale that takes time periods prior to hospitalization and earlier history into consideration. Validity scores correlated positively with scores on five other measures of role participation. Reliability intra-class coefficient scores on the RAPS for the 12 scales ranged from 0.82 to 0.99, with most correlations being above 0.90. The RAPS has been used in research with patients with schizophrenia and major affective disorders (Good-Ellis, 1999).

The social role aspects of the RAPS, in an examination of subscale role clusters associated with the general RAPS score, were influential in nuclear/extended family relationships, social relationships, and leisure activities, indicating that the RAPS role subscales are strong as a reflection of social participation. These areas also had predictive value for successful transition into roles after discharge.

Role Change Assessment

Originally developed by Jackoway, Rogers, and Snow in 1987, the Role Change Assessment (RCA) tool has undergone revision by Rogers and Holm (1999). The current version simplifies the role items and definitions, revises the structure of the measurement of role change, and designs the format for both clinical and research use. This instrument is of interest to clinicians and researchers working with people who are in transition in their lives due to injury, disease, trauma, disaster, job loss, death of a loved one, birth of a grandchild, full-time to part-time employment, remarriage, retirement, and relocation because it looks at the adaptation of individuals in these situations. It is also now designed to focus on the role function of older adults through a semistructured interview. The six role areas include relationships, self-care/home maintenance, productivity, leisure, organization, health and wellness. Scores indicate a shift from past to present with indications of frequency and change value; discussion of roles in the past are included and ranked.

In reliability studies, the average percent consistency of roles at present and 1 year ago was 95%. The average perceived change in the level of role participation was 66%. In a test-retest reliability study of the RCA (n = 11 retirees) comparing initial test day data, 1 day later data, and "past" designated as 1 year ago, the average correlation was 91%. Time value correlation was 93%, while meaning value was 91%. Agreement about changes over the year was 97% if the change was considered positive, 95% if considered neutral, and 65% if considered negative. If this is a norm for "negative" perceptions, then that can be considered a standard if this result stands up over time.

Content validity of the RCA was based on a review of literature, analysis by clinical experts, and input from participants in the pilot study.

Social Skill Tools

There are at least 20 social skill tools currently on the market. It appears that the category of social skill tools has been developed more extensively than that of previously discussed categories of social participation, social networking, and social roles. Three of these tools have been selected for their degree of clarity in focusing on the topic of social skills and on publication in literature, clinical settings, and research studies. Social skills are behaviors enabling interaction with other individuals or groups, which includes the ability to select and modify behaviors appropriate to specific relationships and settings.

Social Skills Rating System

Gresham and Elliott have studied social skills and published their studies with preschool and school children through the 1980s. Then, in 1990, they published the Social Skills Rating System (SSRS) through Pearson's Assessment Publishing Group (Gresham & Elliott, 1990). The general purpose of the SSRS includes assessing children who have problems with behavior and interpersonal skills, detecting problems underlying shyness, and selecting behaviors for treatment in order to plan and prioritize interventions. Since its invention, many additional studies have been undertaken using the SSRS (Gresham, 2000).

This tool examines both positive and negative behaviors. In the positive realm, this assessment tool evaluates cooperation, empathy, assertion, self-control, and responsibility. In the negative sphere, three subscales are included—externalizing problems, such as aggression and weakness in anger control; internalizing problems, such as sadness and anxiety; and hyperactivity, such as restlessness and impulsive acts.

There is structure for multi-rater comparisons and suggestions for intervention and the prevention of negative behaviors. In addition to the tool itself, there are forms for recording, assessment, and intervention plans and reports. The authors indicate that observers using the SSRS can evaluate their social skills program. Purchasers need to indicate qualification information before the tools will be sold.

Social Skills Inventory Manual

Reggio (1989) developed the Social Skills Inventory Manual to measure verbal and nonverbal social competence and emotional intelligence. It evaluates strengths and weaknesses in assessing six domain areas: emotional expressivity, emotional sensitivity, emotional control, social expressivity, social sensitivity, and social control in adults. It requires an eighth-grade reading level and 30 to 40 minutes to complete. The instrument has been used for individual and couples counseling, management and leadership training, and health psychology.

School Social Skills

Brown, Black, and Downs (1984) published *School Social Skills (S-3)* to assess how children relate to others in four categories: adult relations, peer relations, school rules, and classroom behaviors. Ratings are based on observation of student behavior. It is a criterion-referenced measure revealing a student's strengths and deficiencies in an educational setting with behaviors described as prosocial and antisocial. The results obtained from the scale may be used for the purpose of establishing Individual Education Plans (IEPs). The manual provides a valuable description of behaviors under the four categories, examined under 40 subcategories of behaviors and described in detail in a positive manner.

Social Skill Assessment Tools for Specific Groups and Settings

There are a number of additional scales that measure social skills in certain settings, with certain behaviors, for specific populations, and for designated diagnoses. These lists can be further explored on the web, with library search indices, Buros' Mental Measurement Yearbook online, or in Ascher's comprehensive index of assessment tools (2007) (Tables 11-1 and 11-2).

Social Participation Subscales

In some circumstances for assessment, therapists, teachers, and students prefer to use comprehensive assessment tools that include social participation or skill subscales, domains, areas, factors, or dimensions, as preferred by various evaluation tool authors. Some of these subscales can be used separately; however, most are embedded in a

---

Table 11-1

Tools for Assessment of Children's Social Skills

Gardner Social Developmental Scale (Gardner, 1994). (children 1 week to 8 years)

Infant Toddler Social and Emotional Assessment (Carter & Briggs, 2006). (children 12 to 36 months of age)

Preschool Behavior Checklist (McGuire & Richman, 1988). (early childhood)

Preschool and Kindergarten Behavior Scales (Merrell, 2002). (early childhood)

Burks Behavior Rating Scales (Burks, 2006). (children 4 to 18, who are disruptive, impulsive, and withdrawn)

Bell Relationship Inventory (Bell, 2005). (children 11 to 17, to assess object-relation factors)

Test of Playfulness (ToP) (Bundy, 1977, 1993). (for the observation of children)

Social Responsiveness Scale (Costantino, 2005). (children with autism)

Student Behavior Survey (Lachar, Wingenfeld, Kline, & Gruber, 2000). (for assessing school behaviors)

Social Communication Questionnaire (Rutter, Bailey, & Lord, 2003). (autism disorder in children and adults)

Adapted from Ascher, I. E. (Ed.). (2007). *Occupational therapy assessment tools. An annotated index* (3rd ed.). Bethesda, MD: AOTA Press.

Table 11-2

Tools for Assessment of Adult's Social Skills

Social Problem-Solving (D'Zullia & Nezu, 1990). (for social situations)

Social Adjustment Scale (Weissman, 1971). (for mental health or substance abuse)

Interpersonal Behavior Survey (Mauger et al., 1980). (for aggressive/assertive behaviors)

Assessment of Communication & Interaction Skills (Forsyth et al., 1998). (for interpersonal skills)

Adapted from Ascher, I. E. (Ed.). (2007). *Occupational therapy assessment tools. An annotated index* (3rd ed.). Bethesda, MD: AOTA Press.

---

comprehensive scale that incorporates other factors being measured. For example, an early tool including a Social Interaction Scale (SIS) component is the Bay Area Functional Performance Evaluation (BaFPE; Bloomer & Williams, 1979, 1987). It permits separate use of this scale, incorporating observations in 5 situations with a descriptive summary. The SIS component is just one of two areas being examined. Table 11-3 will indicate the portion of each assessment tool that is devoted to social factor evaluation so that the researcher, clinician, or student has an indication of how comprehensive versus how focused the particular tool is on social aspects.

Are there further social scale assessments that are newer on the market than this book? Search the Internet, databases, and indices at the library. These same sources can be used to locate the full references of the assessment tools discussed in this chapter.

Assessment of Social Competence Protocol

In Williamson and Dorman's book on *Promoting Social Competence* (2002), the focus is on information gathering by observing children and interviewing parents and teachers. Observation and interviewing skills need to be developed over time with experience. First, the authors recommend looking at the four aspects of interaction, including instrumental interactions, social emotional interactions, transitions among these two approaches, and appropriate interactions for given settings. The observer needs to determine if the child has acquired a skill but does not use it for some contextual or emotional reason.

The authors (Williamson & Dorman, 2002) suggest the use of some rating scales and questionnaires mentioned earlier, but emphasize the

Table 11-3

SOCIAL PARTICIPATION SUBSCALES, DOMAINS, AREAS, DIMENSIONS, COMPONENTS, AND FACTORS

NAME OF TOOL	FIRST AUTHOR	SOCIAL FACTORS
BaFPE	Bloomer	Social interaction scale
Satisfaction With Performance	Yerxa	Social/community problem solving, general problem solving
Vineland Adaptive Behaviors	Sparrow	Community socialization
Interpersonal Style Inventory	Lorr	Socialization, interpersonal involvement
Qual-OT Assessment	Robnett	Social issues
Community Integration	Willer	Social integration
Katz Adjustment	Katz	Socially expected activities
Philadelphia Geriatric Morale	Lawton	Lonely dissatisfaction
Participation Scale (WHO)	van Brakel	Communication, social and civic life, interpersonal interactions and relations
Transdisciplinary Play-Based	Linder	Social-emotional communication and language
MOHOST	Parkinson	Communication and interaction skills
Children's Assessment of Participation	King	Co-participation
WHO Quality of Life	Division of Mental Health	Social relationship
Sensory Processing	Parham	Social participation

Adapted from Ascher, I. E. (Ed.). (2007). *Occupational therapy assessment tools. An annotated index* (3rd ed.). Bethesda, MD: AOTA Press.

importance of interviews with the child, parent, or teachers. Sample interview questions for parents and children are provided in their book (pp. 72-73). Observations of behaviors in the classroom, cafeteria, and on the playground are recommended. During the interview with the child, problem-solving social situations can indicate where the child needs to develop further skills. Sociometric techniques are suggested, analyzing the children the child would most like to play with, work with, and those least attractive for these tasks.

There are three sample protocols provided for outpatient facilities, for a school-based practitioner, and for a classroom-based teacher. In an outpatient facility, the assessment protocol includes a phone interview with parents, review of records, an interview, and setting goals and objectives.

For the school-based practitioner, the authors recommend that the assessment protocol consist of consultation with the teacher, a review of the record, naturalistic observation, parent interview, and determination of interventions with other school personnel and the parents. As a classroom-based teacher, the assessment protocol can include observation of students, communication with the family, and determination of interventions. Some of the suggested interventions include referral to a social competence group, participation in therapy in pairs, inclusion in special after-school activities, guidance within usual classroom routines, preparation of a social competence program in the classroom curriculum to practice social skills, self-reflection, and social emotional learning (Williamson & Dorman, 2002, pp. 76-78).

An overall consideration for the assessment of social competence, as recommended by Williamson and Dorman (2002, pp. 79-80), is to consider the various environmental contexts and the interplay of settings on social interactions. For example, neighborhood play groups in contrast to classmate play groups, sports chosen by adults versus activities preferred by the child, sleep-away camp or day camp, going to the doctor or dentist office with a supportive family member, physical limitations, lack of nutrition or sleep, and too much television or computer time can all influence a child's behavior in these situations.

Williamson incorporates his "Components of Social Competence" tool (Williamson and Dorman, 2002, pp. 176-177) in an appendix of his book. Four social aspects are rated as rarely, sometimes, and often. They consist of social and play behavior, self-regulation, communication, and social decision-making.

Script: Family Crisis Intervention

Seating Chart

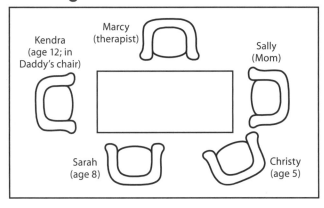

Characters and Situation

Arriving home from 4 days of evacuation due to the direct hit from Hurricane Ike in September 2008, a Houston, Texas family needed help. Although spared from flooding in their large four-bedroom home, two cats had wreaked havoc on the house in their absence, and they had lost power for nearly a week, rendering most of their food supply inedible. Meanwhile, damaged grocery stores, still without power, sold only nonperishable foods for cash (credit card connections and automatic teller machines did not work either). The water supply was declared unfit for consumption and had a brown, murky look. The three girls, ages 5, 8, and 12, would have to remain at home until the damage to their schools was repaired, while Dad is sequestered at work repairing an oil refinery. Mom, diagnosed with obsessive compulsive disorder, is completely overwhelmed and unable to cope. Her church pastor suggested that an occupational therapist might be helpful.

Sally: Age 36, mother of three girls, diagnosed with obsessive compulsive disorder, had given up her job as a social worker when Kendra, her oldest, was born. As a stay-at-home mom, she fills her days with housework, child care, and transporting her children to and from school and to their various after-school activities. Two days each week, she leads Girl Scout meetings in her home, as well as teaching a preschool class each Sunday morning at her church.

Wayne: Age 37, a chemical engineer for a large oil refinery, works long hours and has major responsibilities including being on-call even when home. As a father, he also takes over transporting the children, shopping, and home responsibilities when his wife cannot keep up. Wayne is not present for this meeting.

Kendra: Age 12, copes very well, and helps with the younger children. A gifted fifth grader, she is normally able to handle her studies and numerous after-school activities. However, in this situation, she is bored with staying home, missing school, and not seeing her friends. Without power, computers and cell phones do not work, and even reading is limited to daylight hours.

Sarah: Age 8, considered by Mom a "high maintenance" child, needing to stay busy or she gets into trouble. She is very bright, highly curious, and makes her own fun, often at the expense of household harmony. At school, Sarah attends occupational therapy twice a week for attention deficit disorder.

Christy: Age 5, follows her older sisters around, and they both love getting her into trouble. Without much discipline, Christy is used to getting everything she wants and quickly wears out her caregivers. She had just started kindergarten 2 weeks earlier and had not gotten used to getting up early.

Marcy: An occupational therapist with expertise in both pediatrics and mental health, arrives at the home of this family after her workday has ended, around 6 pm.

Action Begins Here

Marcy: *(rings doorbell, Sally opens the door)* Hi. I'm Marcy. Your pastor said you could use some help.

Sally: *(smiling)* Hello, I'm Sally. We've been expecting you. Come on in.

Kendra: *(kids run up behind Mom)* Who's at the door, Mom?

Sally: (*introduces children, all still in their pajamas*) As you can see, we really need some help.

Marcy: Well, I see you have your power back.

Sally: Thank the Lord, yes. It came on just this afternoon. Now, at least I can heat up Spaghetti-Os. Would you like to stay for dinner?

Marcy: I've eaten, but I'll sit with you if you like. Perhaps we can discuss the situation and what needs to be done.

Kendra: Everything needs to be done. Mom doesn't do anything but sleep all day. I have no clean underwear.

Marcy: Well, until now, the washing machine didn't work. Maybe you should give your Mom a break.

Sally: Yes, and the water is disgusting. I'm afraid anything I wash will turn brown. (*calling*) Christy, Sarah, come get dinner. (*Sally dishes out Spaghetti-Os from a pot in the middle of the table. Kendra brings some bottled water and a box of cookies and opens a can of fruit cocktail. Sarah opens a drawer, gets herself a spoon, sits, begins eating*)

Kendra: Sarah, everyone else needs one, too. Can you get us napkins, too?

Sarah: (*yells*) You do it. I'm eating!

Sally: Kendra, just do it. (*to Marcy*) Sorry about that.

Marcy: I see you are observing dinner time and keeping the kids fed—definitely hard to do without power or fresh food supplies. That's a good sign.

Sally: (*pleased*) Thanks. I just wish the rest of the day was more organized. Without school or Wayne being home, we have no routines.

Marcy: Let's start by telling me about what you did today. When did you all get up this morning? (*looking around the table*)

Sally: Oh, whenever. (*laughs*)

Kendra: I got up first, I think around 8. Christy wanted juice, and I gave her a box. She got her own cereal and dumped it all over the sofa. Sarah and Mom slept 'til practically noon.

Sally: Well, I had a rough night. Christy had a bad dream in the middle of the night. She came to my bedroom screaming, and we couldn't find the flashlight. It's so dark without power, and we're down to our last batteries.

Marcy: That's certainly understandable, but I think you need to have a set routine for everyone. When your normal structure gets interrupted, you need to create a new one. That gives each person some direction for the activities of the day and how the necessary work will get done. Does that sound like a good idea?

Kendra: A really good idea. I don't like playing Mom every morning. I can't wait to go back to school.

Sally: I guess we could do better. I didn't see the point in getting them dressed with no school and no place to go.

Marcy: Routines do more than that. They also give you a sense of well-being, so that helps you feel less stressed out.

Sally: That would be a good thing, for sure.

Marcy: (*takes out a large pad and a marker*) Let's begin with wake-up time. What time would be good to get up? We don't want to get used to sleeping really late, because what will happen when you go back to school?

Sarah: We'll be late. Mom always makes us late anyway. She has to check everything.

Marcy: She does? Well, I heard you sleep late sometimes, too. Don't you?

Sarah: (*with a grin*) Sometimes I do.

Marcy: How about 8 o'clock? (*they discuss and agree on 8:30-9:00am, Marcy writes it down and continues*) Now, what do you do when you first get up?

Christy: I know. Eat breakfast.

Sarah: On school days, we get washed and dressed first. Then, we come downstairs for breakfast.

Sally: This would be more like Saturday, though. No special time to get somewhere.

Marcy: So first we eat, then we get dressed. (*writes it on the schedule*) Who knows how to make their bed?

Sarah: I do.

Kendra: I don't usually take time, cause I'm rushing in the morning.

Sally: I should do it, but….

Marcy: Well, no one's in a hurry for a few weeks now. So, it's a good opportunity to get in the habit.

(*Sarah gets up and runs toward staircase*)

Sally: Hey, we're not finished eating, Sarah.

Sarah: (*yells from upstairs*) I'm going to make my bed.

Sally: Sarah has a problem with not listening. If Wayne were here, he'd give her a "time out."

Kendra: Yeah, but you wouldn't. (*to Marcy*) Mom doesn't discipline. She just yells.

Sally: SARAH! (*no response*)

Kendra: You see??

Marcy: (*smiling*) Let's see how she does. We'll go get her in a minute. So, what happens after breakfast? What's next?

Kendra: Watch TV—now that it works again.

Sally: No, I don't want you sitting bug-eyed in front of the TV all day.

Kendra: Yes, but…we can record shows at night and watch them in the morning. Like Supernanny.

Marcy: You watch Supernanny??

Kendra: I need some help to manage my little sisters. *(to Mom)* Someone has to.

Sally: Kendra, that's mean.

Kendra: Well, you don't, Mom. *(upset and teary eyed)* You stay in bed and expect me to be the Mom. But I'm a kid, too. *(wipes tears)*

Marcy: Could you give me an example, Kendra?

Sally: She's right. I get so overwhelmed sometimes when they all run in different directions, and I'm trying to do laundry or make dinner. I can't deal with their petty arguments.

Kendra: You think I don't get fed up, too? Like this morning. Sarah wanted to play with my Game Boy, and there was almost no battery left. That's my way to de-stress! So I grabbed it away from her 'cause she wouldn't let go. And Mom yells at me and tells me to give it back to her. Sarah just screams and gets anything she wants. It's not fair!

Marcy: *(to Sally)* There's some truth to what Kendra's saying. She needs you to be the Mom. You need to take charge and decide what's fair for Kendra.

Kendra: *(wiping more tears)* Yeah, Mom. I can't wait for Daddy to come home.

Sarah: *(returning to her chair)* Why are you crying, Kendra?

Sally: *(to Sarah)* We were just discussing what happens when you don't listen to Mommy. Didn't you hear me call you before?

Sarah: No. I was upstairs making my bed.

Kendra: Yes you did hear. You never listen!

Sarah: But I didn't hear. I didn't! *(upset voice)*

Marcy: What usually happens when you get up before you finish your dinner?

Sarah: Daddy makes me come back and finish eating.

Sally: *(to Marcy)* She's a slow eater. But she doesn't eat enough, and she's very picky. Wayne likes her to try different foods, and he insists that we all eat together when he's here. So they all know they have to sit here until everyone is finished.

Christy: Can I go play with Muffin and Bunny *(the cats)*? I'm all done.

Marcy: Could you stay while we finish our schedule? I'd really like your ideas, too.

Christy: Okay. I like to play with the kitties.

Marcy: Do you help take care of the kitties?

Christy: No. Mom does. Or Kendra.

Sally: That's another problem. I have to keep the cats locked up on the porch. Since the storm, they've been on a tear. *(shows them torn drapery, scratched sofa, smelly bathmat, broken picture frames, etc)*

Marcy: How could the kids help take care of them?

Kendra: Christy could feed them and change their water. But Mom won't let us help. She's afraid they'll get back in here and hide.

Sarah: Yeah, and it really stinks out there. *(points to porch)*

Sally: I have to change their litter. Something else I can't face.

Marcy: Why don't we put it on the schedule, and we'll go over who's going to do each thing. What chores could the kids help you do in the mornings, while they're home?

Sally: *(surveying the cluttered kitchen, partly unpacked duffel bags, overflowing laundry baskets in the hallway)* Where do I begin? Everything needs to be done. That's where I have problems. Because of my OCD, I have to do it a certain way.

Marcy: I can see why you're overwhelmed, if you can't accept their help. Would you consider teaching them the way you want some things done?

Sally: I could try.

Marcy: Okay. After breakfast, I'm writing chores. *(writes 10:00-12:00pm: chores)* Do the laundry, wash dishes, care for cats, take out trash. What else?

Kendra: I usually vacuum the rugs. The floors need mopping, but not with all this stuff everywhere.

(They divide up the chores. Christy—cats; Sarah—dishes; Kendra—laundry and vacuum; Mom—collect and take out trash, mop floors, generally clean kitchen and bathrooms, fix lunch and dinner.)

Sally: Trash is my biggest problem. So I have to see what's being thrown out. But everyone can fix their own breakfast and clean up. But no food in the family room, okay? *(all nod to agree)*

Marcy: So, we all do chores tomorrow morning. Mom will teach each of you how to do your chore. After lunch, what might be fun as a reward?

Christy: Let's play a game. Like game night on Fridays.

Sarah: I want to go outside. I'm bored being in the house every day.

Kendra: Let's go to the park. Can I meet my friend Jenny there? Please, Mom?

Sally: We could call her. Now that the phone is charged.

Kendra: *(runs toward phone)* Yippeee!

Sally: Not now, get back here. *(smiles in spite of herself)* Just wait until the schedule is finished. Then you can call.

Marcy: Okay, I'm writing down outdoor activity. You can sit down at lunch tomorrow, and if your chores are done, you can decide where you will all go together. But, Mom's in charge. Understand? What she says, goes. *(to Sally)* Are you up for that?

Sally: Well, I do feel much more organized. It's going to be hard, letting go of some things. But I'll try.

Marcy: It looks like everyone is done eating. Let's do one more thing. Make a quick list of what you need to do to get ready for bed. When's bedtime?

Kendra: 10 for me. Sarah and Christy should be earlier.

Sarah: 8:30, because I'm older.

Marcy: *(writes down bedtimes, makes list)* Who takes a shower before bed? *(kids all raise hands)* Okay, where do you shower?

Kendra: I use Mom's shower, because the upstairs bathroom is theirs. Mostly. *(smiles at Mom)*

Sally: We do let Kendra use ours, because they're all bathing at the same time.

Marcy: *(writes)* How about Christy—7:30, Sarah—8:00, Kendra—9:00? Would that work? (Nods yes from all) Now, everyone write on a card— *(hands out cards and pencils)* steps before bed: (1) clear own dishes from dinner, (2) finish homework, (3) take off clothes, hang up or put in hamper, (4) shower, (5) pajamas, (6) lay out clothes for tomorrow, (7) what else?

Sally: Christy and Sarah read a story. Also, we pray.

Marcy: Has everyone finished their list?

Christy: Wait, I'm not done.

Kendra: I'll help her.

Sally: That's okay, Kendra. I'll help Christy finish. You go call Jenny.

Kendra: *(surprised and relieved)* Thanks, Mom.

Marcy: Well, that was a great start. You all have a schedule to follow for tonight and all day tomorrow. It's time for me to leave now. How about I come by tomorrow after work and see how you all did with your routines?

Kendra: Great idea.

Sally: Thanks so much, Marcy. I feel much more relaxed with everything written down. *(gets up, puts schedule on the refrigerator, shows Marcy to the door)* You've been such a blessing. Thanks again for coming. See you tomorrow.

Marcy: Bye, kids. *(byes from all)*
The End.

Discussion

1. Define five specific problems or conflicts facing this family.

2. Which problems were caused by Hurricane Ike?

3. How did Sally's obsessive compulsive disorder affect her ability to deal with this crisis? Give three examples.

4. What strategies did Marcy use to help this family? Give three specific examples.

5. After reading this script, what problems can you predict might happen tomorrow? Describe and justify your predictions.

6. From the point of view of the character you played (or pick one character), how helpful do you feel Marcy's intervention will be? What will be the benefit for you (your character) if her suggestions are all followed?

7. What level of group interaction does this session represent and why?

Learning Activity

Look at Figure 11-3. How can you assess the problem-solving skills that perform this group task successfully? Can you use observational skills to evaluate the social interaction abilities needed for this task? What level of social participation does this group demonstrate?

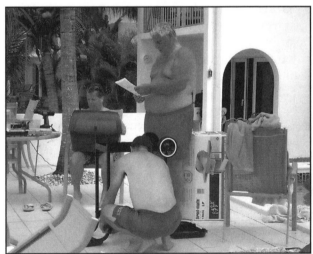

Figure 11-3. Three neighbors collaborating to assemble a new grill.

References

Ascher, I. E. (Ed.). (2007). *Occupational therapy assessment tools. An annotated index* (3rd ed.). Bethesda, MD: AOTA Press.

Avlund, K., Lund, R., Holstein, B. E., & Due, P. (2004). Social relations as determinant of onset of disability in aging. *Archives of Gerontology and Geriatrics, 38,* 85-99.

Barnes, L. L., Mendes de Leon, C. F., Wilson, R. S., Bienias, J. L., & Evans, D. A. (2004). Social resources and cognitive decline in a population of older African Americans and whites. *Neurology, 63,* 2322-2326.

Berkman, L. F. (2007). Social networks, health and aging. Measuring social activity and civic engagement among older Americans. Federal Interagency Forum on Aging-Related statistics. *Gerontological Society of America.* May 8, 2007. Retrieved from www.agingsociety.org/agingsociety/civic

Berkman, L. F., & Syme, L. F. (1979). Social networks, host resistance, and mortality: A nine-year follow-up study of Alameda county residents. *American Journal of Epidemiology, 109,* 186-204.

Black, M. M. (1976). Adolescent role assessment. *American Journal of Occupational Therapy, 30,* 73-79.

Bloomer, J., & Williams, S. (1979). *The Bay Area Functional Performance Evaluation* (research ed.). Palo Alto, CA: Consulting Psychologists Press; 12, 15.

Bloomer, J., & Williams, S. (1987). *The Bay Area Functional Performance Evalution* (2nd ed.). Palo Alto, CA: Consulting Psychologists Press, 1-2, 11.

Brown, L. J., Black, D. D., & Downs, J. C. (1984). *School social skills (S-3).* East Aurora, NY: Slosson Educational Publications.

Cohen, S. (1988). Psychosocial models of the role of social support in the etiology of physical disease. *Health Psychology, 7,* 269-297.

Cohen, S. (1991). Social supports and physical health. In A. L. Green, M. Cummings, & K. H. Karraker (Eds.), *Life-span developmental psychology: Perspectives on stress and coping.* Hillsdale, NJ: Erlbaum Associates.

Cohen, S., Doyle, W. J., Skoner, D. P., Rabin, B. S., & Gwaltney, J. M. (1997). Social ties and susceptibility to the common cold. *Journal of the American Medical Association, 277,* 1940-1944.

Cohen, S., Tyrrell, D. A. J., Russell, M. A. H., Jarvis, M. J., & Smith, A. P. (1993). Smoking, alcohol consumption, and susceptibility to the common cold. *American Journal of Public Health, 83,* 1277-1283.

Cohen, S., & Wills, T. A. (1985). Stress, social support, and the buffering hypothesis. *Psychological Bulletin, 98,* 310-357.

Dalemans, R., de Witte, L. P., Lemmens, J., van den Heuvel, W. J. A., & Wade, D. T. (2008). Measures for rating social participation in people with aphasia: A systematic review. *Clinical Rehabilitation, 22,* 542-555.

Dickerson, A. E. (1999). The role checklist. In B. J. Hemphill-Pearson (Ed.), *Assessment in occupational therapy mental health* (pp. 175-191). Thorofare, NJ: SLACK Incorporated.

Donohue, M. V. (2003). Group profile studies with children: Validity measures and item analysis. *Occupational Therapy in Mental Health, 19,* 1-23.

Donohue, M. V. (2005). Social profile: Assessment of validity and reliability in children's groups. *Canadian Journal of Occupational Therapy, 62,* 164-175.

Donohue, M. V. (2007). Social profile: Interrater reliability in psychiatric and community activity groups. *Australian Occupational Therapy Journal, 54,* 49-58.

Donohue, M. V. (2009). *Social Profile. Unpublished assessment tool.* Retrieved from www.Social-Profile.com

Good-Ellis, M. A. (1999). The role activity performance scale (RAPS). In B. J. Hemphill-Pearson (Ed.), *Assessments in occupational therapy mental health. An integrative approach.* Thorofare, NJ: SLACK Incorporated.

Gresham, F. M., & Elliott, S. N. (1990). *Social skills rating system (SSRS).* Minneapolis, MN: Pearson Assessment Group.

Gresham, F. M. (2000). Assessment of social skills in students with emotional and behavioral disorders. *Assessment for Effective Intervention, 26,* 51-58.

Hemphill-Pearson, B. J. (Ed.). (1999). *Assessments in occupational therapy mental health. An integrative approach.* Thorofare, NJ: SLACK Incorporated.

Hirsch, B. J. (1979). Psychological dimensions of social networks: A multimethod analysis. *American Journal of Community Psychology, 7,* 263-276. Retrieved from Trans.nih.gov/CEHP/HBPsocialconnectmeasures.htm

House, J., Robbins, C., & Metzner, H. (1982). The association of social relationships and activities with mortality: Prospective evidence from the Tecumseh Community Health Study. *American Journal of Epidemiology, 116,* 123-140.

Jackoway, I. S., Rogers, J. C., & Snow, T. (1987). The role change assessment: An interview tool for evaluating older adults, *Occupational Therapy in Mental Health, 7,* 17-37.

Kazak, A. E. (1987). Families with disabled children: Stress and social networks in three samples. *Journal of Abnormal Child Psychology, 15,* 137-146.

Knox, S. (1997). Development and current use of the Knox Preschool Play Scale. In D. Parham & L. Fazio (Eds.), *Play in occupational therapy for children* (pp. 35-51). St. Louis, MO: Mosby.

Kroenke, C. H., Kubzansky, L. D., Schernhammer, E. S., Holmes, M. D., & Kawachi, I. (2006). Social networks, social support, and survival after breast cancer diagnosis. *Journal of Clinical Oncology, 24,* 1105-1111.

Lubben, J., & Gironda, M. (2003). Centrality of social ties to the health and well being of older adults. In B. Berkman & L. Harootyan (Eds.), *Social work and health care in an aging society.* New York, NY: Springer.

Lubben, J., & Gironda, M. (2004). Measuring social networks and assessing their benefits. In C. Phillipson, G. Allan, & D. Morgan (Eds.), *Social networks and social exclusion: Sociological and policy perspectives.* Burlington, VT: Ashgate Publishing Company.

MacDonald, N. M., Bua-Iam, P., & Majunder, R. K. (1994). Clothing purchase decisions and social participation: An empirical investigation of U. S. and U. K. rehabilitation clients. *The Journal of Rehabilitation, 60,* 44-50.

Maier, J., & Klumb, P. L. (2005). Social participation and survival at older ages: Is the effect driven by activity content or context? *European Journal of Aging, 2,* 31-39.

Mendes de Leon, C. F., Glass, T. A., & Berkman, L. F. (2003). Social engagement and disability in a community population of older adults. *American Journal of Epidemiology, 157,* 633-642.

Mosey, A. C. (1986). *Psychosocial components of occupational therapy.* New York, NY: Raven Press.

Oakley, F., Kielhofner, G., Barris, R., & Reichler, R. K. (1986). The role checklist: Development and empirical assessment of reliability. *Occupational Therapy Journal of Research, 6,* 157-169.

Parten, M. B. (1932). Social participation among pre-school children. *Journal of Abnormal and Social Psychology, 27,* 243-269.

Reggio, R. E. (1989). *Social skills inventory (S-3).* Menlo Park, CA: Mind Garden, Inc.

Rogers, J. C., & Holm, M. B. (1999). Role change assessment: An interview tool for older adults. In B. J. Hemphill-Pearson (Ed.), *Assessments in occupational therapy mental health: An integrative approach* (pp. 73-82). Thorofare, NJ: SLACK Incorporated.

Smits Maria, C. H., van Rijsselt, R. J. T., Jonker, C., & Hardy Deeg, D. J. (2004). Social participation and cognitive functioning in older adults. *International Journal of Geriatric Psychiatry, 10,* 325-331.

Stokes, J. P. (2007). Predicting satisfaction with social support from social network structure. *American Journal of Community Psychology, 11,* 141-152.

Utz, R., Carr, D., Nesse, R., & Wortman, C. B. (2002). The effect of widowhood on older adults' social participation. *The Gerontologist, 42,* 522-533.

Willer, B. (1998). *Introduction to the Community Integration Questionnaire.* COMBI: The Center for Outcome Measurement in Brain Injury. Retrieved from www.tbims.org/combi/ciq

Williamson, G. G., & Dorman, W. J. (2002). *Promoting social competence.* Austin, TX: Hammill Institute on Disabilities.

World Health Organization. (2001). *International classification of functioning, disability and health (ICF).* Geneva, Switzerland: Author.

Zunzunegui, M. V., Kone, A., Johri, M., Beland, F., Wolfson, C., & Bergman, H. (2004). Social networks and self-rated health in two French-speaking Canadian community dwelling populations over 65. *Social Science and Medicine, 58,* 2069-2081.

Additional Resources

Dijkers, M. (2000). *The Community Integration Questionnaire.* The Center for Outcome Measurement in Brain Injury. Retrieved from www.tbims.org/combi/ciq

Donald, C. A., & Ware, J. E. (1984). The measurement of social support. *Research in Community Mental Health, 4,* 325-370.

Elliott, S. N., & Gresham, F. M. (1987). Children's social skills: Assessment and classification practices. *Journal of Counseling and Development, 66,* 96-99.

Hemphill, B. J. (Ed.). (1982). *The evaluative process in psychiatric occupational therapy.* Thorofare, NJ: SLACK Incorporated.

Rogers, J. C., & Holm, M. B. (1995). *The role change assessment: An interview tool for evaluating older adults.* Pittsburgh, PA: Unpublished role assessment tool.

Social Participation Interventions

Interventions for Children to Develop Social Participation Roles, Skills, and Networks

Mary V. Donohue, PhD, OTL, FAOTA

This chapter follows up on Chapter 6 and provides suggested interventions that can be used in children's various educational, treatment, and community settings. It will describe approaches to family social participation; social emotional learning; responses to bullies' interactions; and interventions for social competence development for children with learning disabilities, autism spectrum, and developmental disorders, such as self-regulation, communication, pro-social skills, and social decision making.

Children develop social skills gradually in their interactions with others by way of imitation (Bandura, 1977). Both at home and in school, they have the opportunity to take on social roles in groups as they play with other children, parents, and pets. Some people question whether children can form networks; however, children who have similar interests in hobbies, sports, television, books, e-mail, cell phones, and computer game characters often seek each other out in school and in neighborhood settings.

Early Social Environments

Interventions by Parents Affecting Children's Social Development

Parents first need awareness of their role in the social development of their children in the home. *Are they creating sibling rivalry? Are they favoring one child over another? Are they irritable in their interactions with their children, accusing or blaming them? Do they badger or bully their children? Do they use physical means of disciplining their children or physical abuse?* These are some issues raised by Dr. Spock (2001), which he indicates can be styles passed on from one generation to another. Parents need to treat each other with respect so that their children learn mutual respect for each other. Dr. Spock recommends that when children begin to argue or to act in a hostile manner to each other, the parent present must stop what he or she is doing, speak to the child kindly at eye level, talk about how each child is feeling, and how meanness does not solve the disagreement. Helping the children problem solve other options involves using a cognitive approach to finding a solution.

Children need to have fun with their parents (Figure 12-1). A number of parents recommend the Flippy and Friends children's book series (Kelsey & Meese, 2008) to help toddlers and parents laugh together. Appealing in its sing-song rhymes, healthy silliness, and amusing pictures, the Flippy books present a playful tadpole who can become anything he wants to be. Parents laughing with their children is the best part of any day.

If the child is an only child, the parents can introduce this child to other children at a playground so he or she can see and imitate parallel and cooperative play (Spock, 2001). If the parent observes children being bullied in one part of the playground, they can move to another part of the playground or to another park.

Cole, M.B., & Donohue, M.V. *Social Participation in Occupational Contexts: In Schools, Clinics, and Communities* (pp 201-228).
© 2011 SLACK Incorporated

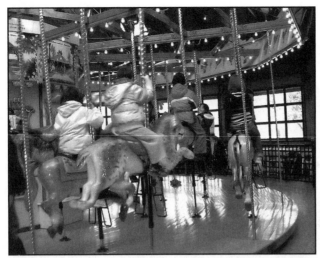

Figure 12-1. Children enjoy the sensory and social participation aspects of a carousel in both a parallel and associative mode interaction.

Parents can begin to invite a child's friends, one at a time, on trips to the zoo, movies, picnics, fishing, or sports in order to provide reinforcement for the friendship and an opportunity to observe the interactions. Invitations to family meals and sleepovers can expand a child's repertoire of social participation. Developing at least one good friendship during the pre-adolescent years is a way to begin relating to others in an enjoyable manner (Spock, 2001). Parents can ask children what after-school activities they would like to join in order to find other children with similar interests who may be potential friends. Family meals together provide opportunity for communication and bonding to the family group. Children who do not have the home environment where meals are shared are twice as likely to smoke and drink, and three times more susceptible to use other drugs, according to a study conducted by the National Center on Addiction and Substance Abuse (Mosher, 2005). Look up LIFT (Linking the Interests of Families and Teachers) on the web for support with parenting.

Intervention of Loose-Part Materials on a Playground: Social Play Increases

Working with teachers on a playground, loose-part materials were introduced to 5- to 7-year-old children in a typical middle-class schoolyard. The materials included car and bicycle tires, hay bales, cardboard boxes, plastic barrels, lengths of tubing, pieces of fabric, foam pieces, crates, and wooden planks. In addition, bags of balls and jump ropes were available. The children's interaction with

these materials on the supervised playground not only increased the creativity of the children, but increased social play with more discussion of the content of their play and more cooperative play. According to the playground monitor and observers, incidents of aggressive behavior on the playground became less frequent with playground duty becoming "more settled" (Bundy et al., 2008).

Teachers reported children "having a great time" and "loving" the materials. Children who became leaders in the activities with loose-part materials were different from the children who had been leaders in the physical games and sports, thus providing a new social opportunity with this added variety of interaction (Bundy et al., 2008).

Social Emotional Learning Programs

Social emotional learning (SEL) is a process of acquiring knowledge about our emotions and the emotions of others, as well as developing the awareness of how we relate to others in our interactions, the impact we have on their emotions, and their response to these interactions. SEL develops in the home, from parents, with siblings, extended family, community participation, and exposure to the media. Adjustment to these environmental factors can be provided in school and community programs. The proliferation of these programs nationwide indicates the extent of the need for such interventions for children. There are a number of approaches to imparting this learning, which are still being researched, refined, and redesigned (Goleman, 1995).

Creating a School Climate for Social and Emotional Education

Cohen (2006) has founded a Center for Social and Emotional Education, now called the National School Climate Center, to develop a positive climate in schools through the creation of social, emotional, ethical, and democratic academic education. The environment Cohen seeks to establish is a school community where children can learn to share and acquire knowledge from each other (Cohen & Devine, 2007).

Here, the climate permits collaborative enterprise in grades from preschool through high school. The needs of all students in the classes are assessed to determine who needs further exposure and more practice for the development of social participation.

The quality and character of school life in this program of social climate development includes

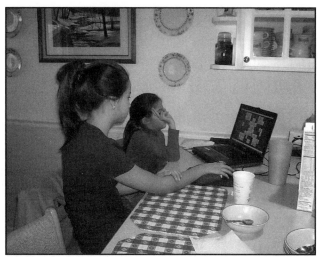

Figure 12-2. Demonstrating a basic cooperative level of participation, these girls assist each other with computer skills and a game.

safety, relationships, teaching, learning, and the environment (Cohen, 2006). The National School Climate Center presents a paper online titled, "The School Climate Challenge," designed to develop school climate policy and practice guidelines for teacher education.

Cohen encourages people to recall days at school when they felt safe, when they loved a class group, admired a teacher treating all with respect, and felt involved in meaningful learning (Cohen, 2006). The total climate in the school becomes the environmental intervention that shapes learning and student development. The result of this type of climate fosters academic achievement, prevents negative interactions among children, and facilitates positive emotional growth in children through a collaborative learning community (2006).

Teachers, clinicians, and group leaders working with children who wish to learn about school climate best practices may request a copy of the 2006 MSS Education report. School climate policy is delineated by a joint effort of the National School Climate Center and the Education Commission of the States through a national policy scan (Cohen, McCabe, Michelli, & Pickeral, 2009), describing the gap between research and policy.

This program recommends a preliminary assessment of the school climate using a tool available through the National School Climate Center. Teachers, students, and parents can then collaborate in a model designed to foster learning by doing joint democratic meetings of students/teachers/parents aimed at fostering connectedness to the school community (Cohen et al., 2009). This process of analysis of the climate assessment, problem solving, and joint planning of change, events, and development of peer panels

with teacher/parent guidance is not only designed to improve school climate but is in itself a process to be used throughout life at home, work, and in the community. Children from grades 3 or 4 onward can be gradually introduced to this process by having class officers, roles, and committees for cooperation with the intent of developing social participation.

Collaborative for Academic, Social, and Emotional Learning

The focus of the Collaborative for Academic, Social, and Emotional Learning (CASEL) as a central clearinghouse is to encourage professionals involved in education to foster social and emotional learning in addition to basic academic skills. They define SEL as a "process through which children and adults develop fundamental emotional and social competencies to recognize and manage emotions, develop caring and concern for others, establish positive relationships, make responsible decisions, and handle challenging situations constructively" (CASEL, 2008).

While there is overlap with the goals of the National School Climate Center, the emphasis at CASEL is more on individual behavioral development in a social setting, whereas the National School Climate Center emphasis is on social climate having an impact on interpersonal interaction. In SEL behavioral training, students learn how to calm themselves when angry, how to approach others to initiate friendly relationships, how to resolve conflicts in relationships respectfully, and how to make ethical and safe choices in school, on the playground, and in the community. The CASEL program points out that the contexts where children feel respected and valued are an essential component in SEL. In this process, safe, nurturing settings where guidance is provided are prerequisites for students to feel comfortable in identifying their emotions to themselves and to others (Zins, Elias, & Maher, 2007; Figure 12-2).

The program designed by CASEL offers training and support workshops at various times of the year at the University of Illinois, Chicago, as well as at national educational and psychological conferences. Free PowerPoint presentations, DVDs free and for purchase, and books on SEL are available at www. casel.org. An example of a PowerPoint presentation provided is "Policy Supports for School-Based Mental Health Promotion: The Case of Social and Emotional Learning (SEL) in IL and Beyond." CASEL also offers workshops for administrators to help them understand and interpret the Illinois Children's Mental Health Act.

Table 12-1

ILLINOIS STATE BOARD OF EDUCATION: THREE MAJOR SEL GOALS AND SEL STANDARDS

SEL GOAL 1: DEVELOP SELF-AWARENESS AND SELF-MANAGEMENT SKILLS TO ACHIEVE SCHOOL AND LIFE SUCCESS.

A. Identify and manage one's emotions and behaviors.

B. Recognize personal qualities and external supports.

C. Demonstrate skills related to achieving personal and academic goals.

SEL GOAL 2: USE SOCIAL AWARENESS AND INTERPERSONAL SKILLS TO ESTABLISH AND MAINTAIN POSITIVE RELATIONSHIPS.

A. Recognize the feelings and perspectives of others.

B. Recognize individual and group similarities and differences.

C. Use communication and social skills to interact effectively with others.

D. Demonstrate an ability to prevent, manage, and resolve interpersonal conflicts in constructive ways.

SEL GOAL 3: DEMONSTRATE DECISION-MAKING SKILLS AND RESPONSIBLE BEHAVIORS IN PERSONAL, SCHOOL, AND COMMUNITY CONTEXTS.

A. Consider ethical, safety, and societal factors in making decisions.

B. Apply decision-making skills to deal responsibly with daily academic and social situations.

C. Contribute to the well-being of one's school and community.

Adapted from Illinois Learning Standards: Social/Emotional Learning. (2008). Retrieved from www.isbe.net/ils/social_emotional/standards.htm

---

Illinois Learning Standards: Social Emotional Learning

An excellent example of a program of intervention in schools for SEL is found on the Web site for the Illinois State Board of Education at www.isbe.net/ils/social_emotional/standards.htm. Three major goals and SEL standards are included in Table 12-1.

On the cover page of the Web site, there are "text page" icons that reveal the subgoals given here above, as well as examples of activities designed to foster the achievement of these goals in school and at home. Some examples of performance descriptors are given in Table 12-2, which correspond with the letters outlined above.

They provide specific examples indicating the processes that can be used as principles or suggestions to bring about change in social behaviors, to consolidate social skills, and to describe social roles for children and adolescents in school and at home. Additional suggested performance descriptor intervention activities can be found on the Web site, providing a model for a learning framework.

The Illinois Learning Standards' three major goals above are programmatically arranged for five levels of intervention: early elementary, late elementary, middle junior high, early high school, and late high school. These levels are presented on the Web site in a well thought-out continuum that provides adequate examples of performance descriptors without incorporating too much detail. This program intervention with its three major goals and learning standards, accompanied by benchmarks and performance descriptors for behavioral change and social activities, is a prototype for other state education departments and local school districts to study and emulate in order to develop the social participation of their students. As rationale, looking back at the studies of Cohen et al. (2009), and Zins et al. (2007), indicates how SEL interventions improve academic levels of children and adolescents in schools, providing a positive community climate.

Caring School Community

Another SEL program that is nationally recognized is the Caring School Community (CSC) (2008a). This is a research-based intervention program for grades K to 6 designed to develop classroom and school-wide community. Their philosophy is similar to that of the National School Climate Center and the Center for School Climate, which believe in the strengthening of connectedness to school as a

Table 12-2

ILLINOIS LEARNING BENCHMARKS AND PERFORMANCE DESCRIPTORS FOR THREE MAJOR SEL GOALS

SEL GOAL 1: DEVELOP SELF-AWARENESS AND SELF-MANAGEMENT SKILLS TO ACHIEVE SCHOOL AND LIFE SUCCESS.

A. Name the emotions felt by characters in stories.

B. Describe situations in which you feel you need help.

C. Describe a behavior you would like to change.

SEL GOAL 2: USE SOCIAL AWARENESS AND INTERPERSONAL SKILLS TO ESTABLISH AND MAINTAIN POSITIVE RELATIONSHIPS.

A. Explain how sharing with and supporting others may make them feel.

B. Describe rules that help students treat each other fairly.

C. Practice sharing encouraging comments with others.

D. Practice self-calming techniques for anger management as a way to de-escalate situations.

E. Describe situations at school in which classmates might disagree and experience conflict (refusing to share supplies, not apologizing for hurt feelings, making false accusations, excluding someone from a group or activity).

SEL GOAL 3: DEMONSTRATE DECISION-MAKING SKILLS AND RESPONSIBLE BEHAVIORS IN PERSONAL, SCHOOL, AND COMMUNITY CONTEXTS.

A. Describe situations when you might feel unsafe and need help, such as bullying.

B. Practice group decision-making with classmates in class meetings.

Adapted from Illinois Learning Standards: Social/Emotional Learning (SEL). (2008). Retrieved from www.isbe.net/ils/social_emotional/standards.htm.

---

motivator to enhance academic work and reduce drug involvement, violence, and delinquency (Blum, McNeely, & Rinehart, 2002). Resnick and colleagues, in their National Longitudinal Study of Adolescent Health, found that students who feel connected to their school are less likely to use alcohol and illegal drugs, to engage in violent or deviant behavior, to become pregnant, or to experience emotional distress and suicidal thoughts or attempts (Resnick et al., 1997).

The CSC program has received recognition from the U.S. Department of Education for its research base and effectiveness. Its premise is that school connectedness builds meaningful student participation. One strategy used by the principal of one school is to bring the sixth-grade children into the junior high a year in advance to observe classes, meet the principal and teachers, and have an opportunity to get to know students from other sixth grades in the district. Disengagement from school, by students in high school, impedes completion of a high school education. Researchers also pointed out that students who connect to the school are also developing skills that they will need to be productive adults in society (CSC, 2008b). This Web site

points out that developing connectedness among children is as important as developing connections between the child, school, and parents.

The CSC Web site states that, "School connectedness refers to the belief by students that adults in the school care about their learning and about them as individuals." Blum and Libbey (2004) emphasize that school connectedness is influenced by individuals, such as students and staff; environment, such as school climate and bonding; and the culture of the school, such as social needs and learning priorities (CSC, 2008a).

In carrying out their research, Blum et al. (2002) stated that,

When middle and high school students feel cared for by people at their school and when they feel like they are part of school, they are less likely to engage in unhealthy behaviors. When they feel connected to school, they also report higher levels of emotional well-being. (pp. 1-20)

Libbey (2004) noted that researchers use a variety of indicators to measure school attachment or connection with some degree of overlap in consistency. These factors include such important variables as academic engagement, belonging, discipline, fairness, liking for school, extracurricular activities, student input in decision making, peer relations, safety, and teacher support. Measuring school connectedness, Blum et al. (2002) based their results on response to statements such as:

× I feel close to people at the school.

× I am happy to be at this school.

× I feel like I am part of this school.

× The teachers at this school treat students fairly.

× I feel safe in my school.

Klum and Connell (2004) found a relationship between school connectedness and academic work. These researchers consider student participation to be a strong predictor of student achievement and social behavior in school. Socioeconomic status was not an intervening variable in their study. They found that students involved in school receive higher grades and have better attendance with lower dropout rates.

The CSC intervention program looks to three theories for a theoretical base of the positive role of connectedness in school. First, they cite the attachment theory of Bowlby, which was described in Chapter 6. In fact, the CSC philosophy and experience has seen children who did not form a caring attachment to their parents learn to work hard in school, avoid negative behaviors, and develop positive milestones of social participation if they meet up with and attach to caring schools and teachers.

A second theory base for the CSC could be the theory of avoidance of deviancy. This theory incorporates four elements: (1) involvement in the school, (2) attachment or affective relationships, (3) commitment to the school, and (4) belief in the values of the school and class group. Development of these components is believed to assist students in moving toward positive behaviors and away from deviant behaviors (CSC, 2008b).

A third theory, social development theory, believes that social interaction helps to develop cognitive abilities through the complexities of social participation. It also indicates that bonding with positive people leads to positive societal rewards, and bonding with negative people leads to situations of delinquency, academic failure, and low-level and problematic lifestyle.

Promoting Alternative Thinking Strategies Enhances Social Participation

An intervention that is often cited as effective in reducing aggression and behavior problems in elementary school is the curriculum titled, "Promoting Alternative Thinking Strategies" (PATHS), based on the Affective-Behavioral-Cognitive-Dynamic (ABCD) model of psychosocial development of social emotional competence. One of the main principles of the ABCD intervention is that awareness of emotions is the basis of a child learning coping skills to regulate his or her behaviors in accordance with social-cognitive understandings he or she has learned. The major introductory lessons include the following:

× The Readiness and Self-Control Turtle Unit

× The Feelings and Relationship Unit

× The Problem-Solving Unit

In getting ready for this program, the image of a turtle is used to slow down impulses, delay gratification, reduce stress, and understand how self-talk can be helpful. In the unit on feelings, the self-awareness lessons include teaching about identifying feelings, labeling feelings, expressing feelings, evaluating the strength of feelings, managing feelings, understanding the difference between feelings and behaviors, reading and interpreting social signs and cues, listening to the outlook of others, having a positive attitude toward life, being aware of nonverbal communication abilities, and using verbal communication skills. Finally, presenting steps for problem solving and decision making gives students more power in controlling their environment.

Originally designed as part of Pennsylvania's Conduct Problems Prevention Research Group work in the 1990s, 198 first-grade classrooms from crime-ridden neighborhoods were randomly assigned to use the PATHS curriculum, with 180 first-grade classes selected as a control group. A 57-lesson curriculum of PATHS was presented to the first group; educators and counselors were trained to use this prevention intervention for preschool through sixth grade.

The study was designed to compare the social competencies of students in both groups (Greenberg, Kusche, & Mihalic, 1998). To assess the changes hoped for, the researchers used teacher interviews to obtain reports on classroom interactions, student interviews to assess sociometric class interactions among students, and observer ratings of classroom atmosphere ranked on a Likert scale. PATHS students were significantly higher than the control group on sociogrammatic reports by student peers. The PATHS students had lower reports of aggression, hyperactivity, and other disruptive behaviors. These results of lower aggressive behaviors were sustained through to the end of fourth grade according to student peer reports.

Kam, Greenberg, and Kusche (2004) studied special education students in 18 classrooms of grades 1 to 3. The classes were randomly assigned to interventions with PATHS curriculum or control classes. The PATHS classes received higher ratings by observers for their general atmosphere and maintained a 3-year lowering in the rates of self-reported feelings of depression. The PATHS classes manifested more positive long-term improvement in external and internal behaviors in contrast with the control group.

Reading, Writing, Respect, and Resolution Program

Currently, a program focused on social and emotional learning strategies and violence prevention has been funded by several grants under the direction of Aber at New York University, and Brown and Jones of Fordham University, for grades K to 5 in 18 New York city schools. The social, emotional, and academic development of children, and the professional development of their teachers are being examined in the process. This program is integrated into the language arts classes in which students read relevant emotional and aggressive situations, write about their own social responses in similar situations, discuss respect of children's emotions in these scenarios, and create resolutions for change of emotional and social responses.

International Social Emotional Learning Program of Reggio Emilia, Italy

The Reggio Emilia Educational Program of Northern Italy, which promotes SEL, has much in common with Montessori educational programs. Seven of its key principles overlap with Montessori approaches, which encourage children to learn about what they are interested in intrinsically. Collaboration with other children is promoted with expression of friendship and affection for one another. There is also close cooperation between parents and teachers in this early childhood program. Parents interact with teachers, closely following the unfolding interests and strengths of the children. While children in the Montessori method often work alone, in the Reggio Emilia approach, communication with other children is facilitated, and interaction and bonding with teachers and parents is stimulated (Reggio Emilia Program, 2008).

It was after World War II that a group of Reggio Emilia teachers, parents, and children began to use this educational approach, enhancing academic and civic learning in order to restore democracy to their community. The founding director, Loris Malaguzzi (1920-1994), was a social constructivist with a progressive educational philosophy. He wanted to develop education based on relationships with people, society, and the environment (Malaguzzi, 1993). In this program approach, children carry out pretend play, sing together, engage in group games, tell stories to each other, read aloud, cook together, play outdoors, and eat sociable meals together. The children bond, initiate, and sustain their own customs (Edwards, 2002). In the United States, Reggio Children/USA is the North American branch of Reggio Children s.r.l., an Italian organization that guides and enriches this educational theory.

Activities for Teaching Emotional Intelligence

Schilling (1996) has organized activities for teachers to use in the classroom in sharing circles. She personifies the amygdala in the brain as the sentry to admission of emotional messages to the brain and the neocortex as the strategist in controlling feelings. It would seem that the sentry and strategist could work together, but the sentry can be triggered so fast that the strategist has no chance to evaluate the situation. The plan in her book, *50 Activities for Teaching Emotional Intelligence,* includes units directed toward self-awareness, managing feelings, decision making, managing stress, self-concept, personal responsibility, empathy, communication, group dynamics, and conflict resolution. This book was inspired by Daniel Goleman's *Emotional Intelligence: Why It Can Matter More Than IQ* (Figures 12-3 and 12-4).

Schilling's book (1996) is composed of components of a number of programs in thousands of schools across the country. Its activities can be integrated into the elementary school curriculum, and while it does take time to implement, it spares the children and the teacher aggravation and time spent on interventions due to emotional problems that would otherwise arise. Five domains on interpersonal and intrapersonal intelligence have been identified that students can use as goals for expanding their emotional IQ: (1) knowing one's emotions, (2) managing emotions, (3) motivating oneself, (4) recognizing emotions in others, and (5) handling relationships. Cartoon-like illustrations in the last pages of this book clearly depict when to use various strategies such as listening, explaining your position, allowing time to cool off, problem solving together, compromising, apologizing, using humor when appropriate, asking for help, and knowing when to walk away from a conflict (Schilling, 1996).

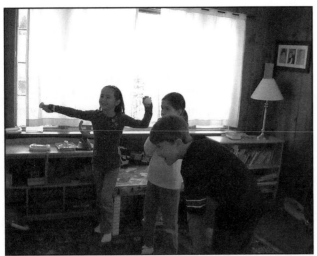 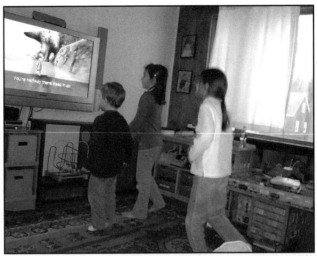

Figures 12-3 and 12-4. Taking turns, role-modeling special swing motions, timing, and regulating emotions lend a social learning component to this video game.

Table 12-3

LIFT: LINKING THE INTERESTS OF FAMILIES AND TEACHERS, OREGON SOCIAL LEARNING CENTER

Teaching Social Skills for nonaggressive interaction—check it out at www.findyouthinfo.gov (also includes information and training for parents).

Table 12-4

CASE STUDY: "MIX IT UP AT LUNCH DAY"

The Southern Poverty Law Center's (SPLC) Report (2006) included news on a day devoted to breaking down social and cultural barriers in school cafeterias across the country. The purpose of this "Mix It Up at Lunch Day" is to break down divisions and misunderstandings in schools and communities. This means leaving one's comfort zone and reaching out. In a middle school cafeteria, students ate lunch with students who they never talked to before. Students asked, "Where you gonna sit?" They chatted, joked, and shared stories and ideas with other kids who they had thought that they could not relate to socially. Some students were shy and scared and needed encouragement. The teachers then agreed to discuss in-class how the lunch day event went.

Social Skills Improvement System

In Chapter 11, the Social Skills Rating System by Gresham and Elliott (1990) was reviewed, and they have now developed a program published in the Social Skills Improvement System (Gresham & Elliott, 2007) with practical strategies for social skills training. It may be used in any setting with more than 40 lessons devoted to cooperation, assertion, responsibility, empathy, and self-control. This program for social skill development is one of the most often cited in clinical and research literature (Tables 12-3 and 12-4).

Conflict Resolution and Peer Mediation

Peer mediation programs in elementary schools have been created to encourage children to work together toward conflict resolution. These programs are designed to foster collaboration in settling disputes responsibly and constructively (Johnson, Johnson, Dudley, & Acikgoz, 1994). Programs require coordination by school administration, school psychologists, special educators, classroom teachers, parents, and children, as well as the training of teachers and children (Daunic, Smith, Robinson, Miller, & Landry, 2000).

Students who are interested in being mediators are reviewed by counselors and teachers and are selected for their potential ability to work with other students constructively. They are then trained by counselors or teachers, who use manuals prepared by the school district or published by the psychologists and special educators who have organized these programs. The Conflict Resolution Unlimited Center (1992) has developed a manual for moderators of programs, videotapes and DVDs for instruction on creative solutions, and a team of instructors in conflict-resolution training who visit schools and school districts to assist in setting up peer mediation programs (Conflict Resolution Unlimited Center, 1992).

Problem-solving approaches have often been used in conflict-resolutions programs; however, some trainers find a transformative approach to be more realistic in achieving reasonable outcomes when disputing children cannot agree on an approach satisfactory to both (Hershman, 2007). In a program called PAZ Peer Mediation, Hershman uses the approach of Bush and Folger (2005) in assisting children to get past their intransigent bitterness and move on. As an example of this approach, Hershman cites the example of two girls who fought on the playground, who could not come to an agreement during a peer mediation session by problem solving cognitively, but who after conversing together with the peer mediators became more empathetic toward each other and walked out the door holding hands! From a transformative perspective, this conclusion was an achievement (Hershman, 2007).

Research carried out examining the results of peer mediation in elementary and junior high school saw school-wide suspensions decrease during a year of the use of peer mediation (Bell, Coleman, Anderson, Whelan, & Wilder, 2000). Referrals to the mediator's office also declined in the second year of the program. In a longitudinal study of 3 years of a program called "Peace Pal," Schellenberg, Parks-Savage, and Rehfuss (2007) found a significant reduction in the school's suspension rate. They attribute this to the intervention of "Peace Talks" that follow a script to promote effective conflict resolution. Based on leadership qualities and a positive attitude, children who were candidates for becoming peer mediators needed to demonstrate compassion, respect, and cooperation. Qualitative aspects of appreciation of the program were included in data collection through questions at the bottom of the written "Peace Treaty," giving teachers, administrators, and parents feedback as to student participants' perceptions of the program. (Schellenberg et al., 2007).

Interventions for Victims of Bullies and Bullies

Babies as young as 3 to 6 months are able to distinguish between good and bad playmates, according to a study by the Yale Infant Cognition Center. In an article published in the journal *Nature*, babies chose helping toys over neutral or bad toys in an activity using a wooden toy trying to climb a hill that was helped or hindered by other wooden toys (Hamlin, 2007). Humans have innate social abilities and skills.

In contrast, it has been found that children with mental illness such as depression included a high percentage of poly-victims, around 86%, with circumstances such as sexual assault, physical abuse, victimization, bias crimes, accidents, family problems, and serious illness (Finkelhor, Ormrod, & Turner, 2007). Children with fragile self-esteem need external support from parents, teachers, school bus drivers, and politicians. An amendment to the No Child Left Behind Act, proposed by representative Carolyn McCarthy to fight bullying in the schools, requires schools to report on school violence; bullying and intimidation were included in the definition of school violence. These and other external interventions to prevent and reduce bullying include metal detectors, cameras in schools and on buses, and school aides on buses and on playgrounds. Grant money from the Federal Safe Schools/Healthy Students Initiative is available to support these interventions. External interventions are supportive; however, programs such as those facilitating SEL provide a school climate that emphasizes and develops internal strengths and skills.

Bullying consists of physical, verbal, and emotional cruelty such as hitting, tripping, shoving, pinching, excessive tickling, threats, name calling, racial slurs, insults, stabbing, choking, burning, rejections, exclusion, isolation, public humiliation, blackmail, terrorizing, dangerous dares, manipulating friends and relationships, sending hurtful or threatening notes or e-mails, or developing a Web site to ridicule someone and to invite others to post negative messages (Wagner, 2008). Situations of bullying can include the bully, a victim, and bystanders. Without intervention toward change, some bullying can go on for years, making school such a tense place that it is not a good learning environment.

Bullying can begin in the home. While international human rights law prohibits corporal punishment of children, and many state laws forbid corporal punishment in schools and prisons, the laws of most states permit parents to carry out "reasonable" corporal punishment (Bitensky, 2006). Some parents have resorted to hiring coaches to guide them in how to organize their interventions with their children at home in dealing with sleeping, television, computer games, and eating food (Kuchment, 2008) without resorting to corporal punishment. Parents need to watch what they say to children. Most bullies come from families where aggression is prevalent (Ascher,

2001). A Swedish study reported that victims of bullying experience low self-esteem and depression as adults (Olweus, 2001).

Sibling rivalry can involve teasing, pushing, and shoving over who chooses what to watch on television or who uses the computer. A survey carried out by Kalman (2008) indicates that children are four times more likely to be hit by a sibling than by a student at school. They are twice as likely to be disparaged by a sibling daily than by a schoolmate. They are also much more likely to go to the emergency room from injury by a sibling than by injury from a fellow student (Kalman, 2008). Letting children try to work out an agreement, rather than intervening too quickly in routine bickering, can enable the child to learn valuable social skills (Adesman & Wolkoff, 2007). Teaching children how to fight and make up is good practice for developing future relationship interactions (Adesman & Wolkoff, 2007). Setting up family ground rules such as no physical aggression, name calling, breaking things, sneaking, stealing, or lying helps prevent bullying habits from getting established (Adesman & Wolkoff, 2007). Parents need to learn to provide a united policy in standing by decisions when confronting issues that arise with their children; otherwise, both at home and at school, some children are bullied for years, enduring kicks, pushes, and curses (Figure 12-5).

In working with children who have been bullied, Kalman (2008) indicates that the most effective way to reduce bullying is by teaching victims how not to be victims. This is one of his major premises in his book *Bullies to Buddies* (2005). His principles help break negative behavior patterns so that victims do not remain in that role. Furthermore, other authors have followed his lead in using bibliotherapy to assist children in learning the psychology and strategies he recommends.

Both of these approaches are used as interventions for victims by other authors of children's books. Cooper's book, *Speak Up and Get Along!*, provides 21 techniques for children to use to respond in situations where they are being bullied (Cooper, 2005). Dialogs are presented as examples of possible ways for children to feel good about being assertive and begin to enjoy school. He emphasizes that all life is social and inserts these 21 techniques into chapters on self-expression, making and keeping friends, ending arguments and fights, stopping teasing and bullying, dealing with blame, and talking back to negative thoughts. This book is lively and positive in its approach to learning how to get along with other people in an affirmative manner.

Similarly, the book *Stick Up for Yourself* is bibliotherapy designed for shy children as a guide to

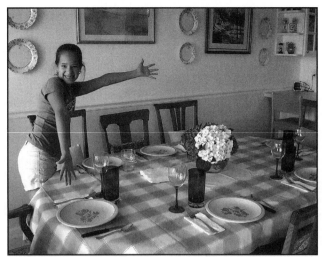

Figure 12-5. "Voila! I've done it...set the table, making my contribution to this family meal," providing the child with an activity for positive behavior.

personal power and positive self-esteem (Kaufman, Raphael, & Espeland, 1999). This book is filled with mini-cases about children who respond to situations to overcome feelings of being picked on by other children. These authors emphasize to the children readers that they are only responsible for their own behavior and that most of the time they can say to themselves that they did their best in a variety of situations. By supporting children in building up their self-esteem, this book prepares previous victims to be more assertive in their posture and stance so as not to elicit bullying. The authors also recommend writing down emotions and situations in a notebook or journal called, "Get Personal" so as to apply each lesson to themselves individually. This book explains the dynamic of getting and using power, making choices, coming to know oneself, and building positive self-esteem. Suggestions for overcoming loneliness and combating moods are interspersed in the cases, which are written to appeal to children using down-to-earth dialog.

Another bibliotherapy self-help book for junior high school children is *Don't Feed the Bully*, written by Brad Tassell (2006). This book is written for victims who are somewhat intellectual, as the vocabulary is challenging. Tassell is an author-comedian who includes humor, sometimes sardonic and other times a chuckle, in a detective-type story that appeals and surprises. It illustrates a plot with a mother behind much of the bullying, a situation that has occurred in real life. The story is gripping enough to engage boys who do not like to read. The appendix (Tassell, 2006) summarizes four basic steps to put into practice in bullying situations:

1. Stay calm

2. Assess the likelihood of violence

3. Have a thick skin and a sense of humor

4. Collect evidence of the time, place, what was said, and who was involved

The author also gives examples of solutions to be proposed to teachers such as:

× The bully and his cohorts are not permitted to talk to victims and are to stay away from victims

× Ask for more supervision on the bus and playground and in the locker room and restroom

× Get other students involved to stand up to the bullies in a united manner (Tassell, 2006)

Interventions for Bullies

The previous interventions were focused on victims of bullying. What interventions can be used for and with bullies to enable them to stop their cruelty to others? The bullies, too, usually have low self-esteem. Bullies need and deserve help; without intervention they will most likely grow up to commit acts of violence (Mestel & Groves, 2001). Some become workplace bullies. Chuck Norris, an icon of the World Combat League, recommends teaching martial arts to keep kids out of prison and away from gangs. He claims that bullies are afraid and insecure kids. By helping them develop security through martial arts, they eventually have no reason to fight.

Friedman (2008) points out that a preteen aggressor's behavior stands in the way of developing positive relationships later in life. Taylor's book *The Pumpkin Goblin Makes Friends* is designed as bibliotherapy for the budding bully (Taylor, 2008). The story is about a monster with a child's heart who picks on neighborhood children until one boy befriends him. The bully realizes how unhappy he has been and how much more enjoyable it is to have friends, rather than make people afraid. Taylor points out that picking on others does not make loneliness and isolation go away. He makes it clear that kindness and respect are best for the bully, too.

A program called *Steps to Respect* consists of two coaching models for victims and for bullies (Taylor, 2008). Hirschstein and Frey (2005) developed the coaching model for bullies to include identification of the problem behaviors, information gathering about the child's history, indication and application of consequences for their behaviors, and generation of a plan for the future, including follow-up meetings. Teachers who used coaching report feeling better prepared to deal with bullying, and they see a reduction of aggression on the playground.

Anger Management Through the Alert Program and Exploring Feelings Program

Williams and Shellenberger's *Alert Program* (1994) and Attwood's *Exploring Feelings Program* (2004) were used and reported on by a collaborative team of special education teachers, psychologists, and occupational therapists, in a Brooklyn, New York public school where higher functioning children with autism spectrum disorder were team taught with typically developing peers (Maas, Mason, & Candler, 2008). Children with spectrum disorders are prone to secondary mood disorders, with anger being a frequently displayed behavior. The major activity components of these two programs are complementary and will be illustrated in Table 12-5.

While this table summarizes the activities, the program was carried out over 10 weeks with 30-minute sessions for activities. During the initial weeks, it was clear that more time was needed for understanding and identification of feelings of anger, especially for children on the spectrum. Sometimes the team did not agree with the child's designations or perceptions but helped the child adapt to the activity through assistance with sticky notes that were prepared for this difficulty in learning. The team believed that, in subsequent months, the children used the strategies in about 75% of the situations where anger began to emerge as a behavior (Maas et al., 2008).

Social Cognitive Intervention and Social Skills Training

Programs for Aggressive Boys

A study by Van Manen, Prins, and Emmelkamp (2004) compared two programs, the Social Cognitive Intervention Program (SCIP) and Social Skills Training Program (SST), as interventions for reducing aggressive behavior in boys 9 to 13 years of age in the Netherlands. The SCIP program treatment components included problem-solving abilities, social cognitive skills, self-control techniques, and the role of emotion in social information processing described in 11 sessions. The Social Skills Program designed by Van Manen consisted of 11 sessions of behavioral training in social skills for children to work on interaction skills with other students. The boys in the study had been referred to outpatient mental health facilities.

Table 12-5

ANGER MANAGEMENT COMPONENTS OF THE ALERT PROGRAM AND EXPLORING FEELINGS PROGRAM

	NAME OF ACTIVITY	TYPE OF ACTIVITY
ALERT PROGRAM		
Sensory focus	*How does your engine run?*	Identifying feelings of low or high energy, and using strategies to self-modulate energy levels
EXPLORING FEELINGS PROGRAM		
Cognitive focus	*Label and color the drawing "How Body Parts Feel"*	Identifying physical impact of anger on the body, then interpreting or restructuring mood
	Label thermometer with levels of anger	Identifying annoyed, frustrated, angry, and furious feelings with physical sensations
Physical tools	*Energy release or relax*	Trampoline, music, stress ball, basketball, etc
Social focus	*Role play feelings*	Interactive scenarios using situations of anger
Visual focus	*Stop Sign*	Remembering to "Stop, Think, and Choose"
Integration focus	*Circle of Connections*	A picture of a circle connecting thoughts, feelings, and behaviors for controlling angry moods
Generalization	*Folder of Strategies*	For children to review with parents

Adapted from Maas, C., Mason, R., & Candler, C. (2008). When I get mad: An anger management and self-regulation group. *OT Practice*, October 20, 9-14.

The Social Cognitive Skills Test was administered. It consisted of six short stories accompanied by pictures. Children are asked questions about their understanding of these socially oriented stories. The treatments were administered in small groups and included role playing and interactive feedback. Groups were perceived to provide a setting for making friends, becoming part of a group, regulating anger, and assisting other students in a helpful manner (Table 12-6).

The evidence from this study indicates that both the SCIP and the SST are efficacious (Van Manen et al., 2004); however, the children in the SCIP treatment program achieved scores of greater improvement on more outcome measures during the post-test and at the follow-up point. It was expected that an analysis of deficits and distortions in cognitive processes would amplify the positive treatment results of SCIP. The researchers expected this contrast and believe that the SST treatment program was as successful as it was because of reinforcement of token economy awards in this behavioral approach. It was concluded that the short-term social cognitive therapy of the SCIP can help to change the negative behavior of aggressive boys (Van Manen et al., 2004).

Programs for Children With Special Social Needs

While the focus of this book is on social issues, before intervening with the social dimensions of behaviors of children with learning disabilities, their physical status of vision needs to be assessed for convergence insufficiency. For example, with children diagnosed with attention deficit hyperactivity disorder, a percentage of those whose vision was tested had difficulty focusing on reading. There are eye exercises that ophthalmologists can give to children to overcome this difficulty.

Interventions for Psychosocial Limitations of Children With Self-Regulation Needs

Gutman, McCreedy, and Heisler (2004) present a thorough process to treat an often neglected aspect of intervention with children who have self-regulation problems. They also address the needs of the parents in relating to their children and to the therapist.

Table 12-6

SOCIAL COGNITIVE INTERVENTION PROGRAM AND SOCIAL SKILLS TRAINING PROGRAM COMPONENTS

SCIP   COGNITIVE BEHAVIORAL TREATMENT COMPONENTS   SELF-CONTROL COMPONENTS

     1. Social information processing   a. Self-observation

     2. Problem-solving abilities   b. Self-evaluation

     3. Social cognitive skills   c. Self-reinforcement

     4. Self-control skills

SST   SOCIAL SKILLS TREATMENT COMPONENTS   SOCIAL SKILLS BEHAVIOR TECHNIQUES

     1. Greeting and listening skills   a. Modeling

     2. Conversation skills attending to verbal and nonverbal cues   b. Role play

     3. Recognizing and verbalizing feelings   c. Prompts

     4. Joining in and reacting to rejection   d. Reinforcement

Adapted from Van Manen, T. G., Prins, P. J. M., & Emmelkamp, P. M. G. (2004). Reducing aggressive behavior in boys with a social cognitive group treatment: Results of a randomized, controlled trial. *Journal of American Academic Child and Adolescent Psychiatry, 43,* 1478-1487.

Table 12-7

PSYCHOSOCIAL DISORDERS OBSERVED IN CHILDREN WITH SELF-REGULATORY NEEDS

1. Dysthymia	Sadness that lasts at least 2 consecutive weeks (American Psychiatric Association [APA], 2000)
2. Mania	Elevated, expansive, or irritable mood (APA, 2000)
3. Physical aggression	Heightened autonomic nervous system; flight/fight response
4. Passive aggression	Unable to regulate social responses; unrealistic parents; tantrum
5. Physical self-injury	Severely low self-esteem; feelings of worthlessness
6. Emotional self-injury	Puts self down as not good enough; negative social comparison
7. Obsessiveness	Rigidly try to control people and things in their environment
8. Perseveration	Unable to transition easily to a new activity or new people
9. Dislike of novelty	Distressed over changes in routine; may refuse to talk
10. Inappropriate social skills	Unable to detect social cues, desire undivided attention, or seek social isolation; walk away while someone is talking

Adapted from Gutman, S. A., McCreedy, P., & Heisler, P. (2004). The psychosocial deficits of children with regulatory disorders: Identification and treatment. *Occupational Therapy in Mental Health, 20,* 1-32.

Several tables, and outlines of components of their system, will provide a succinct overview of their comprehensive program (Table 12-7).

In terms of treatment guidelines for remediation of psychosocial limitations in children with regulatory disorders, prior to intervention, the therapist must build a relationship of acceptance and trust with the child and the child's parents. Children need to feel comfortable enough with the therapist to be themselves. Both physically and emotionally, the therapist needs to get down to the child's eye level (Gutman et al., 2004). Their approach to this intervention includes five components presented in Table 12-8.

In addition to their detailed explanation of therapeutic intervention with the children in therapy, Gutman et al., (2004) describe parental attitudes and behaviors that hinder therapy and the social development of their child. It is essential that the parent be involved in the therapeutic process by gaining some insight that will assist them in changing their perspective and behaviors, as well as the outlook and behaviors of their child. Table 12-9 provides an outline of the problems that emerge in the therapeutic triangle and what indicators may point to their own disorders.

Most parents will be relieved upon finding that a therapist understands their situation, is not judgmental, and provides helpful suggestions. Perhaps, they have observed the problem behaviors in themselves or in their spouse. Once they no longer have to maintain secrecy, a great burden is lifted from their family. These therapists and authors recommend working with the parents by empathetic listening, providing education, clarifying parents' understanding of their child's sensory perceptions, encouraging realistic expectations, helping parents set limits and boundaries in relating to their child, incorporating parents into the therapy carry over at home, and enabling the parents to feel like experts and become advocates for the therapeutic process (Gutman et al., 2004).

Psychosocial Occupational Therapy in Schools

Children with emotional behavioral disorders (EBDs) have, in some instances, lost their student role in circumstances where they are labeled problem students and, for example, are forbidden to use the library. Schultz (2003) describes the process of what she calls "role shifting experiences" for the students using the students' own ability to adapt, moving away from the role of student with bad behavior. Schultz was given the opportunity for the first year in this program to work with the students on individual craft activities. The students selected the activity from among appealing and culturally attractive crafts that were within their competency range. Schultz indicates that it was not any particular activity per se that was therapeutic for the child but rather the opportunity to experience and function within a new role.

In this model, in order to employ the therapeutic use of self, the therapist acts as a facilitator, encouraging self-determination on the child's part. The therapist's intervention includes the expectation that the child can function at a higher level than he or she has been. Social skills are not taught directly but are acquired as required by the activity and the role of the student in carrying out the craft project. Only two guidelines were used in the group for behavioral change: no destructive objects and no aggressive behavior toward oneself or others. When these behaviors occurred, the students were asked to leave the group; gradually, the students became better able to follow these guidelines because they wanted to be with the group (Schultz, 2003). Eventually, the students began to intervene with each other's behaviors so that their projects would be jointly completed without interruption.

Schultz (2003) was adaptable herself in working with the group for a second year within the social studies class. The group did projects of their own design with the theme of the Olympics, which they were proud to display in the hallway. Schultz emphasizes that she offers a minimum of direction, only when needed. Her intervention philosophy is that the adaptive ability enables the child to generalize changes in this role as a student to other roles in the community.

Schultz's principles for change to occur include the following:

- Using real-world activity calls forth an adaptive response in the child

- Identifying the point at which the child has created a therapeutic openness to questions or elicited a confirmation of a step-up in the student role

- Assessing the student's adaptation stance and psychosocial, cognitive, or sensorimotor position to highlight the direction the therapy needs to take

- Exploring processes underway by inquiring about the project's progress

- Moving the focus from too great an emphasis by the child on psychosocial, cognitive, or sensorimotor to one of the other three dimensions

Schultz (2003) expects therapists to help students develop responses and interactions that are more satisfying to the student. She reminds occupational therapists to call on their basic principles of psychology, the therapeutic use of self, awareness of the therapeutic process, and client-centered intervention choices. The focus of occupational therapists on cultural and contextual environments is another asset that can be used for psychosocial intervention in schools (Schultz, 2003). The

Table 12-8

APPROACHES TO INTERVENTION DESIGNED TO IMPROVE PSYCHOSOCIAL SKILLS IN CHILDREN

THERAPEUTIC PRINCIPLES	STEPS IN CLINICAL PRACTICE
Assist the child in identifying problem behaviors	• Explain how behaviors affect others • Provide activity for positive behavior • Grade activities gradually • Address emotional aspects • Suggest carry over to home
Help child identify and manage emotions	• Point out sensory information • Create safe climate for expression • Show how to monitor stimulation • Finding quiet places, using blankets • Beanbag chair for pressure • Child pretends to be a turtle in shell
Help child with impulses, frustration	• Explain impulsivity and intolerance • Discuss why child is frustrated • Teach how to practice thinking first • Explain rules and boundaries • Clarify confusion, disappointment • Teach calming sensory techniques
Help child tolerate transition and change	• Permit time to observe, listen, and ask questions • State clean-up is in 10 minutes • Allow for closure of activity • Acknowledge disappointment • Remind of day, time to resume • Suggest sensorimotor techniques • Use imaginary play-type transition
Help child learn social interaction skills	• Interpret social cues • Match children in dyads initially • Permit one-on-one therapy at first • Suggest new reactions and actions • Mention new ways to ask or speak • Point out times to share, take turns • Indicate how child can help others • Encourage activity with peers • Practice hello, goodbye, listening

Adapted from Gutman, S. A., McCreedy, P., & Heisler, P. (2004). The psychosocial deficits of children with regulatory disorders: Identification and treat ment. *Occupational Therapy in Mental Health, 20,* 1-32.

Table 12-9

PARENTAL PERSPECTIVES AND BEHAVIORS INFLUENCING THERAPY

PARENT'S OUTLOOK	MANIFESTED BY PARENTAL INDICATOR
1. Parental denial in believing in problems	Belief that the school is responsible
2. Parental resistance to therapy	Perceive behaviors as isolated incidents Fail to observe patterns in behaviors Misinterpret therapist's suggestions
3. Parent, child in collusion, hiding problems	Fear of rejection for the child No one is trustworthy at the school May feel anxious, angry, or depressed
4. Parent, child in symbiotic relationship	Lack of boundaries Merging of emotions and identities
5. Unrealistic parental expectations	Believe therapy will solve all May need to grieve child's needs May have similar problems
6. Dysfunction in the family system	Belief that child may be a designated "patient" All family members may have difficulty

Adapted from Gutman, S. A., McCreedy, P., & Heisler, P. (2004). The psychosocial deficits of children with regulatory disorders: Identification and treatment. *Occupational Therapy in Mental Health, 20,* 1-32.

evaluation by the occupational therapist should always begin by asking the teacher about the child's social and emotional behavior.

Occupational Therapy Treatment of an Inpatient Psychiatric Parent-Child Activity Group

Inpatient hospitalization for a child can be traumatic due to being separated from parents, home, and family. Providing an activity group for multiple parents and children can ameliorate this separation, give the therapists a glimpse of parent-child interaction, and begin the therapeutic process by incorporating the parents into that process as early as possible.

Olson (2006) designed and sometimes led this group using activities such as making a sun catcher, painting a model car, doing a puzzle, playing cards, decorating a cardboard box with glue and glitter, making a kite, tracing stencils, making objects out of clay, assembling a dinosaur, and building a picture frame. The parent and child could also go to the gym to play badminton, ping pong, basketball, paddle ball, and netball.

Each child was to engage his or her parent in an activity and not play with other children. Most children and parents found this arrangement to be a relaxing change from visiting in the unit and from the hectic environments in some homes. Parents expressed that the group permitted them to have fun with their child. They also said that kids were different in this group compared to in the unit where they had to follow rules. They felt that stress was taken away, and they felt calm and comforted being with their child doing an activity. During some craft projects, eye contact and smiles between parent and child could be seen. Often, when the pairs tried a new, stimulating activity, the engagement brought out a new playfulness between the parent and child (Olson, 2006).

Olson indicated that, from interviews she had with parents, some had never taken time for leisure activities with their children. The group provides an environment for a positive mood where both parent and child can experience satisfying, neutral activities. They are expected to interact cooperatively, clean up their area at the end of the group, and be open to direction from the group leader. This provided a relief and a needed break from previous negative interactions (Olson, 2006).

Social Competence Intervention Through Children's Activity Group Therapy

In Chapter 11, one of the assessments presented was a social skills protocol evaluation designed by Williamson and Dorman (2002), and described in their book *Promoting Social Competence*. These authors also provide a group therapy protocol for children with special needs. They state that they prefer to work with eight to ten children and two therapists and have found that children should be within 2 to 3 years of age with each other. They caution that the behavioral composition of the group can accommodate a number of special-needs children as long as the focus of the intervention can continue to be the development of social competence, not behavioral management (Williamson & Dorman, 2002). They also indicate that some heterogeneity in the group has proved to be therapeutic.

In designing this group protocol, the authors use a four-segment format, consisting of conversation time as an opener, a short energy-release activity, the day's project, and a review of the session at the end (Williamson & Dorman, 2002). Table 12-10 lays out the suggested format for this social competence intervention group.

While Table 12-10 presents a summary of the activity group program intervention sessions, Williamson and Dorman's book, *Promoting Social Competence*, provides a much fuller delineating of the protocol they designed. Furthermore, they discuss typical negative social behaviors that frequently arise in these groups, suggesting various approaches to individual and group therapeutic intervention by the group leaders. They also engage in astute discussions of the behaviors of discounting the statements of others, interrupting, silliness, boring monologue, bullying, teasing, aggression, excessive competition, inflexible thinking, and motor incoordination (Williamson & Dorman, 2002). These discussions are insightful and invaluable for the therapist wishing to intervene appropriately. It is highly recommended that readers study the original text.

After-School Occupation-Based Social Skills Groups

Occupational deprivation may appear to be a new term, but it describes the vacuum that often exists for school children after their regular school hours. In fact, news releases and an article by Bazyk (2006) indicate that risky behaviors, social aggression, and crimes are most common among children between the hours of 3 pm and 6 pm.

The major needs of these children, according to Bazyk are as follows:

- The need for structured leisure occupations
- The need for SEL
- The need for positive interpersonal connection

A well-designed, organized after-school program can meet these needs by combining the aspects of intervention discussed earlier in this chapter. Some of the provisions in the after-school programs include the protocols presented by Williamson and Dorman (2002); the guidelines provided by social emotional theorists, writers, and group leaders have been incorporated by Bazyk (2006) into the program she created.

Strategies for Intervention With Children With Autism Spectrum Disorder

Autism spectrum disorder has been described by the *Diagnostic and Statistical Manual of Mental Disorders* as a cluster of symptoms including qualitative impairment in social interaction and communication disorders (APA, 2000). Included in the spectrum are Asperger's syndrome and pervasive developmental disorder (PDD). Some examples of interventions for children with autism spectrum disorder that have been studied empirically will be presented here.

Smith, Lovaas, and Lovaas (2002) have studied behaviors of children with high-functioning autism when paired with typically developing versus delayed peers. Extended behavioral intervention for 40 hours per week was performed with children who had significant delay in social interaction and communication. A video of the sessions of paired children focused on interactive toy play, interactive speech, solitary toy play, solitary speech, and self-stimulatory behavior. It was observed that children had significantly more participatory play and interactive speech with typically developing peers when compared to engagement in the same activity with peers who exhibited socially delayed behaviors.

All of the children in the study had the opportunity to rotate partners, alternating their play with typically developing and delayed peers. The videotaping provided the basis for studying these interactions with children with autism spectrum disorder in both scenarios. The pairing strategy can be used in classes, on playgrounds, and at home.

Table 12-10

SOCIAL COMPETENCE ACTIVITY THERAPY GROUP FOR CHILDREN: FOUR SESSION SEGMENTS

ACTIVITY AND CONVERSATION TIME	SAMPLE ACTIVITIES	GOALS
Introduction/opener 15 to 20 minutes	• Discussion of last session • Preview of day's activity • Identity games with peers • Review interaction rules • Identify peer characteristics • Practice conversation	• Remembering focus and listening skills • Listening/discussing session aspects • Sharing personal information • Creating a safe group climate • Learning to know and accept peers • Greeting, mentioning interests, shift from monologue to dialog
Short-term activity 15 to 20 minutes	• Gross motor activities • Hot potato, ball play • Obstacle course • Relays or balloon volleyball	• Release energy • Build cooperation and follow rules • Motor, social, and visual coordination • Practice teamwork and competition
Project activity 30 minutes	• Multiple session activity • Creation of a jungle scene • Playing within jungle • Prepare for celebrations • Plan a magic show • Teaching old games to all • Videotaping a play • Making life-sized portraits	• Development of group continuity • Joint planning/collaboration/sharing • Imaginative, spontaneous acting • Negotiating ideas and follow-up • Designating roles • Communication/responding to others • Observation of nonverbal cues • Listening to the viewpoint of others
Wrap-up/closure 15 minutes	• Cleaning up • Summarizing the session's interactions • Preview of future activities • Eating a snack • Saying goodbye	• Taking on group responsibility • Considering other's opinions, and receiving feedback • Plan continuity and building cohesion • Learning to say please and thank you • Practicing social skills and using indoor voices

Adapted from Williamson, G. G., & Dorman, W. J. (2002). *Promoting social competence.* Austin, TX: Hammill Institute on Disabilities.

Two studies have been carried out by LeGoff using Legos (The Lego Group, Billund, Denmark) as a therapeutic intervention for improving social competence in children with autism spectrum disorders who manifest delay in social skills (LeGoff, 2004; LeGoff & Sherman, 2006). These activities were structured to enhance social performance by means of prompting and cueing social responses. Included in the repertoire of therapeutic interventions were activities with Legos designed to develop collaboration and sharing. These social skill strategies included taking turns, making eye contact, following social rules, using greetings, and attending jointly to the steps undertaken.

After 12 weeks of the Lego therapy, the children's length of social interaction increased from 21 to 36 seconds. After 6 months of Lego therapy, length of social interaction had increased to 1 minute. Children's scores on the Gilliam Autism Ration Scale-Social Interaction Subscale (GARS) increased significantly more during the intervention periods. Even children with more severe social impairment benefited, and outcomes were not correlated with age, gender, or IQ.

The researchers pointed out that the treatment is less intensive than many other interventions for autism spectrum disorder, with only one 60-minute and one 90-minute session per week. Social skills were observed during nonstructured periods as well. It appeared that the Lego play materials were intriguing and engaging. The intervention was carried out in small groups; the strategies employed encouraged the children to share materials in building projects together, thus eliciting interaction. These authors indicate that most of the children appeared to enjoy building and construction. In this study, participants served as their own control.

In the second study, LeGoff and Sherman (2006) measured outcomes for children who had been in their program for 3 years. The groups using Legos as an activity made double the improvement, measured by the Vineland Adaptive Behavior Scales in the Socialization Domain (VABS-SD), as compared to other groups engaged in other activities.

The focus and structure of Lego activities appears to be a positive medium for increasing social skills in children with autism spectrum disorder when interventions to work on collaborative problem solving, joint attention, communication, sharing, and taking turns are designed into the participation plans.

A valuable resource for intervention in children with behavioral and psychological needs has been provided by the American Occupational Therapy Association (Jackson & Arbesman, 2005). Another recommended source suggests social skill activities for children with special needs (Mannix, 1993).

Hippo Therapy for Children With Special Needs

Is riding a horse social interaction? Ask any cat and dog owner if relating to their pet is social participation. These programs of hippo therapy aim to improve behaviors, motor skills, and social interaction (Hernandez, 2008). Approaching the horse begins with a desensitization period of touching, feeding, and brushing the horse in order to "earn" the right to ride the horse as a reward. Therapists, parents, and workers at stables say that they have experienced firsthand that horses can relieve some of the social symptoms of autism, Down syndrome, cancer, brain injuries, heart conditions, multiple sclerosis, blindness, and mental disabilities (Hernandez, 2008).

The horse acts as the rider's therapist along with three handlers of the horse required in equine-assisted programs (Hernandez, 2008). Stable workers and horse handlers perceive horses as an appropriate animal to connect to people because they can detect and express emotions. Horses are herd animals whose social aspects can be seen in the wild as they seek out other horses and a leader to guide them.

Some programs combine hippo therapy with applied behavioral analysis (ABA) to assist the child with all the steps required to be able to ride a horse, including putting on a helmet and practicing balancing a bean bag on the helmet. An example of language development for a child who had never put together a sentence occurred after the child had a few sessions on a horse and said to the handlers, "Ride horse, please."

Cyzner Institute Model: Integrated Education, Relationship, Behavioral, Sensory, and Biomedical Approaches

Cyzner Institute Model integrates relationship, behavioral, sensory, and biomedical approaches into a school for students who have some type of language-based need (Cyzner, 2008). Children may have attention disorders, be nonverbal, or have difficulty regulating emotional reactions or organizing thoughts. The institute is certified by the North Carolina Department of Non-Public Instruction to operate as a nonpublic school.

The children are preschool age through fifth grade. In the behavioral approach, contemporary ABA is used. In the relationship-based approach, developmental and social support for the child and families are incorporated.

Sensory support is tailored to the individual child and allows for sensory breaks during the day so that he or she may learn to assist himself or herself, moving away from external regulation to self-regulation. The biomedical approaches may need to address central nervous system problems, immune system difficulties, digestive abnormalities, biochemical peculiarities, and metabolic and nutritional deficits. Approaches include removing toxic allergy-producing foods, replenishing with needed nutrients, and repairing dietary balance. Some children respond positively to mild hyperbaric oxygen therapy, becoming more alert, attentive, and mentally organized.

The academic process follows the *Manus Academy Series of Teachers' Guides and Workbooks* (Manus, 2007). This is supplemented by pre-educational and coeducational processes of the following:

- ✗ Direct instruction strategies combining positive reinforcement intervention with sensory support, dividing content areas skills into small, sequential goals

- ✗ Sequential instruction in developmental steps, looking for gaps in knowledge or skills, and assuming that learning can be both hierarchical and heterarchical in direction

- ✗ Cumulative instruction integrates new skills into the overall cognitive schema by reviewing its place in the knowledge-based sequence, reviewing how it is related to knowledge gained up to that point

- ✗ Systematic instruction that consists of a review and report structure of daily and monthly discussions of work output and progress with

teachers, occupational therapists, and the director to adjust the overall individual program

Occupational therapists in this school monitor sensory-based and additional behaviors related to the biomedical program and evaluate attention, awareness, hyperactivity, speech and language progress, fatigue, increased mental effort, decline in self-stimulating behaviors, increased tolerance for new foods, and increased emotional involvement (Cyzner, 2008). Teachers and therapists interested in this program will enjoy reading *A Customized Life Approach for Working with Children with Spectrum Disorder* (Cyzner, 2008). The research undertaken to date, which uses the Cyzner Institute Daily Report form, is also described here in detail (Tables 12-11 and 12-12).

Script: Individual Educational Plan

Seating Chart

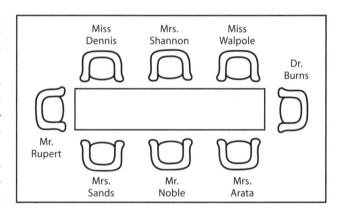

Table 12-11

CASE STUDY: GYM FRIENDS

What could be done to integrate special education children socially into the mix of kids in a middle school?

One special education teacher in South Carolina noticed how other children would sneer or laugh at the awkwardness of her small class of five students as she guided them to the cafeteria. Yet, this teacher believed that her students had interests and abilities that they could share with others in a social situation. This teacher obtained a "Teaching Tolerance" grant from the Southern Poverty Law Center to initiate a program she called "Gym Friends." She organized this with student volunteers who offered to participate in the gym during their after-lunch recess, assisting the school's 20 students with disabilities in learning new sports.

Each volunteer is paired with a student with disabilities to learn one-on-one and to foster peer companionship. Now, these students with disabilities are given high-fives, smiles, and greetings in the halls and the cafeteria, instead of smirks.

Southern Poverty Law Center (2007). Does this child have a friend? Case Study. South Carolina gym friends. *Teaching Tolerance, 32,* Fall, 4.; Fantuzzo, J., Sutton-Smith, B., Atkins, M., Meyers, R., Stevenson, H., Coolahan, K., ... & Manz, P. (1996). Community-based resilient peer treatment of withdrawn maltreated preschool children. *Journal of Consulting and Clinical Psychology, 64,* 1377-1386.

Table 12-12

INFORMATION ON AUTISM SPECTRUM DISORDERS

Autism causes a severely disabling impediment to social participation. Several of the programs described in this chapter try to work with this puzzling social mystery. Autism is difficult to diagnose and challenging to treat. Research is ongoing regarding causes of autism, such as DNA, paternal age, vaccines, and its relationship to gender in boys.

Information on autism needs to be up to date. Some sources available currently that can be researched include the following:

Journals: *Pediatrics; Spectrum; Focus on Autism; Autism Research; Research in Autism Spectrum Disorders; Autism, The International Journal*

Associations: Autism United; Autism Society of America; National Autism Association; Cure Autism Now!; Autism Speaks; Autism Research Institute; Autism Intervention Association Directory Organizations; CDC—Centers for Disease Control; US Autism and Asperger's Association

National Registry: Autism Speaks; The Kennedy Krieger Institute

Data Base: AspergersSyndrome-Families.com; Iancommunity.org

Schools: Alternative Montcalm Programs/Schools

Search the internet for sources on local clinics, programs, and schools for pervasive developmental disorders, autism, and Asperger's syndrome.

What children's psychosocial conditions needing intervention are found in the DSM-IV-TR? Use the criteria in this psychiatric diagnostic guidebook to locate the categories, syndromes, spectrums, and diagnoses found in childhood. What other terms or labels are commonly used for these conditions by practitioners but are not found in the DSM?

Character Descriptions

Alexis Arata: An attractive 7-year-old girl with dark curly hair and a winning smile. She presents uncontrolled behavior problems in school and exhibits signs of attention deficit hyperactivity disorder. The oldest of three children, Alexis has two brothers ages 4 years and 2 months. She is lagging behind in academics but excels at sports and physical activities. (Alexis is not present at the meeting.)

Mrs. Arata: Alexis' mother, age 32, who is married to Manny, a construction worker. From Guatemala, she has no extended family nearby and sometimes feels quite isolated in her small rented house. She has trouble controlling her daughter's overactive behavior since the birth of her second son, and with Manny always working, feels overwhelmed with child-care responsibilities.

Miss Dennis: Alexis's second grade teacher, young and self-assured, but not very experienced in dealing with students with attention deficit disorders or any other disability. She has alerted everyone at the meeting that Alexis has a behavior problem and needs discipline, not therapy.

Dr. Burns: School psychologist, responsible for intelligence, personality, and learning disability testing for all elementary school children in the rural school district.

Mr. Rupert: School principal in his early 40s, tall, dark hair, dressed in a suit, very much in charge of the meeting. He has responsibility for all discipline as well as administering all special services to students. He has called this meeting because of a disciplinary issue with Alexis.

Miss Walpole: Pediatric occupational therapist in her late 20s, working for all schools in the rural district. She has some expertise in sensory integration interventions, and she is often called upon to help students with disabilities to adjust to mainstream classes.

Mr. Noble: Gym teacher, who also leads recreational activities during recess. He, like the other teachers, takes his turn monitoring during lunch time and after school.

Mrs. Shannon: Reading specialist, who has been working individually with Alexis. At age 56, she is the oldest and most experienced member of the team. She has short gray hair and wears thick glasses. It is clear that she loves working with troubled kids, and she is very nurturing. As the only provider of special services, she is responsible for recording the proceedings at Alexis' Individual Educational Plan (IEP) meeting.

Mrs. Sands: A parent who volunteers as a safety monitor after school each day. Her duties involve gathering groups of children according to their school bus routes, escorting them from inside the school to the front courtyard, and getting them safely onto the correct school buses for the ride home.

Situation Description

Alexis was identified by her second grade teacher as significantly delayed in academics, especially reading. The first IEP was held at the beginning of second grade, and a comprehensive evaluation report was discussed. During first grade and part of second, Alexis took Ritalin for ADHD, but a month ago she had a "bad" reaction to the drug and her parents discontinued it. Now, they are afraid for her to take any other drugs, but they have noticed a higher level of hyperactivity since the Ritalin was discontinued. At the previous IEP, the team had decided to send Alexis for extra help with the reading specialist as well as providing her with extra physical activities with Mr. Noble in the gym.

The current meeting was triggered by an incident of uncontrolled behavior after school. The goal of this meeting is to re-evaluate the plan based on Alexis' problem behaviors as well as to review her progress toward the initial goals. The meeting begins at 4 pm, and all are seated around a long rectangular table at the front of the second grade classroom.

Action Begins Here

Mr. Rupert: (looks at his watch) I guess we can get started. Mrs. Arata, have you met everyone?

Mrs. Arata: (holding a sleeping baby in her lap, looks around) I don't remember everyone, no.

Mr. Rupert: Perhaps we can all introduce ourselves. Why don't we start with Miss Dennis.

Miss Dennis: (nods to Mrs. Arata) We've already met at the parent-teacher conference. I'm Alexis' classroom teacher.

Mrs. Shannon: Hello Mrs. Arata. I'm the reading teacher. I started working with Alexis after the last meeting, so we haven't met. What an adorable baby you're holding.

Mrs. Arata: (smiling) Thank you.

Miss Walpole: I'm the occupational therapist. Mr. Rupert asked me to come because Mrs. Shannon suggested that Alexis might need my services.

Dr. Burns: I'm Dr. Burns, the school counselor. We met at the last IEP.

Mr. Noble: Physical education (waves at Mrs. Arata), we talked a few days ago by telephone.

Mr. Rupert: All right. (with a stern expression) You all know the reason we're here today. That reason is no laughing matter. This is Mrs. Sands (indicates the person to his right), one of our volunteer safety monitors. I've asked her to attend so she can describe firsthand what happened after school 2 days ago while Alexis was waiting for the bus. Mrs. Sands?

Mrs. Sands: Alexis gave us a real scare. I still don't know why she bolted. How do I begin?

Mr. Rupert: We generally have all the students lined up according to their bus number, outside in the front courtyard. They usually go in order, but on Tuesday, Alexis' bus was late, and her group had to wait longer. Mrs. Sands, please tell us what happened next.

Mrs. Sands: Alexis' group was already outside but the bus was late, so I had them sit on the steps to wait. Then we, that is, me and the other monitors, continued escorting the next groups to board their buses. Then, I heard the loud screeching of brakes. When I turned to see what happened, I saw Alexis bolting across the busy street, and a car almost hit her. I immediately stopped what I was doing and called her to stop when she reached the sidewalk, but she just kept on running. Mr. Noble happened to be on duty at the other side of the courtyard, and he took off after her, but he couldn't catch her.

Mr. Rupert: What happened then?

Mrs. Sands: We called the police. They finally found her 2 blocks away, in a stranger's yard, playing with a dog she'd never seen before. If that dog had been vicious…

Mrs. Arata: No one told me about any dog. Was she chasing the dog?

Mrs. Sands: I doubt it. The dog was tied up to a post on the front porch.

Mrs. Arata: Alexis loves animals. She's always wanted a dog.

Mr. Rupert: Let's not get side tracked. The point is, Alexis broke the rules and didn't respond to Mrs. Sands' instructions to stop. The fact is, she could have been killed. That's why we asked you, Mrs. Arata, to drive her to school and pick her up each day or to keep her home.

Mr. Noble: Well, it didn't happen exactly like that. I called Mrs. Arata to inform her what happened, and she wasn't able to get away to pick up Alexis. So, we put Alexis on her bus, which was late as we've said, and asked Mrs. Arata to meet Alexis at the neighborhood bus stop.

Mr. Rupert: Mr. Arata dropped Alexis off yesterday, and he came to see me. He explained that you have just one car and that you (nods to Mrs. Arata) need to stay home all day while he's working. So, I asked that Alexis be kept at home until we resolve this behavior problem. Most of our second graders follow instructions, and we've never had this kind of incident before.

Miss Dennis: I was surprised that Alexis showed up at school yesterday and today. Has there been any problems with catching the bus?

Mr. Rupert: Not that I know of, *(looks at Mrs. Sands, who shakes her head "no")* but that's not the point. The school can't be responsible for a student so out of control that she takes this kind of risk. That's why we have rules and safety monitors.

Dr. Burns: So, we understand about the car situation, but why wasn't Alexis kept home, as Mr. Rupert requested?

Mrs. Arata: Mr. Rupert called and told me this, to keep her home, but Manny wouldn't do it. He says his daughter has to go to school. He'll drive Alexis to school on his way to work, but she'll have to come home on the bus.

Dr. Burns: What issues does Alexis present when she's home all day? How do you control her behavior at home?

Mrs. Arata: She's difficult to have at home with a baby and a toddler. Sometimes, she runs outside, and I can't chase her and leave her brothers alone. But she always comes back. So, I wasn't that surprised when she did it at school. She gets frustrated with me and her brothers. I think she just needs to calm down. When Manny gets home, he, you know, gives her a talking to, and she listens better to him.

Dr. Burns: Does anyone know why she bolted on Tuesday? *(a long pause)*

Mr. Noble: I can guess. The other kids tease her a lot. She never defends herself verbally. Sometimes, she does things purposely to get a reaction from them. She spits at them or growls like an animal. They just laugh at her. She probably reached her limit.

Mrs. Arata: It's true. When Alex comes home from school, she feels very bad sometimes. When she tells me what they do, it makes me cry. Last year, she didn't have so many problems, and she had more friends in school.

Dr. Burns: *(reading a report)* I notice that Alexis used to take medication last year. Is she still taking medication for attention deficit disorder?

Mrs. Arata: She had to stop a month ago because she got very sick from it. The doctor said she may be allergic to her medicine. My husband doesn't want her to take it anymore anyway. We're keeping Alexis away from sugar instead… trying to control her diet.

Dr. Burns: It would have taken a month or so for some medications to work their way out of her bloodstream. That might explain the sudden change in Alexis' behavior. What other discipline issues does the team notice? Any other incidents?

Miss Dennis: There is definitely an increase in Alexis' disruptive behaviors in class. She gets distracted easily and has a hard time staying in her seat. I'm in the middle of a lesson, and suddenly I'm aware that Alexis is wandering around at the back of the classroom picking things up, making noises, and bothering the other students. This just started a few weeks ago, and I'd hoped it was only temporary.

Mrs. Shannon: I'm listening to this discussion, and I have to say this is not the Alexis I know. My sessions with her are mostly individual, and in that situation she stays engaged in the reading and writing tasks and seems to pay attention quite well. She enjoys talking about the stories we read, and she's making progress with her comprehension.

Mr. Noble: Now that you mention it, Alexis used to sit with a group of kids at lunch. But lately, when I've monitored lunch, she sits by herself. No one wants to be around her. The other day, when a new kid sat by her, Alexis did strange things to gross her out, like chewing with her mouth open or spitting out water… so, finally, the new kid moved to another table.

Mrs. Arata: That's strange for Alexis. That sounds more like my 4 year old when he eats. He makes a mess at the dinner table just to get our attention. Since the baby came, I guess both of them get less attention from Mama and Papa.

Mr. Noble: Now gym's a different story. Alexis plays a mean game of soccer, and she's one of the best runners and jumpers. *(laughing)* Guess that's why nobody could catch her.

Mr. Rupert: Anyone else observe problem behaviors? *(silence)* Okay, so we have two issues here regarding Alexis. The first involves discipline—how can we make sure Alexis follows rules and instructions to prevent any further safety risks? And, second, how can we improve her academic performance?

Dr. Burns: If I could suggest a third issue, a social one. It sounds like Alexis could use some help with social participation as well. Running into traffic doesn't sound like a useful response to being teased or bullied. Perhaps some counseling could help her learn to use words instead of actions and to speak more assertively.

Miss Walpole: Has Alexis been evaluated for social skills and social maturity?

Miss Dennis: No, but I wish someone would test her. She doesn't work with other kids very well when we do group assignments. When she's listening to me, which isn't often these days, she just speaks out without taking turns.

Mr. Rupert: Okay, let's all think about the social/discipline issue, and we'll get back to it. In the meantime, let's change course and review her academics. Miss Shannon, you have provided the only special education service to date. How's Alexis doing with reading?

Mrs. Shannon: I'll begin with Alexis's first educational goal. *(reads from her report)* Alexis will raise her reading level from first grade to beginning second grade level within 5 months. To meet this goal, Alexis will attend remedial reading sessions three times each week for 30 minutes.

Miss Dennis: If I could interject here—Alexis leaves my classroom during the regular reading times, which is a relief because she was very disruptive to the other children. Now, I wish she'd go every day, because she only gets distracted and can't seem to participate anyway.

Mrs. Shannon: Perhaps you're right. Alexis spends three afternoon sessions each week reading and answering questions to test her comprehension. She does focus better with individual attention, and her answers are usually correct. I've noticed, however, that her handwriting on the test papers lacks control and clarity. I've asked that the occupational therapist be consulted for her handwriting. That's why Miss Walpole came today.

Miss Dennis: I've noticed the poor handwriting, too. She's very slow with writing, and she doesn't always finish her worksheets on time. How does she do with homework assignments, Mrs. Arata?

Mrs. Arata: She resists doing the homework when she first comes home, and I hate to stop her from playing outside with her brother. But after dinner when we sit her down at the kitchen table, she tries hard to get the worksheets done. I wish I could help her more. Manny's English isn't so good, and he gets frustrated trying to help her. But I'm always busy with the little ones.

Mrs. Shannon: Could we put that topic on hold for now? I'd like to get back to the first goal. Although she tries really hard, she often can't focus, so she has not yet reached the second grade level as we had hoped. Because spelling and handwriting are also issues, I think if Alexis had more time in special education classes, she could work on all of the skills at once. The second goal in reading is vocabulary. Alexis has raised her grade level to beginning second grade level in just 4 months—when tested orally, that is. The writing really seems to slow her down.

Mr. Rupert: Let me ask you, Miss Walpole, what can you do with the handwriting issue?

Miss Walpole: We have tests for fine motor skills and eye-hand coordination. But I'd also recommend that we test her sensory systems and her postural responses. Alexis needs good trunk stability in order to improve her fine motor control for eye-hand coordination.

Mr. Rupert: What does everyone think?

(all agree to go ahead with the sensory testing)

Mr. Rupert: Very good. Let's make that a goal for our next meeting. You can send us a report of your results, and we'll include handwriting intervention in Alexis' academic goals. *(Mrs. Shannon writes this goal into the IEP goal list)* How does the team feel about increasing Alexis' reading sessions to 5 times per week?

(all agree; Mrs. Shannon adds this goal also)

Mr. Rupert: All right. Now, back to the first issue—discipline. What can we do about obeying the rules? Following instructions? Any ideas?

Miss Dennis: What about behavior modification? We've done that for other special needs kids, like giving gold stars when they get through a lesson without getting distracted or when they complete their worksheets on time.

Dr. Burns: That might work, but how can we apply it to discipline outside the classroom? In behavior modification, there should be a positive reinforcement for good behavior and a negative one for bad behavior.

Mrs. Arata: Can you explain more about what you mean by positive reinforcement and negative reinforcement? How does that work?

Dr. Burns: *(looking pleased that he's been asked about his area of expertise)* Well, a positive reinforcement might be giving Alexis something she likes, kind of like a reward. When she finishes her homework, she gets a special dessert, like ice cream. When she doesn't, no ice cream. Kind of like Miss Dennis' gold stars.

Mrs. Arata: Okay. I could do that, but not with sugar. That just makes her crazy, right?

Dr. Burns: Then something else that would seem like a reward. For example, your attention, looking over her work and praising her—telling her she did a good job. *(Mrs. Arata nods, she understands)* What else does Alexis like that would represent positive reinforcement? Anyone? What could we use during school?

Mr. Noble: How about extra recess time? She loves gym and really gets into the physical activities. In fact, she even wins the admiration of the other kids when she wins a running race or scores a goal in soccer. These are the same kids that avoid her at lunch or tease her after-school.

Mr. Rupert: *(with interest and respect)* Very good idea. How might that method work for her behavior problems like bolting into traffic? Can there be a positive reinforcement and negative reinforcement for that?

Mr. Noble: We could tell her if she doesn't follow rules or instructions, she doesn't get to go out for recess. Would that be a negative consequence?

Dr. Burns: Yes, exactly. She can get extra gym time for good behavior, such as following instructions. However, the best time to give reinforcement would be directly following the positive or negative behavior. If Alexis follows the rules after-school, who's going to supervise her extra recess time? She may not remember it by the next day and may not connect the behavior and its consequence.

Miss Dennis: During the day it could work, though. If Alexis sits through a whole lesson and doesn't distract other kids, she could get more recess time. If she gets distracted and is disruptive, she doesn't go to recess at all.

Miss Walpole: Well, that might be true in behavior modification, but with kids who have attention deficits, sitting inside and missing the opportunity to get the sensory input that comes from all that physical activity can actually make her behavior worse. Physical activity and the sensations that go with it, vestibular, proprioceptive, and tactile sensory input, can ease physical tension and make Alexis more able to sit still, concentrate, and focus on learning. Occupational therapy sessions that use sensory integration interventions can do the same thing in a more controlled way.

Mr. Rupert: We haven't established that Alexis has any sensory problems that would require therapy. Can you evaluate her for that, too?

Miss Walpole: Of course. That's what I was suggesting before.

Mr. Rupert: What does everyone think?

Miss Dennis: *(addressing Miss Walpole)* When you put it that way, I can see that occupational therapy might help address the attention issue as well as handwriting. It wouldn't hurt to have her evaluated.

(all others agree)

Mrs. Shannon: Shall I write that down as a goal also? *(nods all around)* When can we expect a report from the occupational therapist?

Miss Walpole: Not more than a month. I would need to meet with Mrs. Arata to do a Sensory Profile, also. Can we set that up today? *(she nods, yes)*

Mr. Noble: What about the social issues? Shouldn't the kids who tease Alexis during lunch and after school also get "negative reinforcement"?

Mrs. Sands: Hey, I'm just a volunteer. Not a disciplinarian. I don't have training in behavior modification.

Dr. Burns: That's true. But you could report bullying to us professionals when you see it happening. In

a way, everyone needs to be aware of what's happening with Alexis socially, who's teasing or bullying, and how she reacts.

Mrs. Sands: I could do that.

Dr. Burns: In fact, I think the social issue should be addressed somewhat differently. Alexis could use a few sessions in counseling to talk about her feelings, where they come from, and to learn some more effective ways to deal with bullying, like using assertiveness responses. And she should be reinforced for exhibiting socially appropriate behaviors. For example, she could be rewarded for sitting with other kids during lunch without behaving in ways that push them away, like the spitting you mentioned, Mr. Noble. And when she exhibits good teamwork during sports, make a point to recognize that and help her learn how she can cooperate with her teammates when working toward a goal.

Mr. Rupert: Does the rest of the team agree that Dr. Burns will provide some counseling sessions? *(all agree)* Let's summarize today's session. I guess we've come up with some good ideas for interventions for Alexis: occupational therapy evaluations for handwriting and sensory deficits, increased special reading sessions to continue progress in academics, counseling for social skills and behaviors, and behavior modification for disciplinary and other social participation issues. Mrs. Shannon, I'll ask you to follow up with the written report for today and the goals we've set for the rest of the school year. All of us will identify the positive social and learning behaviors we expect of Alexis, and we'll use positive reinforcements of praise, extra recess time, and gold stars. We will withhold these "rewards" for Alexis' bad behavior. Please give your individual social and behavioral goals to Mrs. Shannon for the report. Anything else? *(no responses)*

Mr. Rupert: Let's talk to each other and compare notes informally during each week. Anyone who has significant problems please alert me immediately, and we'll call another meeting. Good work everyone. This meeting is adjourned.

The end.

Discussion

1. Referring to this and prior chapters, what principles of group interaction does this meeting represent? How would you describe the team structure?

2. Who was the designated leader, and how would you describe his role?

3. Who else took on some of the leadership responsibilities, and what did he or she do?

4. What member roles did you identify during the discussion?

5. What level of interaction did this group demonstrate and why?

6. What was the goal of this group and how was it accomplished?

7. How will the child, Alexis, benefit from this team approach?

8. What disagreements or conflicts could you identify, and how were they resolved?

9. What different explanations did members have for Alexis' deviant behavior?

10. If you were the leader of this group, what would you have done the same and what would you have done differently? Why?

References

Adesman, A., & Wolkoff, S. R. (2007). Oh brother! What causes sibling rivalry, and what can calm it. *Newsday, December 23*, G10, G11.

American Psychiatric Association. (2000). *Diagnostic criteria from diagnostic and statistical manual-IV-TR (DSM-IV-TR)*. Washington, DC: Author.

Ascher, L. (2001). *What parents can do to help.* The Allentown Morning Call: Henry J. Kaiser Family Foundation, CA.

Attwood, T. (2004). *Exploring feelings: Cognitive behavior therapy to manage anger.* Arlington, TX: Future Horizons.

Bandura, A. (1977). *Social learning theory.* New York, NY: General Learning Press.

Bazyk, S. (2006). Creating occupation-based social skills groups in after-school care. *OT Practice, September 25*, 13-18.

Bell, S. K., Coleman, J. K., Anderson, A., Whelan, J. P., & Wilder, C. (2000). The effectiveness of peer mediation in a low-SES rural elementary school. *Psychology in the Schools, 37*, 505-516.

Bitensky, S. (2006). We need child 'whisperers.' *Newsday, November 30*, A41.

Blum, R. W. & Libbey, H. P. (Eds.). (2004). School connectedness: Strengthening health and education outcomes for teenagers. *Journal of School Health, 74*, 229–99.

Blum, R. W., McNeely, C. A., & Rinehart, P. M. (2002). *Improving the odds: The untapped power of schools to improve the health of teens.* Minneapolis, MN: Center for Adolescent Health and Development. Retrieved May 20, 2010 from www.sfu.ca/cfrj/fulltext/blum.pdf

Bundy, A. C., Luckett, T., Naughton, G. A., Tranter, P. J., Wyver, S. R., & Ragen, J. (2008). Playful interaction: Occupational therapy for all children on the school playground. *American Journal of Occupational Therapy, 62*, 522-527.

Bush, R. A. B., & Folger, J. P. (2005). *The promise of mediation* (2nd ed.). San Francisco, CA: Jossey-Bass

Caring School Community. (2008a). *Caring school community.* Retrieved from www.devstu.org/csc/videos/index.shtml

Caring School Community. (2008b). *School connectedness and meaningful student participation.* Retrieved from www.ed.gov/admins/lead/safety/training/connect/school_pg3.html

Cohen, J. (2006). Social, emotional, ethical and academic education. Creating a climate for learning participation in democracy and well-being. *Harvard Education Review, 76*, 201-237.

Cohen, J., & Devine, J. (2007). *Making your school safe: Strategies to protect children and promote learning.* New York, NY: Teacher's College Press.

Cohen, J., McCabe, L., Michelli, N. M., & Pickeral, T. (2009). School climate: Research, policy, teacher education and practice. *Teachers College Record, 111*, 180-213.

Collaborative for Academic, Social, and Emotional Learning. (2008). *What is SEL?* Retrieved from www.casel.org/basics/index.php

Conflict Resolution Unlimited Center. (1992). Retrieved from www.cruinstitute.org

Cooper, S. (2005). *Speak up and get along!* Minneapolis, MN: Free Spirit Publishing.

Cyzner, L. E. (2008). A customized life approach for working with children with spectrum disorder. *OT Practice, 13*, CE1-CE8.

Daunic, A. P., Smith, S. W., Robinson, R. R., Miller, M. D., & Landry, K. L. (2000). Implementing schoolwide conflict resolution and peer mediation programs: Experiences in three middle schools. *Intervention in School and Clinic, 36*, 94-100.

Edwards, C. P. (2002). *Three approaches from Europe: Waldorf, Montessori and Reggio Emilia, in early childhood research and practice.* Retrieved from www.ecrp.uiuc.edu

Finkelhor, D., Ormrod, R. K., & Turner, H. A. (2007). Poly-victimization: A neglected component in child victimization. *Child Abuse and Neglect, 31*, 7-26.

Friedman, R. (2008). The school bully deserves help. Retrieved from rfriedman@newsandexperts.com

Goleman, D. (1995). *Emotional intelligence: Why it can matter more than IQ.* New York, NY: Bantam Books.

Greenberg, M. T., Kusche, C. A., & Mihalic, S. F. (1998). *Blueprints for violence prevention. Book 10: Promoting alternative thinking strategies.* Boulder, CO: Center for the Study and Prevention of Violence.

Gresham, F. M., & Elliott, S. N. (1990). *Social skills rating system (SSRS).* Minneapolis, MN: Pearson Assessment Group.

Gresham, F. M., & Elliott, S. N. (2007). *Social skills improvement system (SSIS).* Retrieved from www.ags.pearsonassessmentd.com/group.asp

Gutman, S. A., McCreedy, P., & Heisler, P. (2004). The psychosocial deficits of children with regulatory disorders: Identification and treatment. *Occupational Therapy in Mental Health, 20*, 1-32.

Hamlin, K. (2007). Social evaluations by preverbal infants. *Nature, 358*, 749-750.

Hernandez, C. (2008). Therapy on 4 legs. *Newsday, January 27*, G1, G4-G6.

Hershman, L. (2007). *PAZ Peer Mediation.* Retrieved from www.mediate.com/articles/herhmanL1.cfm

Hirschstein, M., & Frey, K. S. (2005). Promoting behavior and beliefs that reduce bullying: The STEPS TO RESPECT program. In S. R. Jimerson & M. J. Furlong (Eds.), *The handbook of school violence and school safety: From research to practice.* Mahwah, NJ: Lawrence Erlbaum Associates.

Jackson, L. L., & Arbesman, M. (Eds.). (2005). *Occupational therapy practice guidelines for children with behavioral and psychosocial needs.* Bethesda, MD: AOTA Press.

Johnson, D. W., Johnson, R. T., Dudley, B., & Acikgoz, K. (1994). Effects of conflict resolution training on elementary school students. *The Journal of Social Psychology, 134*, 803-817.

Kalman, I. (2005). *Bullies to buddies: How to turn your enemies into friends.* Retrieved from www.thewisdompages.com/book.html

Kalman, I. (2008). *Worried about bullying in school? Survey reveals it's much worse in the home!* Retrieved from presslist@bullies2buddies.com

Kam, C. M., Greenberg, M. T., & Kusche, C. A. (2004). Sustained effects of the PATHS curriculum on the social and psychological adjustment of children in special education. *Journal of Emotional and Behavioral Disorders, 12,* 66-78.

Kaufman, G., Raphael, L., & Espeland, P. (1999). *Stick up for yourself.* Minneapolis, MN: Free Spirit Publishing.

Kelsey, D., & Meese, J. (2008). *Home of Flippy the tadpole and all of his friends.* Retrieved from www.flippyandfriends.com

Klum, A. M., & Connell, J. P. (2004). Relationships matter: Linking teacher support to student engagement and achievement. *Journal of School Health, 74,* 262-273.

Kuchment, A. (2008). When kids attack. *Newsday, April 14,* 80.

LeGoff, D. B. (2004). Use of LEGO as a therapeutic medium for improving social competence. *Journal of Autism and Developmental Disorders, 34,* 557-571.

LeGoff, D. B., & Sherman, M. (2006). Long-term outcome of social skills intervention based on interactive LEGO play. *Autism: The International Journal of Research and Practice, 10,* 317-329.

Libbey, H. P. (2004). Measuring student relationships to school: Attachment, bonding, connectedness and engagement. *Journal of School Health, 74,* 274-283.

Maas, C., Mason, R., & Candler, C. (2008). When I get mad: An anger management and self-regulation group. *OT Practice, October 20,* 9-14.

Malaguzzi, L. (1993). For an education based on relationship. *Young Children, 49,* 9-12.

Manus, R. (2007). *Manus curriculums: Unleashing the power of practice.* Unpublished manuscript.

Mannix, D. (1993). *Social skills activities for special children.* West Nyack, NY: The Center for Applied Research in Education.

Mestel, R., & Groves, M. (2001). Bullyproofing kids. Prevention programs seek to help victims—and aggressors. *Newsday, May 1,* B10.

Mosher, K. (2005). Family meals bolster health. *The City Paper, September 26,* 3.

Olson, L. (2006). *Activity groups in family-centered treatment.* New York, NY: Haworth Press.

Olweus, D. (2001). Bullyproofing kids: Prevention programs seek to help victims—and aggressors. *Newsday, May 1,* B10.

Reggio Emilia Program. (2008). *Infant and children educational schools.* Retrieved from www.lifeinitaly.com/potpourri/children-education.asp

Resnick, M. D., Bearman, P. S., Blum, R. W., Bauman, K. E., Harris, K. M., Jones, J., ... & Udry, J. R. (1997). Protecting adolescents from harm: Findings from the national longitudinal study on adolescent health. *Journal of the American Medical Association, 278,* 823-832.

Schellenberg, R. C., Parks-Savage, A., & Rehfuss, M. (2007). Reducing levels of elementary school violence with peer mediation. *Professional School Counseling, 10,* 475-481

Schilling, D. (1996). *50 Activities for teaching emotional intelligence.* Torrance, CA: Innerchoice Publishing.

Schultz, S. (2003). Psychosocial occupational therapy in schools. *OT Practice, September,* CE-1-8

Smith, T., Lovaas, N. W., & Lovaas, O. I. (2002). Behaviors of children with high-functioning autism when paired with typically developing versus delayed peers. *Behavioral Interventions, 17,* 129-143.

Spock, B. (2001). *Dr. Spock's the school years.* New York: Pocket Books.

Tassell, B. (2006). *Don't feed the bully.* Santa Claus, IN: Llessat Publishing.

Taylor, A. (2008). *The pumpkin goblin makes friends.* Austin, TX: The Emerald Book Company.

Van Manen, T. G., Prins, P. J. M., & Emmelkamp, P. M. G. (2004). Reducing aggressive behavior in boys with a social cognitive group treatment: Results of a randomized, controlled trial. *Journal of American Academic Child and Adolescent Psychiatry, 43,* 1478-1487.

Wagner, F. (2008). Online thugs. *Back to School West,* August, 28.

Williams, M., & Shellenberger, S. (1994). The Alert Program for self-regulation. *Sensory Integration Special Interest Section Newsletter, 17,* 1-3.

Williamson, G. G., & Dorman, W. J. (2002). *Promoting social competence.* Austin, TX: Hammill Institute on Disabilities.

Zins, J. E., Elias, M. J., & Maher, C. A. (Eds.). (2007). *Bullying, victimization, and peer harassment. A handbook of prevention and intervention.* Binghamton, NY: Haworth Press.

Additional Resources

Fantuzzo, J., Sutton-Smith, B., Atkins, M., Meyers, R., Stevenson, H., Coolahan, K., ... & Manz, P. (1996). Community-based resilient peer treatment of withdrawn maltreated preschool children. *Journal of Consulting and Clinical Psychology, 64,* 1377-1386.

Illinois Learning Standards: Social/emotional learning (SEL). (2008). Retrieved from www.isbe.net/ils/social_emotional/standards.htm

Kalman, I. (2007). *School psychologist warns anti-bully lawsuits will bankrupt our schools.* Retrieved from www.mail.bullies2buddies.com

Kalman, I. (2008). *Expert advisory: Workplace anti-bullying laws.* Retrieved from miriam@bulliestobuddies.com

Linking the interests of families and teachers (LIFT). (2009). *Find Youth Info.* Retrieved December 29, 2009 from www.findyouthinfo.gov

National School Climate Center. (2008). *School climate.* Retrieved from www.schoolclimate.org/climate/index.php

Norris, C. (2006). Chuck Norris—Actor, director cult icon. Retrieved from www.dailynews.att.net/cgi-bin/news?e=pri&dt=061019&cat=frontpage

Shafii, M., & Shafii, S. L. (Eds.). (2001). *School violence. Assessment, management, prevention.* Washington, DC: American Psychiatric Publishing, Inc.

Southern Poverty Law Center. (2006.) Millions of students 'Mix It Up' across the nation. *SPLC Report, 36,* December.

Southern Poverty Law Center (2007). Does this child have a friend? Case Study. South Carolina gym friends. *Teaching Tolerance, 32,* Fall, 4.

chapter 13

Interventions for Adolescents to Develop Social Participation Roles, Skills, and Networks

Mary V. Donohue, PhD, OTL, FAOTA

Some interventions with adolescents aimed at their social lives are on a continuum with children's social goals in areas such as building self-esteem as a basis for successful social interaction and as a precaution against bullying or being bullied. This chapter will discuss interventions of issues specific to adolescence, as well as those that need expansion from childhood developmental efforts in the social sphere. One section will examine adolescent violence, another will examine interventions for growth of positive peer relationships in school and in the community, and finally, a section about interventions within comprehensive programs in mental health, with spectrum disorders, and within the forensic system will be included. The chapter closes with a learning activity case session of a high school student government discussing prom plans for that year.

Introductory Issues

Identity in Adolescence and DSM Relational Disorders

One of the looming issues for adolescents is finding their identity, exploring their potentials, and seeing who they are in relationships with other people. This was the major premise of Erikson's book, *Identity: Youth and Crisis* (1968). The work of adolescence is to move from identity confusion to developing productive, relational, and recreational roles in

society. The new *Diagnostic and Statistical Manual (DSM)* has a number of social issues including relational disorders, cross-cultural issues, gender identity, and sexual orientation. However, it is currently under consultation, in planning, and in preparation in work/study groups of psychosocial and statistical professionals (Carey, 2008). Distinctions in social connotations associated with various diagnoses will be found in the new DSM-V (2009-2011). Current readers are encouraged to follow the DSM development and debate as it relates to adolescents' issues of social/relational identity, since many mental health issues emerge during adolescence.

CDC Community Guide to Social Environment: Adolescents

The Centers for Disease Control (CDC) publishes an online Community Guide for the public. One article that was previously published in a medical journal discusses a model for linking the social environment to health (Anderson, Scrimshaw, Fullilove, & Fielding, 2003). The CDC encourages communities to examine social determinants of health. People are reminded to look at neighborhoods, workplaces, city environments, and social relationships such as people's positions within social hierarchy, varying treatment of social groups and social networks. These settings exude a climate felt keenly by adolescents, which they often feel locked into socially. For example, if they live in a high-crime neighborhood (a setting with high unemployment, without after-school

Cole, M.B., & Donohue, M.V. *Social Participation in Occupational Contexts: In Schools, Clinics, and Communities* (pp 229-250).

Table 13-1

SOCIAL EMOTIONAL LEARNING

In Chapter 12, the section on social emotional learning held a prominent position. In this chapter, readers can look back at the variety of social emotional learning programs across the country and evaluate which ones are appropriate to be carried on from childhood into adolescence. There are many adolescents who have never been exposed to these types of programs and may need an introduction to social emotional learning adapted to their developmental level. Discuss this in class with your teacher and classmates. Wellness Reproduction publishes a cartoon poster depicting facial emotions that would appeal to adolescents. Perhaps your class can purchase one.

---

programs, or without shelters for homeless people), their overall psychological health is affected by these social circumstances. Of all age groups, adolescents reflect the neighborhood in which they are developing, and the CDC's site fosters social support systems that include social activities, mentoring programs, and recreational opportunities, such as scouting, community sports, YMCA/YWCA/YHCA, and job corps programs. Public health facilities for adolescents (ball fields, art, drama, and dance centers) engage youth who might otherwise lack goals and a place in society.

The CDC site also suggests universal school-based programs for adolescents to reduce violence (CDC, 2008). They consider juvenile violence to be a substantial public health problem, as evidenced by 1.56 million incidents of violence by adolescents 12 to 20 years of age in just the year 2003. Juvenile perpetrators during the past 25 years have represented about 12% of the population, but they carry out about 25% of serious acts of violence. Knowing that adolescents are exposed to traumatic experiences, the CDC recommends cognitive behavioral therapy to reduce psychological harm (2008).

Social exposure and attitudes without norms can lead to risky sexual behaviors that require interventions of information, training, and support at the individual, small group, and community levels, in order to prevent HIV, STDs, and pregnancy. In order to change attitudes and beliefs, counseling is needed for risk reduction. Listening to positive popular leaders, community action projects, religious groups, and social networks greatly reduced the number of adolescents engaging in unprotected sex, according to 19 studies carried out by a team of Community Preventive Services reviewers (CDC, 2008; Task Force on Community Preventive Services, 2007; Table 13-1).

Violence in Adolescence

School Assessment and Intervention in Violent Climates

In 1995, 15% of homicides were committed by adolescents under 18 years of age according to the U.S. Federal Bureau of Investigation (U.S. Department of Justice, 1996). Unfortunately, most murders of teenagers predominantly occur among economically deprived, cultural minority youth. Shafii and Shafii (2001) describe how difficult it is for professionals to carry out assessment, management, and treatment of youth with a potential for violence at school. Scales used to assess adolescents include behavioral checklists, parent and teacher rating scales, aggression, and depression rating scales (Shafii & Shafii, 2001). Interviews are also recommended with the adolescent, parents, siblings, peers, and school personnel in order to examine academic performance, behavior, attitude, peer friends, and general social relationships. The Shafiis present a range of options for management and treatment, including family therapy, peer group therapy, individual psychotherapy, medication, inpatient hospitalization, and residential treatment on a long-term basis (2001).

Layne, Pynoos, and Cardenas (2001) describe a pilot psychotherapy program they designed for the teenagers they label as "wounded adolescents"—teens who have suffered a violent injury or who have witnessed the injury or death of a family member or close friend. They assessed high school students for exposure to trauma, emotional distress, and impact on their development. Examples include youth who saw a hanging, drowning accident, driving homicide, earthquake, amputation, police confrontation, murder-suicide, aggravated assault, rape, or gang shootings (Layne et al., 2001). Many of these traumatic incidents caused social relationship rupture, loss, estrangement, shock, and disability. Group content and process is delineated by these authors who provide a group therapy case over six sessions in a school-based intervention, including the goals and process of each session (Layne et al., 2001). Group issues include the social aspects of a desire to break off a relationship before the injury and trauma and being "stuck" in the relationship afterwards as a caregiver. Awareness brought on by a gunshot injury led to emotional fear in a teen's family because he was involved in a gang and the gang members discounted and ridiculed this frightening incident. Flashbacks due to post-traumatic stress need to be addressed in the group or individually.

Bomb and Gun Threats

If your child's school district were plagued by a string of bomb threats, what do you believe should be done? Parents naturally express fear and anger, demanding more security and that the administration try harder to find out who the perpetrators are. Parents question whether there is effective communication between students and faculty. Parents express that their teenagers are afraid to go to school. Some parents would keep students home until there is reasonable assurance of safety. School security is disrupted in such incidents, and instruction is difficult to carry out when a string of evacuations have occurred. Administrators begin to investigate, creating further ripples of insecurity and gossip. After the Virginia Tech massacre, the Federal Education Department gave schools permission to "act first" in emergency situations and discuss responses later (Albanese, 2008).

In looking for solutions to school shootings, "cooperative learning" has been recommended by Aronson (2000). Of course, some schools have relied on metal detectors, surveillance cameras, guards, and teacher concerns. In his book, *Nobody Left to Hate*, Aronson, a social psychologist, points out that often high schools are places of taunting, bullying, discounting, sarcasm, verbal and physical abuse, humiliation, threats, social stereotyping, isolation, and revenge (2000). Hostile environments in schools can cause shootings (Aronson, 2000). As indicated in Chapter 12, all students need to be taught social skills of cooperation and assertiveness with a basis in self-esteem. A teaching method based on a form of cooperative learning where all small group members' information needs to be heard, respected, and remembered in order to pass the course shifts the students' focus from hostility to tolerance (Aronson, 2000). While this method may not be able to be applied in every course, Aronson recommends that it be incorporated into some courses for all students. A reviewer of Aronson's work, Chance (2000), states

that few schools have tried this intervention, giving the impression that society does not truly care about the climate in our schools.

Online Risks

Related to climate in schools is the climate on the internet. Zimmerman (2009) reports that the suicide rates reported this year by the CDC (2008) have indicated that for girls 15 to 18, the incidence of suicide has risen 30% in recent years, while the suicide rate for girls 10 to 14 shot up 76% in 2004. Psychologists report that the frequency of self-harming behaviors, such as cutting and burning, has also risen. Emotional struggles have become public when the internet is used to share and air crises. Girls are socialized to be caregivers, as well as to excel in academics and athletics, and still be thin, sexy, and beautiful (Wiseman, 2003). If a girl e-mails a friend about things not going so well, it can soon be spread all over the internet through instant messages, e-mail, and social blog sites. Viewing the film "Mean Girls" can give a glimpse into the book, *Queen Bees and Wannabes: Helping Your Daughter Survive Cliques, Gossip, Boyfriends and Other Realities of Adolescence* (Wiseman, 2003).

Examples of cyberbullying that adolescents have experienced online from "e-bullies" include a bully deleting all of a student's buddies, receiving a barrage of derogatory messages, and receiving a harassing e-mail about a friend in a private chat room (Jackson, 2006). Some adolescents love the anonymity of the web and take advantage of that situation to confront fellow teens they envy or are annoyed at without experiencing the personal confrontation in reality. Teenagers are often overly intimidated, not wishing to tell their parents about the bullying because their parents might prohibit them from being online. Social needs to belong and to be accepted sometimes also glue the teenager to the computer. This type of social networking is traumatic for sensitive teens. A group called WiredSafety provides a network of Teen Angels in a program designed to provide alternate friends in protective online communities. Teen Angels have been trained by the FBI to run this program, educating younger kids. They also ran a WiredSafety.org Summit where they discussed problematic musical lyrics, computer hacking, and sexual predators. Participants of the Summit were also informed that cyberbullying can be punished by charges of felony (Jackson, 2006). In one instance, an adolescent was charged with a written threat to kill.

One guidance director searches for teenagers' blogs and alerts parents to ask their adolescents to show them their blogs. Teenagers may be computer savvy but socially immature as evidenced by what they post publicly on their blogs. Parents need to be informed that if teens change behaviors, do not want to go to school, say everyone is picking on them, are silent about what is going on at school, are distracted, or are losing possessions, parents need to ask open-ended questions about their day, lunchtime, and walk home to encourage adolescents to communicate openly about their school climate (Williams, 2003).

Is talking online to unknown people always a risk? Mitchell, Wolak, and Finkelhor (2008) have studied types of people in online situations and have come up with four categories: people known in person previously, unknown people met through friends, unknown people met in a chat room, and unknown people met in other places online. These researchers are looking for traits and interactions that put people at risk on the web. They reported that teens who were both bloggers and interactors online and who posted personal information were most likely to experience sexual solicitation, as well as other offline interpersonal victimization or harassment (Mitchell et al., 2008).

Polyvictimization

Hazing incidents, targeting victims for bullying, humiliation, or abuse, reflects not just on the school climate but on the parents and educators who need to instill a climate of caring in the home. As indicated in the paragraph on risky online behaviors, the same teens had been victims of abuse offline. Finkelhor, Ormrod, and Turner (2007) conducted a national longitudinal study regarding multiple forms of victimization and found that 18% of youth experienced four or more kinds of victimization in 1 year. It was found that these teens reported feeling symptoms of traumatization due to these negative interactions.

Allan and Madden (2008) studied hazing in 11,480 students at 53 colleges and universities. Their Web site for hazing research reports that more than half of college students in organizations, clubs, bands, and teams have been subjected to hazing before attending college (Allan & Madden, 2008). Aspects of social participation of a negative type include isolation from people outside the hazing group by being required to have contact only with the in-group. During this time, students have been experiencing verbal abuse, humiliation, sleep deprivation, sexual exposure, nakedness, and alcohol games. Participation in some of these activities can be dangerous in cases of sexual assault and alcohol poisoning through group coercion (Sharp, 2009). Brutality and aggression can lead to psychological scarring affecting future relationships in dating, marriage,

parenting, and the workplace (Sharp, 2009). Allan emphasized that we need to find better ways to support students who are experiencing fear in reporting the behaviors of their peer group and eventually carrying on socially negative traditions inflicted on incoming students despite college policies on initiation activities (Aull, 2006).

Having an identity as a homosexual as an adolescent may be more acceptable now than in previous years, with some "coming out" with their discovered identity by age 13. There are instances in the news of school faculty not knowing how to relate to teenagers in some emerging situations of identity and sexuality due to the complexity of the implications involved (Setoodeh, 2008). While tolerance is expected of classmates and teachers, some adolescents who are "coming out" flaunt their cross-sexual clothing with disastrous results. Gay bias crime can be elicited by troubled teens who need guidance from counselors as to how to interact with others safely without being provocative of conservative classmates.

Parental maltreatment was studied by Teicher, Samson, Polcari, and McGreenery (2006) who examined more than 500 participants aged 18 to 22 using the Verbal Abuse Questionnaire. Parental verbal aggression resulted in irritability, depression, anxiety, and anger-hostility. This verbal aggression was associated with moderate to high scores on the questionnaire, similar to having seen domestic violence in the home, and higher scores than those connected to family physical or sexual abuse. Experience of many forms of maltreatment as a child continued to be powerful, in terms of recall, as high scores of abuse on the questionnaire.

Some adolescents have difficulty in giving up an abusive girlfriend or boyfriend because of social insecurity. Murray (2001) has written a book about emotionally abusive relationships, and this book is recommended as it uses examples from both the abused and the abusers.

Drugs and Drinking

The federal Improving America's Schools Act and the Safe and Drug-Free School and Communities Act (Office of Safe and Drug-Free Schools, 2009) have been the inspiration and incentive for many local and state programs organized to provide mental health, character, and civic education for students in order to counteract the drug culture, which is an epidemic in many communities. Some schools have gone beyond drug education programs and now use dogs to search for drugs (Lam, 2009). Some parents use drug-test kits to detect drug use in their adolescents.

Serious drugs killing teens, such as heroin, are bringing together social and medical agencies as well as police, politicians, and teachers to share information (Altherr, 2008). One high school student recently indicated that adults do not understand that at any time of day, in any hallway in school, students can encounter someone who could sell them drugs (Horsley, 2008). Previously the use of heroin was easily identified by a sickly appearance with track marks on the addict's body. Pure heroin is now less expensive, snortable, can be more easily hidden, and is quite readily available. Emergency room statistics attest to the commonality of overdose. Heroin seizures in some localities have doubled in recent years (Horsley, 2008). Funding for treatment is needed. Recently, Nassau County, New York became the first in the nation to pass a law requiring extensive social participation by police in notifying schools when an arrest due to heroin possession is made nearby (Russo, 2009). Heroin is highly addictive, so the law further requires schools then to notify parents of any heroin arrests before it is too late to rescue the adolescent, if possible. The community needs to be united in its network of cooperation to fend off the marketing of cheap, powerful heroin and the increasing access to prescription opium-related drugs.

Social influences on drinking practices in college students, often free of parental guidance for the first time, put these students in the category of continuing adolescents in terms of experimentation with alcohol. On some campuses, designated as "party schools," binge drinking begins on Thursday night and continues throughout the weekend. Some presence of social disapproval is considered capable of assisting people in keeping their imbibing under better control (Cheever, 2008). Among adults, it is no longer so acceptable to become drunk. *Will this trend filter down to high school and college students?* Adults say that seeing someone who is drunk provides a social stigma that helps to prevent excessive imbibing (Cheever, 2008).

Addressing concerns about alcohol abuse or dependence, Alcohol Answers provides evidence-based treatment and support. Readers can go online to www.alcoholanswers.org to answer questions provided for self-evaluation. The mission of this organization is to educate the public about the disease of addiction, to help reduce the stigma and discrimination of people with addiction disorders, and to act as a conduit connecting people in need to treatment providers.

Emotional Illiteracy

This chapter began by discussing social emotional learning as it has been organized in programs designed to fill the vacuum of homegrown social development. In 1995, Goleman described the results of emotional illiteracy among adolescents as an alarming deficiency in teenage guidance by parents, teachers, and counselors. Learning how to cooperate, how to disagree but compromise, and how to problem-solve social situations can help adolescents and society avoid many social problems that have been described previously. Whether the problem is an emotional malaise, aggression, depression, anorexia, bulimia, or addiction, teenagers need to learn the skills to share what they are feeling. However, first, they must develop insight into what they are experiencing. The social emotional learning programs need to be designed for teenagers as well as for children. With that element in place, the challenge of responsibility needs to be added for social and emotional maturity to develop in adolescents. As Goleman (1995) quoted Aristotle: "Anyone can become angry—that is easy. But to be angry with the right person, to the right degree, at the right time, for the right purpose, and in the right way—this is not easy."

Interventions in the Community and in School

Citywide Programs

In order to find solutions for school violence, a whole community needs to be involved. Many people can recall the communities that have been struck by violence, but few people know that Philadelphia, New Haven, Chicago, Boston, and Hawaii have extensive programs in place to intervene with school violence and that it takes more than a village to remedy these issues. Of course, some of the violence begins in homes and is transported from there to the school. The reduction of domestic violence is an important place to begin (Fink, 2001; Finkelhor et al., 2007). These authors indicate that physical abuse of wives is passed on by mothers who become batterers of children. The trauma seen in communities where there are shootings and murders either causes the normalization of these experiences in youth or terror resulting in post-traumatic stress disorders (Fink, 2001). Teen boys in these communities speak of what they will become in the future, "if they make it" alive. Some children feel that they are worthless garbage. In these areas, there are many single-parent homes or two-parent homes where the adults have difficulty communicating with each other (Fink, 2001). This is why social emotional learning is so essential if academic learning is to occur in schools. Children need to be spoken to about values, emotions, and problems.

In Philadelphia, truancy hearings were increased from 2 times a month to 12 times a month and were decentralized so that both parents and adolescents could be present at the hearings.

Because guns were used in 80% of the murders of children and adolescents, the mayor and police department pursued those who sold guns to minors and installed metal detectors in schools. A 30-hour training program for those youth found carrying guns included a trip to the morgue, 40 hours of community service, and assignment to a mentor. Out of 50 teens in the first program, only three had follow-up offenses. Clusters of counselors, school nurses, principals, and assistant principals began to meet monthly to discuss cases as a group. Specific group members were asked to do follow-up interventions. The Department of Human Services (DHS) began to assign the label of medical neglect if parents were not following recommendations, and the DHS threatened to remove the child from the home. The Youth Homicide Committee worked toward reducing the number of kids who could not attend school because they were out on bench warrants. When this Committee saw that the most homicides and instances of youth acting-out occurred between 3 pm and 8 pm, they had the Department of Recreation develop 150 after-school programs in recreation centers. Sixty attorney mentors were assigned to neglected youth to address problems early on before they needed to appear in court (Fink, 2001).

In New Haven, Police Mental Health Collaborators work with youth who have been traumatized so that they have some opportunity to communicate their distress. In Arizona, volunteers go to visit families traumatized by crime while investigations are underway. Some cities have set up school-based mental health clinics, for psychiatrists and clinical psychologists to act as consultants in carrying out on-site interventions (Fink, 2001). Chicago's Violence Prevention Strategic Plan perceives violence as a public health issue and brings the mental health community into the schools to undertake a number of projects with violent youth.

In Boston, the city was able to reduce the number of murders of children under the age of 18 to zero for 2.5 years (Fink, 2001). This was achieved, in part, by a policeman and a probation officer patrolling together in the evenings to pick up adolescents who were breaking their probation. A combination of FBI-like information, street workers, community volunteers, and the courts cooperated to reduce the prevalence of drugs and worked around bureaucratic blockades to enable changes to take place (Fink, 2001).

In Hawaii, Head Start and Healthy Start programs jointly identified 90% of high-risk families of newborns, through systematic hospital-based screenings, and continued to visit their homes to lower risky situations. As a result, child abuse has been reduced by 80%.

Fink believes that parenting education is essential to enable parents to raise children with love so that they do not become teenagers filled with hate and violence.

School-Based Sessions on Emotional Intelligence for Adolescents

Two valuable workbook programs designed for intervention with high school students that provide structured sessions around emotional questions, issues, and dramatizations are entitled *Talking With Kids: Guided Discussions for Teaching Emotional Intelligence* (Palomare & Cowan, 1998) and *Discussion-Provoking Scripts for Teens* (Sorenson & Nord, 2002). The first workbook consists of 78 sessions, each one-page long, focused on the larger categories of self-awareness of emotions, self-management, relationship skills, and listening. There are guidelines for the teacher or counselor in processing the group strategies for gradual exposure of emotional awareness and regulation. The topics are designed to appeal to adolescents, with titles such as, "A Way I Show I'm a Good Friend," "How I Help Out at School," and "A Time I Felt Left Out."

The second workbook provides 33 scenarios that are one-page long, accompanied by another page with processing questions and discussion notes. Topics include "Among Friends," "Working to Please," "Legalities and Moralities," and "Home and Family." Scenarios are aimed at questions such as "Partners?" "Who's Disgusting?" "Late Nights?" "It Couldn't Happen to Me," "Not Old Enough," and "Who Cares?" These topics and scenarios are well-developed for thought-provoking discussion (Figures 13-1 and 13-2).

Peer Mediation and Conflict Resolution Programs

In Chapter 12, programs in peer mediation and conflict resolution were described as they have been used in elementary and middle schools. The National Crime Prevention Council (NCPC) recommends the strategy of peer mediation be employed in high schools as well (National Crime Prevention Council, 2009). The Council emphasizes the need for training the students to prepare for the use of this strategy. First, teachers, administrators, and staff

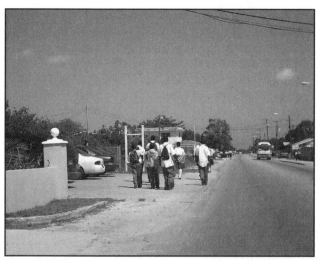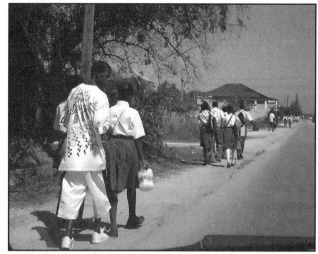

Figures 13-1 and 13-2. Teens hanging out on the way home from school.

need training; then, they need to organize training for students, along with student input. It is suggested that administrators, teachers, and staff team up to train students. One high school in Ohio was so successful in resolving disputes that they intend to expand the program to their middle schools (National Crime Prevention Council, 2009).

The Center for Research on Counseling and Personnel Services of Greensboro, North Carolina, reported on a survey they gave to four groups: faculty, students in eight homeroom classes, trained student mediators, and students who had used the mediation program to resolve a conflict incorporating this conflict-resolution strategy. Those individuals who were directly involved with the program expressed greater satisfaction than those who had no personal experience with the program. Theoretically, responders projected that the prospect of a peer-mediation strategy was appealing, yet they had not used it. One rationale for this neglect of the program was ascribed to a lack of information about the program (ERIC, 1998).

Theberge and Karan (2004) carried out a study to ascertain what problems arose in a junior high school where only 12% of students used the peer-mediation program, despite the fact that 95% of the students indicated that they knew about the conflict-resolution program. Some of the reasons that emerged from this survey included the following:

- Students' attitudes and feelings about mediation, such as distrust, desire for privacy, concerns about confidentiality, and perception of mediation as not "cool"
- Students' approach to conflict, such as a desire for immediate resolution; relying on friends for help; or aggressive types of conflict with teasing, name-calling, and threatening

- Students' attitudes and feelings in school, such as dealing with teen emotions, power imbalance, boy-girl interactions, or a lack of respect of and by teachers
- School climate, such as the lack of community, lack of bonds with adults in school, concerns about safety, the exercise of power by teachers and administrators through discipline and rules, or overcrowding
- Structure and organization of the mediation program, such as a lack of understanding of how it works, limited resources, a lack of time slot and space for meetings, lack of information, or no program to teach mediation skills
- Societal issues, such as cultural differences, or viewpoints of mediation as divergent from mainstream culture, which prefers separation and divorce to mediation

A good source of information about conflict resolution/peer mediation is Safe & Responsive Schools of Indiana at www.indiana.edu/~safeschl, which provides more than 20 general references to peer mediation curricula, information on workshops, videos, and DVDs (Safe & Responsive Schools, 2002).

Peer Support Programs for Social Inclusion in High Schools

Service learning programs designed by Carolyn Hughes (Hughes & Carter, 2008), professor in the Department of Special Education and Human and Organizational Development at Vanderbilt University in Nashville, Tennessee, have been funded by a federal grant to establish the Metropolitan Nashville Peer Buddy Program. In this program, typically developing teens are trained in service learning classes to accompany and work with teens who have learning disabilities and spectrum disorders. After training, buddies accompany their teen peers to at least one class a day. This program encourages both buddy development and citizenship, along with personal and social skills for the peers who need coaching and role modeling, in order to facilitate social inclusion in high schools.

Inclusion speaks to Maslow's need for love and belonging (1943), which all teens crave and which students with disabilities need both opportunity and immersion to achieve. The Individuals with Disabilities Education Improvement Act (IDEA; 2004) calls for incorporation of as many students with disabilities as possible, to allow them to have access to standard education courses and to mingle with peers without disabilities, in order to learn social skills in a nonstaged environment. The buddies are taught to be open, friendly, and accepting of their peers.

One teen with severe autism responded so well to her peer buddy that she began to make eye contact with her, to laugh with her, to look for her to come in the room, and to initiate conversation, even though her vocabulary only increased from 4 to 11 words (Hughes & Carter, 2008). Parents of teens with disabilities notice their teen is less isolated on the weekends and is invited to go out with peer buddies, who also call to chat in the evenings. One peer buddy pointed out that students with disabilities sat at a table by themselves before the institution of the peer buddy program, but that subsequently when they went outside, they began to talk to people they normally would not approach (Hughes & Carter, 2008).

Peer buddies point out the practicality of a service learning project as an academic course. They also report that they have learned life skills, participated in citizenship, and developed friendships with other teens who they say are more like them than different.

When peer buddies greet students with disabilities in the hall and invite them to their lunch table, a spirit of community develops in the school as a whole (Hughes & Carter, 2008).

Parents and teachers observe that students with disabilities engage in conversation more, feel more confident, and can speak up for themselves (Copeland et al., 2004). Programs need organization and collaboration from counselors, students, teachers, special education teachers, parents, and administrators in order to be successful.

Meaningful social relationships developed as peer-supported strategies in learning provided a basis for interaction (Carter, Cushing, & Kennedy,

2009). Research on social interaction for students with disabilities shows that both people in the peer partnership improve their academic skills (Cushing & Kennedy, 1997). Lasting friendships also develop (Hunt, Soto, Maier, & Doering, 2003). One study (Salisbury, Gallucci, Palombaro, & Peck, 1995) observed that with peer support, there was more emphasis on commonalities among students in contrast to differences among students, thus building up the culture of classroom membership in terms of fostering a spirit of belonging.

Supported Education for Adolescents With Psychiatric Disabilities

Gutman and Schindler (2007) describe a program of supporting the educational progress of high school, GED, and college students by being paired with occupational therapy graduate students who know how to organize and structure studying, homework assignments, presentations, and term papers. This program helps to intervene in the vicious cycle that can occur when people with psychiatric disabilities cannot succeed in school on their own. Appropriate accommodations, such as going to classes part-time, make it possible for patients to go to therapy sessions and meet with their doctor for medication adjustment. The occupational therapy students use activity analysis, synthesis, and sensory and intellectual strategies for their level of study. Using as many senses as possible during study facilitates learning. The occupational therapy students sometimes provide tutoring, advisement regarding selection and registration, and small group classes on how to study efficiently and effectively, how to develop social and behavioral skills useful in interacting with faculty and fellow students, and how to access resources for papers and presentations in class.

Efforts toward building social skills are vital because psychiatric illness often includes social isolation on the part of the individual. Gutman and Schindler (2007) recommend having the individual supported in this program keep a journal of social participation, recording social opportunities, initiation of social interaction, description of activity participation, reasons for declining invitations, and feelings following participation or withdrawal. This journal can be reviewed by the individual, with his or her support person, for discussion and coaching. Role playing can be used to facilitate future situational participation. Progress in social participation can be a barometer of mental health recovery. It needs to be balanced schedule-wise with the individual's academic needs (Gutman & Schindler,

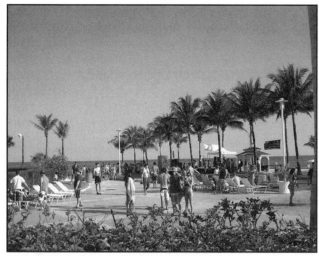 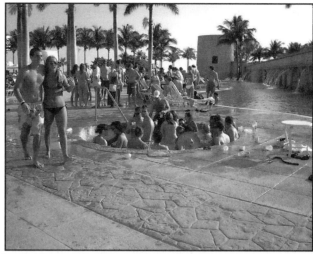

Figures 13-3 and 13-4. Spring break attracts groups of high school and college students to travel together to popular destinations.

2007). In assessing social interaction with the individual's teachers and other authority figures, the supporting student needs to evaluate the possible need for anger management, stress reduction, and social skills practice (Gutman & Schindler, 2007).

It is also recommended that support students work with the individuals to learn to identify feelings and emotions so that they can become aware of when they may be experiencing a relapse and need additional treatment. Signs and symptoms can be recorded in a diary and reviewed with his or her psychotherapist or doctor (Gutman & Schindler, 2007). This article can be read in full in order to understand how the support student can work within a mental health facility to assist individuals as they are discharged and transition back into the community and campus (Gutman & Schindler, 2007).

College Campuses

College campuses often sponsor related programs encouraging peer educators to work with other students needing support after choosing a "specialty" area, such as alcohol and other drugs, gender and sexuality, healthful eating and stress, sexual assault education, and sexual health (Events NYU, 2008). Graduate assistants in dormitories serve as support personnel in orienting freshmen to campus life, college studies, and independent living after leaving home. It is expected that these programs ease the way for homesick, isolated, and troubled youth to learn how to become involved in social activity participation with campus clubs and events (Figures 13-3 and 13-4).

Linking the Interests of Families and Teachers for Adolescents

Linking the Interests of Families and Teachers (LIFT) was mentioned earlier for children, but it is also a program designed for adolescent social competence in peer interactions. This program is known for both adolescent and parent training (Ralph et al., 1998). It has been able to improve social skills and encourage assertiveness, social efficacy, and initiative.

The interventions have included classes in problem solving, social skills training, and behavior modification on the playground. The adolescent program was aimed at reduction of opposition, deviance, and social ineptitude. The parent program worked on disciplining and monitoring teenagers in an appropriate manner. Research measured improvement by parents in the program intervening with their teenagers by problem solving and conflict resolution (Ralph et al., 1998). These youth were less socially avoidant than those in a control group and became more socially interactive with peers.

Just4Teens: Safety First— A Reality-Based Approach to Drugs

Just4Teens offers a program discussing drug use with teenagers. It consists of a DVD video by and for youth dealing with a range of drugs. It includes a Facilitators' Guide and booklets titled, *Safety First*, *Beyond Zero Tolerance*, and *Making Sense of Student Drug Testing*. The booklets are available upon request, and the DVD is $15. Teachers and group leaders can learn how to incorporate interactive and educational techniques for drug prevention into the classroom (Drug Policy Alliance, 2008). This program, sponsored by the state of New Mexico, avoids the scare tactics of the past 25 years, which have not worked using "just say no" messages. The philosophy of this program is controversial for some people as it perceives random student drug testing as an invasive policy that erodes trust between students and adults. Drug Policy Alliance (DPA) is another organization that also calls for reform of national and international drug policies so that students do not fear prosecution if they call for help for someone experiencing an overdose (International Drug Policy Reform Conference, 2009). The DPA also works to stop the overkill of SWAT teams following UPS home deliveries of drugs sent to innocent people in drug-smuggling schemes.

Another balanced, community-based approach to youth substance abuse is the Substance Abuse and Mental Health Services Administration (SAMHSA), in collaboration with the Office of National Drug Control Policy (ONDCP), with their Drug-Free Communities program. The federal government has encouraged this program by providing millions of dollars in grants to reduce substance abuse throughout the nation (ONDCP, 2007).

Building Racial Tolerance Through Social Interventions

In studies designed to establish social relationships between culturally diverse people, psychologists have been able to arrange that pairs of people experience a reduction in the awareness of bias within hours. It was also found that after a 4-hour session of structured interactions, answering a list of questions, barriers were broken down. Sample questions included asking about attaining fame in an area of one's choice and changing how an individual was raised.

Then, in a second intervention, the pair competes against another pair in timed strategic games. In a third interaction, the pair talks about what they are proud of in their cultural group. Finally, they take turns, while wearing a blindfold, being guided through a maze by their partner. These basic activities build relationships, according to social psychologists (Aron et al., 2004). Tests of saliva stress hormones show reduced anxiety during future encounters with the new cultural group. Furthermore, the new relationship can last for months. These researchers have further indicated that just being in a classroom with other interracial pairs interacting can minimize levels of bias. One concept of social

participation that the Arons espouse is "including close others in the self" by making themselves a part of others' lives (2004).

Interventions of Volunteering, Parent Education, Support Groups, and Bibliotherapy

Some schools encourage outreach into the community by volunteer work or after-school employment designed to expand the horizons of teenagers, educating them as to the areas of work they might select and enjoy later in life. Volunteering at a nursing home, hospital, after-school program, scouting, Big Brother/Big Sister, or adult day care center; helping seniors who live alone; coaching Little League; tutoring in math or reading; or working in a supermarket, gas station, pet store, or hardware store can enable teens to perceive the realities of life and to communicate with people in the community. This type of program expands democracy in the community, giving people of both ends of the age spectrum a feeling of connectedness. Intergenerational interactions increase self-esteem and feelings of connectedness and build up social participation and networking in the community (Bleiberg Seperson & Arfin, 2008). Promoting these social systems builds up the bedrock of our democratic society.

Evening workshops for parents designed to improve their interactions with their adolescent youth can focus on listening to their teen, moral and ethical behavior, being consistent, holding ground, and avoiding arguments (News From Campus, 2009). Parents find these meetings to be insightful and supportive of their roles at home, becoming acquainted with the impact of facial expressions, tone of voice, and undermining sarcasm.

There are times when group support in the community or at work is positive, emerging in an informal manner. It has been found that when a small group of people decide to stop smoking, they make it easier for each other. In addition, this sometimes pressures other smokers to join in the effort so as not to feel ostracized (Christakis, 2009).

Writing Therapy, an Intervention for Changing Teens and Their Changing World

An English class of at-risk teens who defined themselves socially by their ethnic background began writing about their daily experiences in a journal in order to mirror their thoughts and responses to the violence and chaos in their surroundings. After reading the diary of Anne Frank and Zlata Filipovic's diary of a child growing up in Sarajevo during wartime, as well as books and stories about the Freedom Riders of the 1960s, they named themselves the *Freedom Writers.* They raised money to bring Zlata Filipovic and Miep Gies, who sheltered Anne Frank, to speak to them in their classroom. Ninety percent of these adolescents of deprived backgrounds graduated and went on to further education in trade schools and community and 4-year colleges. Few of these students had expected to achieve a high school diploma or even survive in their neighborhood. Together, they wrote the book, *The Freedom Writers Diary: How a Teacher and 150 Teens Used Writing to Change Themselves and the World Around Them* (Gruwell, 1999).

Comprehensive Intervention Programs—Mental Health, Spectrum, and Legal

Engaging Psychiatrically Hospitalized Teens With Their Parents: A Parent-Adolescent Activity Group

Olson (2006) designed a parent-adolescent activity group as a multifamily group meeting once a week. In this group, adolescents are involved in an activity of their choice, carrying it out with their parent parallel to the other families. The adolescent is given a choice of an activity that he or she enjoys, wishes to explore, or in the past completed with his or her parent successfully. Aspects of the group process are at work in the group as families observe how other families interact. Seeing another parent and adolescent having experiences similar to theirs can be the most powerful intervention (Olson, 2006). While the group is meeting, adolescents and parents can be observing, talking, and doing the activity side by side. Even the observation of a negative interaction in another family can be instructive as a model of what not to do, or the negative behavior occurring in their family interaction could be embarrassing enough to provoke insight and a correction of direction. If a parent is critical of the youth and is not listening, the emergence of this behavior is valuable in adjusting the relationship.

In this chapter of Olson's book, she delineates eight aspects of the role of the leader and provides two case examples illustrating how this parent-adolescent participation can stimulate building a relationship through activity bonding or helping a teenager to develop independence (Olson, 2006).

Social Responsibility Training: Character Development Systems

Social responsibility training (SRT) works with social emotional aspects of development, such as those used in schools with children, but with the added dimension of responsibility, now that the youth is no longer a child and needs to be addressed with greater maturity (SRT, 2007). SRT is planned as a comprehensive solution for school disengagement, designed to empower at-risk adolescents and their families, and aimed at enabling students to stay in school.

Established in 2001, the training has been standardized successfully in more than 60 school districts in 17 states (SRT, 2007). This curricula is pulling together partnerships of schools, parents, community agencies, and justice systems in a collaborative manner.

Social environmental risks of students involved in the SRT program included criminal behavior in neighborhoods, minimal school satisfaction, minimal teacher and friend support, negative friends' behavior, weak home/academic environment, low school behavior expectations, and no social environmental assets. As far as individual adaptation to risky environments, the school engagement of these high school students was weak, and there were problems with avoiding trouble, low happiness assets, and poor academic performance assets (Lasater et al., 2005).

The SRT Web site (www.characterdevelopmentsystems.com) provides a 6-minute video introduction, articles to be downloaded, and a PowerPoint presentation providing a history of work and achievement from 2001 to 2007. First, there is a presentation of the cost to society of doing nothing for adolescents in crisis. Just one high-risk youth dropping out of high school can cost more than $1 million in terms of incarceration expenses (SRT, 2007). The positive attempt here is to build foundations of character in order to increase high school graduation rates.

SRT provides a visual model of interaction of mainstream classrooms, alternative schools and behavior management, parents and family, special education, community corrections, treatment settings, native and inner-city youth cultural programming, and the courts (SRT, 2007).

The focus of SRT is to empower the adolescent to discover who he or she is as individuals, uncovering what his or her problem is, when they arise, and

---

Table 13-2

STEPS TO CREATING FAMILY FREEDOM

1. Draw up family communication ground rules

2. Weekly family action steps to remedy problems and challenges; enhance family strengths

3. Develop a family agreement, indicating responsibilities, benefits, and consequences for each family member

4. Develop Individual Action Plans to meet family responsibilities

Social Responsibility Training. (2007). *Project Report 2001-2007.* Retrieved May 18, 2010 from www.characterdevelopmentsystems.com

---

what can be done to move on. Classes are open-ended and are designed for the individual. The classes are set up to provide positive team support for successful behavioral change. Trained coaches are part of the program and are assigned 10 to 15 youth. The SRT workbook series addresses steps to life mastery—how to get along in life and how to change behaviors of shoplifting and substance use. Other classroom tools include drawing situations and feelings, peer feedback, role play, contemplation, and video clips. These small classes and individualized programs increase completion rates of the following school year by 50% for suspended and expelled students and decrease the long-term suspension/dropout rate of high-risk high school students by 50%. Overall, this program provides support for parents and families by creating community-wide collaboration. The implementation of SRT consists of a five-step process:

1. Assessing needs

2. Program design

3. Staff training

4. Ongoing program support

5. Ongoing evaluation

Workbooks for parents are provided to work on personal responsibility in a 3-day program devoted to character and freedom and the steps to life mastery. A subsequent workbook enables parents to move at their own pace through 30 exercises, with results of homework presented and discussed in class. These guidelines review the work of the high schoolers and dilemmas confronting parents of teenagers. These interventions with parents reinforce the efforts of their teens. The steps to creating family freedom is outlined in Table 13-2.

Since 2001, the SRT program has empowered 15,000 students, as well as their parents and families, through the process of using schools, alternative schools, juvenile and adult court settings, detention, re-entry programs, and social services (SRT, 2007).

It has been pointed out that up to 30% of American youth and families are not thriving. Community empowerment and accountability is the cornerstone of these programs, which are aimed at helping people help themselves. The foundation of the program is a cognitive-behavioral intervention, which in the first year, motivated about 70% of the students to make substantial changes in their lives and to remain in school. In addition to students dropping out of school, there are "invisible" others who are at risk: alienated, failing many classes, using drugs or alcohol or depressed by home, school, and community circumstances, without hope of getting out of the spiraling cycle of life decline. The organizers of the SRT program believe that most American communities need the support, skills, and accountability the SRT can provide (SRT, 2007) (Table 13-3).

The above investigators studied how well the SRT program supported youth school success during the first 3.5 years of the program in a Montana senior high school.

- 68% graduated successfully or were still attending senior high school

- 16% were positively engaged in other settings (e.g., GED, Job Corps, and treatment)

- 15% were unsuccessful: dropped out or expelled

Lasater and Beckett (2007) carried out a study of the results with high-risk students in a Georgia alternative school program. The year-end status for high school students consisted of the following:

- 51% successfully returned to the original school

- 18% continued enrollment in transitional school

- 19% transferred to another school or withdrew

- 10% were expelled or sent to detention or prison

Table 13-3

THE SIX LIFE ISSUES ADDRESSED BY THE SOCIAL RESPONSIBILITY PROGRAMS

1. Evaluation of self in belief, attitudes, behaviors, defense mechanisms

2. Evaluation of relationships with others and plans to heal the relationships

3. Strengthening of positive behaviors and habits regarding responsibilities

4. Positive identity formation by exploring the real self and establishing goals

5. Building self-worth, self-respect, and social participation skills

6. Decreasing hedonism by learning how to delay gratification and pleasure-seeking behavior

Adapted from Lasater, L., Robinson, K. D., Willis, T., Meyer, C. L., Jahns, N. R., Bush, L., ... & Duffey, K. R. (2005). *Using social responsibility training (SRT) to support youth school success.* Retrieved from www.CharacterDevelopmentSystems.com and www.CharacterDevelopmentSystems.com/img/making-a-differnce.pdf

Pre- and post-test comparison ratings were made by teachers ranking students into three groups—high, medium, and low in social responsibility. The highest group improved from 66% to 71% ratings of social responsibility scores. The medium group gained the greatest ground with 18 points of improvement in social responsibility rankings, from 45% to 63%. The students with the lowest rank in social responsibility improved 8 points, from 22% to 30%. While the highest group did not improve much, the medium and low groups' ratings increased significantly (Lasater & Beckett, 2007).

Small Learning Communities: Institute for Student Achievement

Learning communities provide hands-on support in high schools that are part of the Institute for Student Achievement's (ISA) partnership programs. In this model, a team of teachers works with the same group of 100 students throughout their 4 years of high school so that teens become well known to educators. The teachers come to know these teens as students and as people. They are able to develop caring and close relationships with their students so as to work with commitment in achieving greater performance (Kern-Rugile, 2006). This program was begun on Long Island, New York, and has spread to other states. Both educational and emotional tools are part of the program, which aims at preparing students for their futures. ISA programs have achieved a 90% graduation rate. A Web-based program is incorporated where teachers can post projects, homework assignments, and lesson plans. Students, parents, and faculty like the communication created by this opportunity known as "Teacher Ease." The personal attention provided by this program has brought some students from below grade level to where they are now, helping to teach classes.

Social and Mental Health Help for Juvenile Offenders

The National Mental Health Association (NMHA) has created *A Compendium of Promising Practices* to be used as interventions for adolescents in the juvenile justice system (2004). This is a free guide that highlights current treatment that is evidence based and aimed at assisting community leaders, advocates, and family members with the individual needs of their teenagers. These services incorporate the physical, emotional, social, and educational needs of teens in the juvenile system as they often have more mental health needs than the typical adolescent. The best research-based treatment programs can reduce recidivism rates of these youth from 25% to 80% (NMHA, 2004).

The American Academy of Child and Adolescent Psychiatry has developed a set of guidelines for incarcerated youth who have no interventions for their mental health problems (Vieira, 2005). These guidelines have been set up for psychiatrists and other clinicians who need assistance in consultation, management of role conflicts, prescribing psychotropic medications, or the use of seclusion and restraints. The guidelines are designed to assist in monitoring youth who threaten or attempt suicide. They also provide assistance in dealing with the juvenile correctional facilities and their staff.

Homeless kids and runaways can be referred to The Bridge program for someone to talk to, breakfast and lunch, a place to shower and do laundry, classes to earn a GED, job counseling and training, medical checkups and dental care, and transitional housing (Bridge Over Troubled Waters, 2010). Called The Bridge Over Troubled Waters, this Boston-based organization can be contacted for information as to the availability of such programs in others cities. They point out that the kids' needs can include a desire to leave the streets, talk to someone who cares, and make changes in their life. This program has been working for 40 years.

In Hempstead, New York, a devoted youth social worker tries to save young people from the street in a group center called STRONG Youth. Her main message is to try to keep young people away from violence. She works with youth to help them resolve conflicts peacefully. Her work is dangerous at times, but she says that it is not possible to be a good social worker behind a desk. Without being out in the community, she says that she would not see what is pulling them into various situations (Rivera, 2008). She makes house calls, goes to where the teens hang out, visits hospitals and jails, even going to homicide scenes. She works with the teenagers to role play potentially violent circumstances at parties. She coaches the kids as to what to do in a shooting scene.

In a consortium devoted to supporting young adults before crime becomes a way of life, John Jay College of Criminal Justice in Manhattan partners with the city's Center for Economic Opportunity and the Department of Correction to provide the Justice Corps. This is a modification of the national youth corps movement designed to insert young people back into communities that they damaged in some way (Fahim, 2009). The program is designed to build self-worth by helping youth build up their community by making a contribution. Participants in the program are paid $8.50 to $9.50 an hour while looking for long-term jobs. The program provides experience in transitional employment leading to regular work.

Centers for Adolescent Health Promotion

In Los Angeles, a joint venture of ACLA and Rand Health has undertaken many projects funded by a variety of grants at the Center for Adolescent Health Promotion—affiliates and community partners for youth needing after-school activities and programs, cognitive behavioral interventions for trauma and bullying in schools, physical activities for girls, preventative health care for youth, education in family communication, teen HIV and STD risk reduction, firearm storage at home, and interventions for the effects of terrorism, violence exposure, drugs, neighborhood deterioration, sexual practices, smoking, and food interventions (RAND Center for Adolescent Health Promotion, 2009).

For others wishing to work with adolescents, the University of Minnesota School of Nursing has a program within the Center for Adolescent Nursing, at the graduate and doctoral levels, preparing nurses to care for maternal and child health. They serve as a national hub for professionals specializing in adolescent health. This program is open to people of a number of disciplinary backgrounds (Nursing for Adolescents, 2009). The program is aimed at individual, community, and population levels of health concerns for adolescents. The goals of this program are to amplify scientific knowledge, management and communication skills, policy and advocacy, and methodological and analytical skills in adolescent health issues.

Peninsula Counseling Center on Long Island has a grant from the New York State Office of Mental Health in a 5-year preventive program to identify kids with signs of stress, trying to intervene with and for them as early as possible. Originally, they set out to assist families in trouble with problems and are now observing their 95th year of serving the community. Helping youth assume responsibility has assisted in building community. This center encourages national community service as a way for youth to give back in thanks for their education and upbringing (Amon, 2008).

Special High Schools for Adolescents With Spectrum Disorders

Montcalm School for Girls and Montcalm School for Boys, located in Van Wert, Ohio, have both been established to provide special education for youth with spectrum disorder diagnoses. Their curriculum includes alternative programs to assist adolescents with these diagnoses with their struggles in the social realm. These are therapeutic boarding schools that accept students nationally and internationally (Montcalm School for Girls/Boys, 2008), and employ a Starr Private Treatment Program. This alternative program is structured for youth with social disorders. In a strength-based environment, this program integrates the power of interpersonal communication, peer group treatment, and learning through the principles of positive peer culture. The intervention is aimed at developing healthy relationships and taking personal responsibility for choices (Montcalm School for Girls/Boys, 2008).

Recently, in Westbury, Long Island, New York, an area known as the NIMBY (not in my back yard) capital of the country, citizens and parents asked the village zoning board to approve plans for a residential high school for teenagers with high functioning autism and Asperger's syndrome. Called the Westbrook Preparatory School and housed in a former convent, it will soon begin serving a dozen youth because the community believed that these challenged kids deserve a place to learn (Brockland, 2010). This effort is also supported by an organization called Congregations, Associations, and Neighborhoods (CAN), set up in the spirit of social networks and social capital.

Online, The Help Group maintains an index of related resources for adolescents with spectrum disorders at www.thehelpgroup.org. ADD Consults are another online source with a helpful directory at www.addconsults.com.

Social Interaction Using Augmentative and Alternative Communication

Lillenfeld and Alant (2005) presented a case of the social interactions of an adolescent in a peer training program using augmentative and alternative communication for a severe disability (AAC). This study compared the interactions of the adolescent with his classroom peers before and after a peer training program in psychosocial participation. The program brought about an increase in the frequency of communications from the teenager, and changes were noted in his discourse structures and functions.

Adolescent Psychiatric Inpatient and Partial Hospitalization Programs

Several examples of inpatient and partial hospitalization programs for adolescents will be described here. When teens experience acute symptoms of psychiatric disorders, emotional illness, or substance abuse or dependence that disrupt their social relations with their family, peers, and teachers, they can be referred for hospital-based treatment. The goals of these programs are to develop responsibility in a supportive therapeutic setting. If the adolescents can live at home, they can use the services of a partial hospitalization program in order to set up support system networks in their community. In this way, they can continue to develop their roles as student, family member, team member, and religious observer, while volunteering in a community-based setting.

Some examples of adolescent psychiatric treatment programs can be found here:

- × www.south-oaks.org in Long Island, New York
- × www.sjmercyhealth.org for St. Joseph Mercy Health System in Ann Arbor, Michigan

- × www.tenbroeck.com/TBResources/ for Ten Broeck Hospital in Louisville, Kentucky
- × www.ccca.dmhmrsas.virginia.gov/ for the Commonwealth Center for Children and Adolescents, Staunton, Virginia
- × www.highfocuscenters.com/adolescent_psychiatric_services.html in northern New Jersey

For locations near you, search on the Web for adolescent psychiatric hospital programs.

Troubled Teens—Currie's *The Road to Whatever*

Older teens tend to feel greater social pressure to excel in academics, sports, mature social relationships, and many forms of community participation and service, especially as they move beyond high school to colleges, universities, vocational training programs, and employment or other community roles. The current economic situation forces new graduates to compete for fewer available jobs, and the high cost of everything makes many aspects of the transition to adulthood more difficult. A recent study (Currie, 2004) looks at the perceptions that adolescents and young adults have about the social roles available to them, what the future holds, and why they often feel ambivalent about becoming responsible adults. Interpreting the results of hundreds of interviews with middle-class youth who had experienced serious trouble, such as drug addiction or institutionalization for violent, reckless, or self-destructive acts, Currie (2004) concludes that once an adolescent gets caught in a downward spiral, the social institutions in the United States offer very little help and support. He blames a "pervasive culture of exclusion and neglect... that helped to propel these teenagers into the perilous state of not caring very much about what happened to them" (p. 48). Within this negative culture, four themes emerge:

1. *Inversion of responsibility*—Teens describe coming from homes in which parents have abdicated responsibility for authoritative or nurturing roles, leaving teens to care for themselves and "exposing them to a multitude of perils in an increasingly risky world" (Currie, 2004, p. 50). In these "sink or swim" families, when teens survive, they also learn much that is of value in coping with life.

2. *The problem of contingent worth*—Social contexts of school, peers, and families that measure worth by certain narrow standards (i.e., grades, competition in sports, or "whatever arena is considered important for status and prestige") (p. 68). Within this context, teens face a no-win situation

in which doing well is never quite good enough because winning means being better than everyone else, a nearly impossible standard of social worth.

3. *The intolerance for transgression*—An equally narrow definition of moral acceptance in which there is little tolerance for even legitimate mistakes. This is reflected in policies such as "zero tolerance" for possession or use of illegal drugs or involvement in episodes of criminal activity. Religious contexts often reflect the same intolerance for any type of deviance, demanding sexual abstinence and complete avoidance of any activity considered sinful. Currie (2004) found that many troubled teens felt labeled as bad because of one mistake, an impossible standard of perfection.

4. *The punitive reflex and the rejection of nurturance*—Reflects society's lack of tolerance for "normal deviance" so that minor lapses in meeting social and moral expectations result in rejection (e.g., expulsion from school), withdrawal of both physical and emotional support (by parents telling teens to "get out" of the house), and health care professionals giving prescription medications instead of guidance for mental health issues (Currie, 2004).

This research study concludes that, for teens to gain support before the really serious trouble begins, the culture surrounding them must change from one of neglect and punishment to one of support and inclusion.

A Word About Tough Love

Tough love is a movement that originated in the 1970s by weary parents who felt victimized by their wayward teens. The tough love philosophy appealed to them because they had lost all parental authority and felt the need to set some boundaries for their own safety and well-being. Burney, a spiritual teacher who counsels such parents, explains that tough love teaches parents how to avoid enabling their teen's self-destructive behaviors, a role that psychologists have labeled *codependency*. Enabling teens to practice any form of addiction or other compulsive behaviors (sex, gambling, eating disorders) includes supporting them financially, providing food and shelter, making excuses for them, or any other action or inaction that allows them to continue the behaviors. Tough love teaches parents to set limits out of respect for themselves. Parent support groups practicing tough love thrive to this day (Tough Love Parenting, 2008).

The tough love philosophy pervades most teen residential rehabilitation programs, including wilderness programs, behavior modification centers, and emotional growth boarding schools (Szalavitz, 2006). Several hundred public and private facilities serve wayward American teens, with little or no regulation, no admission criteria other than statements and payment by parents, and very few published studies of their effectiveness (Szalavitz, 2006). The National Institutes of Health, in a "state of the science" consensus statement, concluded that "get tough" treatments "do not work and there is some evidence that they may make the problem worse." Currie's (2004) study concurs with this conclusion.

Summary

Both Chapters 12 and 13 have presented a variety of programs for the service professional to understand and use in current or future settings. Usually, social learning programs are broad based and are intended for all children and adolescents as part of their psychological and social repertoire of participation growth. They have varying perspectives, providing educators and health caregivers with a great choice of social participation approaches. Other programs that have been reviewed in Chapters 12 and 13 are designed for children and adolescents with special social needs or problems that require intervention designed specifically for the individual situation and environment. Future service professionals in education and health care should assess which suggested programs meet the needs of the individual or group and should discuss these with a professor, supervisor, or colleague, as well as with the individual or group receiving education or intervention.

Can you now distinguish between social learning programs and social intervention programs?

Script: Teen's "Road to Whatever" Group

Scenario

This script represents an imagined conversation between some of the "troubled teens" interviewed for the Currie (2004) study, whose ideas contributed to his recognition of a need for cultural changes in the service structures that serve adolescents when they encounter problems.

In this idealized scenario, Katie, a new graduate in occupational therapy, was awarded a state educational grant as part of Obama's stimulus package to create an alternative educational program for teens who fail to fit into the formal educational approach. To begin, Katie and Marvin, the school counselor and her partner on the "inside," have invited all students who dropped out of high school in the past year to participate in this "focus group." They are seated in bean bag chairs in one corner of the gym on a Saturday afternoon in January.

Seating Chart

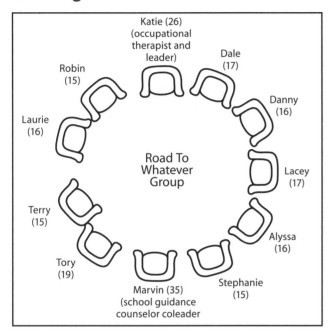

Characters

Danny: (age 16) Fell in with violent kids and was sent to juvenile hall for beating up and robbing another boy for a trivial slight.

Terry: (age 15) Drinks a fifth of gin a day. His idea of fun is driving stolen cars at reckless speeds while being chased by a cop. He uses methamphetamine and has tried heroin. Fell in with militant racist kids in a suburban town, but did not care about their "trip"—just did not care.

Laurie: (age 16) Ex-cheerleader, tried Terry's weed and could not remember what else she took, but overdosed and ended up in the detoxification unit of the community hospital.

Tory: (age 19) Once an addict, now coordinator of services for the homeless.

Robin: (age 15) Mother and father argued a lot and had their own issues. Parents did not know the difference between a minor offense and a major one. Mother repeatedly threw her out of the house until she learned to live on the street or in the back of a car.

Stephanie: (age 15) Lived alternately with each divorced parent, neither could deal with her behavior and had little or no rapport with her. Her friends got her high on heroin and brought her unconscious to the hospital. Now, she is unable to follow a conversation and cannot focus long enough to fully understand what someone is saying to her.

Dale: (age 17) Smart enough to explain all of the physiological effects of drugs like crystal meth and how much it takes to kill you. He is tall with specs, feared by other kids because of his bad temper and volatility, and has "gone off" on teachers at school, which got him expelled.

Alyssa: (age 16) Conflicts are common within her home, causing her to become nonemotional and look right through people. Her parents had their own problems (workaholic, alcoholic) and forced her to take care of younger sisters when she was too young. She did not always do the right thing, but always felt abandoned and unsafe in her home. In high school, she turned to drugs, then attempted suicide.

Lacey: (age 17) Sexually assaulted by an older guy after a few dates. In therapy, she was labeled a problem child. Why was she attracted to men who abuse her? She is a pretty blonde, now about 7 months pregnant. Even when she is at home, she always has feelings of abandonment.

Katie: (age 26) Trained occupational therapist leading this group meeting, the purpose of which is to better understand what caused them to get into trouble and for them to come up with their own creative solutions within their homes, school, and community. The program invites all kids who dropped out of high school and gives them a place where they are accepted and can belong.

Marvin: (age 35) School counselor and coleader for this group.

Action Begins Here

Katie: Thank you all for coming. This is Marvin, whom some of you have met. He'll be helping me to lead this discussion.

Marvin: Hello, everyone. It's nice to see you back at school. Today, we'll be turning things upside down. Instead of students, you'll be our teachers. We are here to learn something from each of you.

(a few groans)

Katie: Now don't worry, any of you, because Marvin's rules will apply to every one of our conversations. We all agree that anything said here will be confidential. Nobody's going to call the police or use what you say against you. Can we all agree on that?

(grumbles, mostly nods)

Marvin: I know some of you have messed around with drugs. You've probably told me lots of stuff that could get you into trouble if you were still a student, but my records are confidential. And you're not students anymore. Today, we want you to be honest with us; otherwise, we can't come up with solutions that will actually help you.

Dale: Nothin' will help us anyway. So I don't much care. What do you want to know?

Terry: Yeah, Dale knows a lot about drugs and trafficking. You can make a lot of easy money.

Robin: Tory can tell you more than I can about homeless people. She works with them now. That's how we met.

Katie: I know you all have interesting stories to tell. Why don't we all introduce ourselves, and each of you tell the group what you've been doing since you dropped out of school. Who wants to start?

Danny: Mine's easy. I've been locked up in juvenile hall 'til about a month ago. Now, I'm temporarily staying with my mom. Now that she understands I'm not going back to school, we don't fight so much. But it's so *b-o-r-i-n-g*, I can't think of nothing to do but sleep.

Stephanie: At least you got a place to live. I'm sleepin' in a car most nights. My mom can't handle me at all.

Robin: Guess your Mom booted you out, too?

Stephanie: And my dad, depending on which parent I'm living with at the moment.

Katie: *(writing notes)* I hear that both Stephanie and Robin have some problems with parents, and we'll get back to you for more details in just a minute. We wanted to start with an overview so that you all could begin to know something about each other, too.

Danny: Why don't you just make us wear name tags. Like detention?

Marvin: We thought of that. Would you like to? I'll get markers. *(he stands)*

Danny: Naah. I was just—you mean you actually would do it?

Marvin: Sure, why?

Danny: It's just, no one usually listens.

Katie: It's good you said that, 'cause I wanted all of you to know that here we will listen—we want to listen to all of you.

Lacey: Yeah, right.

Katie: You don't believe me.

Lacey: I believe you. Today, you'll listen. But next week… maybe not.

Robin: That's what you say, but I'm not falling for it. I'm with… what's your name?

Lacey: Lacey.

Marvin: *(returns with name tags and markers)* Guess you need these after all. *(hands Lacey and Robin tags and markers)*

Katie: Look, Lacey and Robin, I hear you saying that your parents didn't listen to you and that has you upset, but Marvin and I would really like to show you that you can trust us. We have a project to plan, and we need your help to make sure what we plan will actually help kids like you. So, we are different from other adults, like parents, teachers, or police. Right?

Lacey: Different how? Like the therapists they sent us to? I told Dr. Burns my feelings about being raped and beat up. And all he could ask is, "What's wrong with you?" Like it was my fault, 'cause I wear short skirts and low necklines? 'Cause I dated an older man? Now I'm having this kid I don't want, and who's gonna help me take care of it? You?

Terry: I know folks who'd pay big money for a kid. To adopt it… didn't you know you could sell it? Specially if it's a girl and she has pretty blonde hair. *(raises eyebrows, flirting—looks to Dale for approval)*

Lacey: SHUT UP, CREEP! I'll…

Marvin: I have to intervene here. I'm not judging any of you, and I have to ask that you also don't judge each other. Outside with your other friends you can say what you want, but in this group, we treat each other with respect. So, we'll take a different road, here. We'll listen and maybe offer suggestions that might actually help.

Terry: Yeah, whatever. *(makes a face at Dale, who smirks, stifling a guffaw)*

Marvin: Dale? Did you have something to say?

Dale: I been here before—in counseling and in drug rehab, too. They don't listen to the reasons why you did something. Just stop doing drugs. Take methadone. Like we just do drugs cause we're bored. No, we get labeled as problems—failures, unable to cope without getting high every day. It's bullshit, that's what.

Marvin: We've met before, I know. So you're upset with me for not helping you more in counseling?

Dale: You could say that. If I cared. Which I don't anymore.

Katie: *(writing notes again)* So a few of you have some issues with the kind of therapy you got. Is that accurate? Lacey? Dale?

Lacey: Right. And, yes, I could use some help with my… situation. Is it true, some people would pay me to adopt my baby?

Katie: I'm writing that down too, Lacey. *(writes, then looks around the circle)* Who haven't we heard from yet?

Alyssa: *(raises her hand, shyly)* Me, Alyssa. I... maybe I'm the only one here who actually tried to OD... you know, to off myself. I survived, but I'm not sure I'm glad. No one listened to me in the hospital either. They didn't want to know the reasons. Just take the pills. Like there's nothing and no one around me that drove me to do it. It's all my problem. Lacey and Dale got it right—they don't care so why should we? *(she manages to say all this with almost no emotion, looking straight ahead)*

Dale: See, that's what I mean. She didn't even get good advice on drugs. I could have told you what would work—what you'd have to do so you'd really die. But then, you can find it on the web, too.

Marvin: No, Dale. That's not what she needs. But I think you know that, right?

Dale: *(smirks)* Busted.

Marvin: Don't tell me, Dale. Tell her. Do you really think you should help Alyssa commit suicide?

Dale: Sorry, Alyssa. I don't know you, really. You probably have lots of talent to contribute to the world.

Tory: I was going to say that, only more sincerely. Alyssa, I used to be an addict, never heroin, but I did slam crystal meth, like you told me you did. But then I found some people I really liked living on the street. And I took them to my Dad, who's a lawyer, and he helped them find loans and places to live. And now I help them, too. If you don't have a job and you want to do something for other people, there's a lot of homeless people, and I'm looking for an assistant. It doesn't pay much, but it has its rewards.

Alyssa: Yeah, whatever.

Tory: *(looking offended)* Well, it's just a suggestion.

Katie: That's the second time I've heard that word "whatever" said today. What does it mean, Alyssa? What made you say it?

Alyssa: Tory doesn't know me, either. She didn't hear me out. How when I was 5, my parents were AWOL—gone. Well, there but not there. I had to make my sisters lunch cause Mom was working and Dad was passed out drunk. I was FIVE, and I'm taking the vodka bottle away from my 3-year-old sister. Tory thinks I don't do enough to help other people. That's all I've ever done.

Katie: So, it's not that Tory doesn't have a helpful idea. It's just that you wanted her to listen first.

Alyssa: That's right. *(shows the first sign of real emotion—tears well up)* Not just Tory. I'm sorry, I'm not mad at you. *(makes eye contact with Tory)* Sure, I'd like to have a job where I could actually do some good, but at home it didn't matter what I said. Mom never listened either, or Dad, or any of the doctors at the hospital.

Katie: Well, it's almost time to end for today. You all have given us, me and Marvin, some important information about the kinds of problems that made you get off track with your education and your life. I don't know about you, Marvin, but I have more questions than answers after our discussion. We definitely need to continue these discussions next week.

Marvin: *(sums up)* I agree, we've only begun to understand your point of view about the difficulties high school students like you have experienced. We'll continue to need your input with this planning phase of our project. So, all of you are welcome to attend every Saturday and bring your ideas and concerns. And just a reminder, we keep anything said during this group confidential. Next week, same time, same place.

The End.

Discussion

1. What legal constraints might apply to this group? Look up medical, educational, and psychiatric legal policies regarding confidentiality on the internet.

2. What conflicts can you identify between members, both leaders, and participants? How were these addressed?

3. When leaders responded to trust issues, what techniques from Chapters 1 and 3 can you identify?

4. Do you agree with the therapeutic interventions used by the occupational therapist and school counselor? Why or why not?

5. How would you respond to Dale's comment that "Nothing will help us anyway"?

6. What resources might be available to help Lacey with her pregnancy, upcoming birth, and parenting issues?

7. What social support does the group provide to prevent Alyssa from resorting to suicide?

8. What levels of social participation can you identify in this group? Which of the five levels (Donohue) are most often demonstrated?

References

Albanese, L. (2008). Parents demand answers. *Newsday,* *November 13,* A9.

Allan, E., & Madden, M. (2008). *Hazing in view: College students at risk.* Nashville, TN: National Collegiate Association.

Altherr, S. (2008). Fighting drugs in Smithtown. *Newsday,* *December 18,* A32.

Amon, R. (2008). A long view on mental health. *Newsday,* *September 21,* G2.

Anderson, L. M., Scrimshaw, S. C., Fullilove, M. T., & Fielding, J. E. (2003). The Community Guide's model for linking the social environment to health. *American Journal of Preventive Medicine, 24,* 12-20.

Aron, A., McLaughlin-Volpe, T., Mashek, D., Lewandowski, G., Wright, S. C., & Aron, E. N. (2004). Including close others in the self. *European Review of Social Psychology, 15,* 101-132.

Aronson, E. (2000). *Nobody left to hate. Teaching compassion after Columbine.* New York, NY: W. H. Freeman.

Aull, E. (2006). Study: Hazing widespread. *Portland Press Herald, August, 7,* Retrieved from www.pressherald.mainetoday.com/news/state/060807hazing.shtml

Bleiberg Seperson, S., & Arfin, P. (2008). Separating generations a bad idea. *Newsday, December 15,* A31.

Bridge Over Troubled Waters. (2010). *You don't have to be on your own. Bridge can help.* Retrieved from www.bridgeotw.org

Carey, B. (2008). Psychiatrists revise the book of human troubles. *New York Times, December 18.* Retrieved from www.nytimes.com/2008/12/18/health/18psych.html

Carter, E. W., Cushing, L. S., & Kennedy, C. H. (2009). *Peer support strategies for improving all students' social lives and learning.* Baltimore, MD: Paul H. Brookes Publishing Co.

Centers for Disease Control. (2008). *Violence; sexual behavior. Guide to community preventive services.* Retrieved from www.thecommunityguide.org/violence/sexualbehavior

Chance, P. (2000). Gunning for a solution to school shootings. *Psychology Today, September/October,* 74.

Cheever, S. (2008). Drunkenfreude. *New York Times, December.* Retrieved December 18, 2008 from www.proof.blogs.nytimes.com/2008/12/15drunkenfreude

Christakis, N. (2009). Peer pressure. *THE WEEK, January 9.*

Copeland, S. R., Hughes, C., Carter, E. W., Guth, C., Presley, J., Williams, C. R., & Fowler, S. E. (2004). Increasing access to general education: Perspectives of participants in a high school peer support program. *Remedial and Special Education, 26,* 342-352.

Currie, E. (2004). *The road to whatever: Middle class culture and the crisis of adolescence.* New York, NY: Holt & Company.

Cushing, L. S., & Kennedy, C. H. (1997). Academic effects on students without disabilities who serve as peer supports for student with disabilities in general education classrooms. *Journal of Applied Behavior Analysis, 30,* 139-152.

Drug Policy Alliance. (2008). *Innovative Drug Prevention DVD, Just4Teens, Now Available to Teachers, Counselors, and Prevention Specialists in New Mexico.* Retrieved from www.drugpolicy.org/news/pressroom/pressrelease/pr100108b.cfm

ERIC Document Reproduction Service. (1998). No. ED 415 455, Report No. CG 028 225. Greensboro, NC: Center for Research on Counseling and Personnel Services.

Erikson, E. (1968). *Identity: youth and crisis.* New York, NY: W. W. Norton.

Events NYU. (2008). *You can become a peer educator- Apply now!* Retrieved from www.events.nyu.edu/?cmd=showevent&cal12&id=187246

Fahim, K. (2009). Seeking to intervene with young adults before crime becomes a way of life. *NY Times, March.* Retrieved from www.nytimes.com/2009/03/04/nyregion

Fink, P. J. (2001). Problems with and solutions for school violence. In M. Shafii & S. L. Shafii (Eds.), *School violence. Assessment, management, prevention* (pp. 231-250). Washington, DC: American Psychiatric Association.

Finkelhor, D., Ormrod, R. K., & Turner, H. A. (2007). Polyvictimization and trauma in a national longitudinal cohort. *Development and Psychopathology, 19,* 149-166.

Goleman, D. (1995). *Emotional intelligence. Why it can matter more than IQ.* New York, NY: Bantam Books.

Gruwell, E. (1999). *The Freedom Writer's diary: How a teacher and 150 teens used writing to change themselves and the world around them.* New York, NY: Doubleday.

Gutman, S. A., & Schindler, V. P. (2007). Supported education for adults and adolescents with psychiatric disabilities: Occupational therapy's role. *OT Practice, 12,* CE1-CE8.

Horsley, W. R. (2008). Fighting off heroin's resurgence. *Newsday, December 16,* A37.

Hughes, C., & Carter, E. W. (2008). *Peer buddy programs for successful secondary school inclusion.* Baltimore, MD: Paul H. Brooks Publishing Co.

Hunt, P., Soto, G., Maier, J., & Doering, K. (2003). Collaborative teaming to support students with severe disabilities in general education classrooms. *Exceptional Children, 69,* 315-332.

Individuals with Disabilities Education Improvement Act. (2004). 20 U.S.C. § 1400-1485 (2004).

International Drug Policy Reform Conference. (2009). *About the event.* Retrieved from www.reformconference.org/

Jackson, C. (2006). E-bully. *Teaching Tolerance, Spring, 50,* 51-55.

Kern-Rugile, J. (2006). Institute for Student Achievement: Small learning communities that enable students to achieve big results. *Newsday, October 5,* B6.

Lam, C. (2009). Tension over tipline. *Newsday, May 11,* A8.

Lasater, L., & Beckett, J. A. (2007). *Character development results with high-risk students in a Georgia school alternative program.* CrossRoads Success Academy, Eastanollee, GA. Retrieved from www.CharacterDevelopmentSystems.com/pubs/georgi-report-07

Lasater, L., Robinson, K. D., Willis, T., Meyer, C. L., Jahns, N. R., Bush, L., ... & Duffey, K. R. (2005). *Using social responsibility training (SRT) to support youth school success.* Retrieved from www.CharacterDevelopmentSystems.com and www.CharacterDevelopmentSystems.com/img/making-a-differnce.pdf

Layne, M., Pynoos, D. & Cardenas, E. (2001). Trauma and grief component therapy for adolescents (TGCT). Retrieved August 2008 from the National Child Traumatic Stress Network (NCTSN) at www.nctsnet.org

Lillenfeld, M., & Alant, E. (2005). The social interaction of an adolescent who uses AAC: The evaluation of a peer-training program. *Augmentative & Alternative Communication, 21,* 278-294.

Maslow, A. (1943). A theory of human motivation. *Psychological Review, 50,* 370-396.

Mitchell, K. J., Wolak, J., & Finkelhor, D. (2008). Are blogs putting youth at risk for online sexual solicitation or harassment? *Child Abuse & Neglect, 32,* 277-294.

Montcalm School for Girls/Boys. (2008). *Alternative programs.* Retrieved from www.montcalmschools.org/alternativeprograms

Murray, J. (2001). But I love him: Protecting your teen daughter from controlling, abusive dating relationships [Kindle version]. Retrieved from www.amazon.com/But-Love-Him-Controlling-Relationships/dp/0060957298

National Crime Prevention Council. (2009). Retrieved from www.ncpc.org/topics/bullying/strategies/strategy-peer-mediation-in-high-school

National Mental Health Association. (2004). *Mental health treatment for youth in the juvenile justice system: A compendium of promising practices.* Retrieved from www.nmha.org/children/justjuv/index.cfm

News From Campus. (2009). *Malverne Schools 12. Why do kids do what they do? Malverne parents get expert advice at a district-sponsored workshop.* January 3, 2009. Retrieved from www.malverne.k12.ny.us

Nursing for Adolescents. (2009). *Adolescent nursing, University of Minnesota.* Retrieved from www.nursing.umn.edu/Adolescent_Nursing/home.html

Office of National Drug Control Policy. (2007). *Drug free communities support program.* Retrieved from www.ondcp.gov/dfc/

Office of Safe and Drug-Free Schools. (2009). *Reports & resources.* Retrieved from www2.ed.gov/about/offices/list/osdfs/resources.html#online

Olson, L. (2006). *Activity groups in family-centered treatment. Psychiatric occupational therapy approaches for parents and children.* New York, NY: Haworth Press.

Palomare, S., & Cowan, D. (1998). *Talking with kids. Guided discussions for teaching emotional intelligence.* Torrance, CA: Innerchoice Publishing.

Ralph, A., Hogan, S. J., Hill, M., Perkins, E., Ryan, J., & Strong, L. (1998). Improving adolescent social competence in peer interactions using correspondence training. *Education & Treatment of Children, 21,* 171-194.

Rivera, L. (2008). A 'first responder' against violence. *Newsday,* September 15, A15.

Russo, M. (2009). New law to combat rising heroin use. *Lynbrook/East Rockaway Herald,* January 1, 3.

Safe & Responsive Schools. (2002). *Resources, conflict resolution/peer mediation.* Retrieved from www.indiana.edu/~safeschl/resources_mediation.html

Salisbury, C. L., Gallucci, C. I., Palombaro, M. M., & Peck, C. A. (1995). Strategies that promote social relations among elementary students with and without severe disabilities in inclusive schools, *Exceptional Children, 62,* 125-137.

Setoodeh, R. (2008). Young, gay and murdered. *Newsweek, July, 19.* Retrieved from www.newsweek.com/id/147790

Shafii, M., & Shafii, S. L. (Eds.). (2001). *School violence. Assessment, management, prevention.* Washington, DC: American Psychiatric Publishing, Inc.

Sharp, D. (2009). High school rife with hazing, Maine study finds. *Associated Press, April 16.* Retrieved from www.news.yahoo.com/s/ap/20090416/ap_on_re_us/hazing_study

Social Responsibility Training. (2007). *Project Report 2001-2007.* Retrieved May 18, 2010 from www.characterdevelopmentsystems.com

Sorenson, D. L., & Nord, D. A. (2002). *Discussion-provoking scripts for teens.* Minneapolis, MN: Educational Media Corporation.

Szalavitz, M. (2006). The trouble with tough love. *The Washington Post, January 29,* B01. Retrieved February 18, 2009 from www.washingtonpost.com/content/article/2006/01/28/AR2006012800062

Task Force on Community Preventive Services. (2007). Recommendation for use of behavioral interventions to reduce the risk of sexual transmission of HIV among men who have sex with men. *American Journal of Preventive Medicine, 32,* S36-S37.

Teicher, M. H., Samson, J. A., Polcari, A., & McGreenery, C. E. (2006). Sticks, stones, and hurtful words: Relative effects of various forms of childhood maltreatment. *American Journal of Psychiatry, 163,* 993-1000.

Theberge, S. K., & Karan, O. C. (2004). Six factors inhibiting the use of peer mediation in a junior high school. *Professional School Counseling, 7,* 283-290.

Tough Love Parenting. (2008). *How parenting child development helps make you closer to your kids.* Retrieved May 18, 2010 from www.parenting-child-development.com

Vieira, C. L. (2005). *New mental health help for juvenile offenders.* Bradley Hospital: A lifespan partner. Cvieira1@lifespan.org.

Williams, D. (2003). *Mix it up at lunch hard to swallow for some. Teaching tolerance.* Retrieved from www.tolerance.org/teens/stories/article.jsp

Wiseman, R. (2003). *Queen bees and wannabees: Helping your daughter survive cliques, gossip, boyfriends and other realities of adolescence.* New York, NY: Random House.

Zimmerman, E. (2009). Teen angst turns deadly. Why girls are killing themselves. *Psychology Today, January/February,* 30.

Additional Resources

ADD Consults. (2009). *ADHD Directory Complete List.* Retrieved from www.addconsults.com/directory/listingall.phpe3

Alcohol Answers: Evidence-based treatment and support. (2009). *For the alcohol dependent person.* Retrieved January 7, 2009 from www.alcoholanswers.org

Brockland, B. (2010). *A pleasant suburban surprise.* Retrieved from www.saintbrigid.net/convent/nextsteps.html

Center for Adolescent Nursing, University of Minnesota School of Nursing. (2009). Retrieved from www.nursing.unm.edu/Adolescent_Nursing/home.html

Character Development Systems, LLC. (2007). *Social responsibility training. A comprehensive solution for school disengagement. A PowerPoint presentation.* Retrieved from www.characterdevelopmentsystems.com.

Commonwealth Center for Children and Adolescents, Stanto, VA. Retrieved from www.ccca.dmhmrsas.virginia.gov

Diagnostic and Statistical Manual of Mental Disorders (5th ed.). Washington, DC: American Psychological Association.

Eisenberg, M. (2008). Family meals and substance use: Is there a long-term protective association? *Journal of Adolescent Health, 43,* 2.

Help Group. (2009). *Specialized schools: Helping children with autism.* Retrieved from www.thehelpgroup.org/index.php

High Focus Centers. (2005). *Adolescent Psychiatric Services.* Retrieved from www.highfocuscenters.com/adolescent_psychiatric_services.html

Holmes, B. (2008). Rom-coms 'spoil' your love life. *BBC News.* Retrieved from www.bbc.co.uk/2/hi/uk_news/scotland/edinburgh_and_east/.stm

Klass, P. (2009). *Another awkward sex talk: Respect and violence.* Retrieved from www.nytimes.com/2009/04/14health/14klas.html

Levitt, D. (2009). Making overtures. *Psychology Today, January/February,* 11.

Linking the interests of families and teachers (LIFT). (2009). *Find Youth Info.* Retrieved December 29, 2009 from www.findyouthinfo.gov

National Collaborative for Hazing Research and Prevention. (2010). *Research.* Retrieved from http://www.hazingstudy.org/research.php

National Crime Prevention Council. (2009). *Strategy: Peer mediation in high school.* Retrieved from http://www.ncpc.org/programs/circle-of-respect/understanding-bullying-and-cyberbullying/bullying/strategies/strategy-peer-mediation-in-high-schools/

National Research Council and Institute of Medicine (2009). Report: Tween, teen years crucial to health. *Newsday, January 6,* A27.

Partnership for a Drug Free America. (2009). *Parent resource.* Retrieved from www.drugfree.org

RAND Center for Adolescent Health Promotion. (2009). *Archived projects.* Retrieved from www.rand.org/health/centers/adolescent/archive/

South Oaks Adolescent Partial Hospital Program. (2009). *Child & adolescent center for excellence.* Retrieved from www.south-oaks.org

St. Joseph Mercy Health System. (2010). *Mercy health system.* Retrieved from www.mercyhealth.org

Taylor, D. (2006). NAMI Letter. *National Association for the Mentally Ill, October.*

Ten Broeck Hospital, Louisville, KY. (2009). Ten Broeck resources. Retrieved from www.tenbroeck.com/TBResources/

The Help Group. (2010). *Schools, Camps & Programs.* Retrieved from http://www.thehelpgroup.org/programs.htm

Tracy, J. (2008). Whooping it up? It's only natural. *Newsday, August 13,* A27.

Tuttle, S. (2008). Make. It. Stop. *Newsweek, August 1,* 2.

U.S. Department of Justice. (1996). Uniform crime reporting program press release 10/13/96. Retrieved from www.fbi. gov/ucr/ucr95prs.htm

Wired for Safety. (2010). *WiredSafety.* Retrieved from www. WiredSafety.org

chapter 14

Adult Interventions to Promote Social Participation

Marilyn B. Cole, MS, OTR/L, FAOTA

Adults within the mainstream of society have already developed social competence and may be participating within a wide variety of social roles and relationships. Barriers to social participation can emerge in adulthood because of the following factors:

- Physical or mental health conditions

- Life stressors such as death of a spouse or child or loss of employment

- Changes in social context, such as place of residence or socioeconomic status

- Predictable life transitions, such as midlife crisis, empty nest, or retirement

- Lifestyle changes by personal choice or otherwise

When barriers exist, interventions are needed to develop or re-establish social roles and to reintegrate individuals into their preferred social groups or communities. The interventions covered in this chapter fall into the following categories: social skills training, community reintegration, social support groups, work-related interventions, and friendships and family relationships.

Social Skills Training

Social skills training is a form of behavior therapy used by teachers, therapists, and trainers to help people who have difficulties relating to other people

(*Encyclopedia of Mental Disorders*, 2009). Originally designed for mental health settings, social skills training emerged in the late 1980s, when many large state hospitals were closing due to a lack of funding, to assist chronic patients in re-entering their communities. Social skills training uses principles of behaviorism, such as modeling, shaping, social learning, role playing, and reinforcement, to teach basic interpersonal communication in small units (Bellack, Mueser, Gingerich, & Agresta, 2004; Liberman & Fuller, 2000). Social skills are behaviorally defined as "interpersonal behaviors that are normative and/or socially sanctioned" (Bellack et al., 2004, p. 3), and include the following:

- Dress and behavior codes

- Rules about what to say/not to say

- Expression of affect/emotion

- Social reinforcement (approval, disapproval, support)

- Interpersonal distance

The early social skills training programs were designed for people with schizophrenia, a persistent mental illness that typically involves a lack of social skills, making it difficult to establish and maintain social relationships, fulfill social roles (worker, spouse), or have one's basic needs met. Many of the intervention strategies described here are applicable for schizophrenia as well as other groups with cognitive or social impairments such as cerebral palsy, mental retardation, autism, or head injury.

Cole, M.B., & Donohue, M.V. *Social Participation in Occupational Contexts: In Schools, Clinics, and Communities* (pp 251-272).
© 2011 SLACK Incorporated

Table 14-1

GROUP SESSIONS FOR DEVELOPING FRIENDSHIP AND DATING SKILLS

- Expression of positive feelings
- Giving compliments
- Accepting compliments
- Finding common interests
- Asking someone for a date

- Ending a date
- Expressing affection
- Refusing unwanted sexual advances
- Asking partner to use a condom
- Refusing pressure to engage in high-risk sexual behavior

Adapted from Bellack, A., Mueser, K., Gingerich, S., & Agresta, J. (2004). *Social skills training for schizophrenia* (2nd ed.). New York, NY: Guilford Publications.

The goal of social skills training is to establish social competence, which includes the following assumptions:

- Usefulness and effectiveness of social skills are situation specific
- Appropriateness is culturally and situationally determined
- It requires the ability to perceive and analyze subtle social cues
- Skills, rules, and needed judgments can be learned.

Morrison (1990) has been credited with identifying the component skills for social competence, beginning with some of the social participation basics described in Chapter 3. These expressive and receptive abilities, both verbal and nonverbal, make up what has been called *social intelligence,* a combination of knowledge, judgment, interpretation, and performance (Bellack et al., 2004).

Social skills training programs currently flourish in hospital and community health settings where they are planned and led by occupational therapists and others within a group format. Many clients place high priority on the establishment or continuation of social roles such as job performance, friendships, and family relationships. For example, an occupational therapist in a mental health walk-in clinic used a client-centered approach by asking her group of four young women with schizophrenia to choose which social skills they would most like to work on. Not surprisingly, they chose conversational skills, job skills, and intimate relationships. She uses Bellack and colleagues' (2004) curriculum to structure ongoing group sessions focusing on these skills. The sessions related to establishing intimate relationships are listed in Table 14-1.

Although designed specifically for people with schizophrenia, the skills in Bellack's curriculum can

Table 14-2

BELLACK'S SOCIAL SKILLS CATEGORIES

- Conversation skills
- Conflict management skills
- Assertiveness skills
- Community living skills
- Friendship and dating skills
- Medication management skills
- Vocational and work skills

Adapted from Bellack, A., Mueser, K., Gingerich, S., & Agresta, J. (2004). *Social skills training for schizophrenia* (2nd ed.). New York, NY: Guilford Publications.

be modified to serve a broad range of mental and physical disability populations. Other categories of Bellack and colleagues' (2004) social skills training are listed in Table 14-2. The premise of the social skills model is that social competence involves both a learned repertoire of behaviors and the application of judgment for their appropriate application in natural settings. Generalization of skills depends upon clients carrying out homework assignments and practicing the skills in vivo. Group discussions about the outcome of skill-use serves to reinforce learning and application of new behaviors, as well as providing emotional support.

Liberman

Liberman's (Liberman et al., 1993) Social and Independent Living Skills (SILS), also designed for people with serious mental illness, uses a

---

Table 14-3

LIBERMAN'S SOCIAL AND INDEPENDENT LIVING SKILLS MODULES

- Medication management module
- Recreation for leisure module
- Workplace fundamentals module
- Substance abuse management module
- Involving families in mental health services

- Symptom management module
- Basic conversation skills module
- Community re-entry module
- Friendship and intimacy module

Adapted from Liberman, R., Wallace, C. J., Blackwell, G. A., Eckman, T. A., Vacaro, J. V., & Kuchnel, T. G. (1993). Innovations in skills training for the seriously mentally ill: The UCLA social and independent living skills modules. *Innovations & Research, 2,* 43-59.

"structured educational method designed to compensate for cognitive deficits and symptoms" (Liberman & Fuller, 2000). This program applies cognitive behavioral theory in the acquisition of basic living skills, with some similarities but a broader format than that of Bellack and colleagues (2004). The SILS Modules listed in Table 14-3 include both social and activity skills organized by occupational performance areas within work, leisure, self-care, and community participation.

Generalization of skills, a concern for most clinical settings, has been studied by Liberman and Fuller (2000). They found evidence that living skills learned in the clinic were maintained 2 years after discharge for individuals with schizophrenia when environmental support is promoted. Environmental opportunities and support are accomplished through in vivo homework assignments and helping the client to identify opportunities in which to use specific skills. Positive reinforcement, also deemed necessary for generalization, can be fostered through self-reinforcement techniques and by tangible reinforcement by peers or trainers (2000, p. 4).

Linehan

Linehan's (1993a) dialectic behavior therapy (DBT) was developed specifically for people with borderline personality disorder (BPD). This persistent mental disorder has historically been resistant to both psychotherapy and medication. Therapists will rarely encounter clients with BPD unless they present with a coexisting physical or mental disorder. Because their symptoms are ego-dystonic (i.e., they deny that they have a disorder at all), they rarely seek therapy specifically addressing BPD and usually refuse it if offered. People with BPD can be encountered everywhere, in schools, families, communities, and the workplace, recognizable because of their history of failed and troubled interpersonal

relationships, their patterns of crisis and emotional turmoil, and their fragile grasp of reality, which undoubtedly interferes with their social participation despite often extraordinary talent, intelligence, or skill.

In teaching the skills of dialectic thinking, Linehan (1993a) challenges clients with BPD to transcend polarities (a black-and-white view of self and the world) and to see reality as complex and multifaceted. Dialectic thinking represents a compromise between the acceptance of objective and subjective truth, a kind of gray area that encompasses neither extreme of good or evil, but can encompass all of the realities of being human. The target behaviors of dialectic behavioral therapy are (1) decreasing suicidal behaviors, therapy interfering behaviors, behaviors that interfere with the quality of life, and behaviors relative to post-traumatic stress, and (2) increasing behavioral skills and strategies and respect for the self. Some of the specific lesson plans for therapy sessions are listed in Table 14-4.

The training manual that accompanies Linehan's text provides guidelines for therapists and group leaders, including handouts for sessions and homework sheets. For example, the Interpersonal Effectiveness Homework Sheet asks the client to describe a problem situation that arose between group sessions. It gives the following five examples:

1. Your rights or wishes were not respected.

2. You want another to give you something, do something, or change in some way.

3. You needed to say no or resist pressure.

4. You wanted your point of view to be heard and respected.

5. You had a conflict with another individual.

The client must describe the prompting event and his or her response then identify what factors reduced or interfered with interpersonal effectiveness such as

---

Table 14-4

LINEHAN'S DIALECTIC BEHAVIOR THERAPY TRAINING UNITS

DIALECTIC BEHAVIOR THERAPY CATEGORIES	INDIVIDUAL SESSION EXAMPLES
1. Dialectic strategies	Entering the paradox, use of metaphor, Devil's Advocate Technique, extending, activating your wise mind, making lemonade, allowing natural change, dialectic assessment
2. Core strategies I: Validation of...	Emotion, behavior, cognition, and "cheerleading" (support client strengths)
3. Core strategies II: Problem solving	Behavior analysis, insight (interpretation), didactic information, solutions analysis, orienting, making a commitment
4. Change procedures	Contingency: Reinforcing target behaviors, using aversive consequences, observing limits, being consistently firm
	Skill building: Training, practice, exposure-based learning, cognitive restructuring
5. Stylistic strategies	Balancing communication, interacting with the surrounding community
6. Specific task strategies	Explaining dialectic behavior therapy rationale, repairing relationships, telephone calls and e-mail, crisis strategies, addressing suicidal behavior, therapy interfering behavior, ancillary training, relationship strategies

Adapted from Linehan, M. (1993b). *Skills training for treating borderline personality disorder.* New York, NY: Guilford Press.

---

skills-lacking, worrying thoughts, interfering emotions, internal indecision, or environmental barriers.

This exercise works well with students and serves as an example of how to consider the many facets of a social situation when analyzing and interpreting social behaviors. This homework, in working with clients, would be openly discussed with the group as part of the preparation for therapeutic behavior change.

Concern in the rehabilitation community about the generalization of social and living skills training to the clients' everyday lives has generated multiple research efforts. Recognizing that social skills alone would not produce successful social participation for posthospitalized clients with schizophrenia, Liberman and colleagues used a role play format to train client groups in social problem solving (Liberman, Eckman, & Marder, 2001). They identified the following five steps in social problem solving:

1. Identify the problem (in a videotaped segment)

2. Generate alternative solutions

3. Weigh the pros and cons of each solution

4. Select a feasible solution

5. Implement the selected alternative

Table 14-5

SITUATIONS FOR SOCIAL PROBLEM SOLVING

Restaurant situation: Waitress brings the wrong order.

Shopping situation: Salesperson refuses to refund your money for a returned stereo that does not work.

Home situation: A friend changes the TV channel right before the big game begins.

Work situation: After arriving on time for a job interview, you are told that the interviewer has left for the day.

Adapted from Liberman, R., Eckman, T., & Marder, S. (2001). Rehab rounds: Training in social problem solving among persons with schizophrenia. *Psychiatric Services, 52*, 31-33.

Some examples of problems used for the role plays are listed in Table 14-5. In the 2001 study, while both experimental and control groups could successfully identify social problems (step 1), group members who experienced the role play training improved their social problem solving by 19% to 23% in steps 2 through 5.

Using a social support approach, Tauber, Wallace, and Lecomte (2000) enlisted indigenous community supporters to assist people with severe mental illness with appropriate applications of learned social skills. After receiving 6 months of social skills training, each participant selected someone from his or her own community to perform the role of supporter for an additional 6 months. While participants' basic psychopathology did not change, those with supporters made significant improvements in interpersonal functioning, global functioning, and level of life satisfaction. Similarly, Liberman and colleagues used in vivo amplified skills training (IVAST) to promote generalization of independent living skills (Liberman, Glynn, Blair, Ross, & Marder, 2002). IVAST calls for specially trained case managers to provide each client with individual teaching of behaviors and to promote their use in community settings. The client's family members, staff in community agencies, and others became involved in continued support and reinforcement for client use of learned skills. This technique, although labor intensive, documented improvements in social adjustment for clients transitioning to independent living in their communities.

Ability to maintain employment is recognized as an essential ingredient for sustained ability to live independently for people with persistent mental illness (and others). Dickerson, Bellack, and Gold (2007) measured both social competence (skills) and social cognition (problem solving) among two groups of employees with mental health diagnoses: those with a history of poor vocational functioning and those with a history of good vocational functioning. This study defines social competence as the expressive component involving social skills and their appropriate use, while social cognition involves the receptive abilities, including emotional and social cue perception; verbal memory, reasoning, attaching meaning, and generation of response alternatives; and selection of appropriate content, nonverbal communication, and balance. Not surprisingly, the group with poor vocational functioning lacked effective social competence and social cognition in equal measure when compared with the group histories of good vocational functioning.

Generalization for Linehan's DBT has also been studied. Cloud (2009) reports that today more than 10,000 therapists practice DBT using Linehan's techniques, which are shown to have been effective in numerous clinical trials for reducing intentional self-injuries as well as days of hospitalization for people with BPD. The incidence of this disorder has increased since Linehan first developed her approach in the early 1990s. In a 2008 survey, the incidence of BPD is 5.9% of the U.S. population, with an estimated 75% of these committing self-destructive acts like cutting or burning themselves, becoming over-medicated, and committing suicide at nearly twice the rate of people with mood disorders (Harned et al., 2008). Currently, Linehan's DBT remains the only intervention shown to be effective for this disorder's propensity for troubled and stormy interpersonal relationships (Cloud, 2009).

Community Reintegration

The goal of most disability-based social skills training is to assist clients with the transition from dependent care to independent living in the community. Basic communication and an understanding of the social norms of everyday situations is a minimal requirement for getting needs met through community services. For example, driving or taking public transportation to a shopping area, using money or credit cards to purchase needed items at a store, and ordering food from a restaurant all require the use of basic social rules and routine interactions according to local customs or norms. Adults who have an acquired brain injury, such as a concussion, stroke, or a persistent mental illness, may need training and practice to re-establish such routines in order to live independently in the community.

Community integration has been defined as a "process of becoming part of the mainstream of family and community life, participation in normal roles and responsibilities, and being an active and contributing member of one's social groups and society as a whole" (Dijkers, 1998, in Dudgeon, 2009, p. 182). Integration presumes membership, while participation as a goal goes further to include active and dynamic sharing with others in desired social groups in community locales such as home, schools, businesses, parks, clubhouses, churches, public transportation, and other public buildings or areas.

In recent years, therapeutic interventions for community integration have moved from client centered to community centered (Fazio, 2008). While health is still a personal issue, one's health status and functional well-being involve a dynamic interaction between personal and community factors (Dudgeon, 2009). In other words, participation in life situations relies heavily on the client's social skills and cognition in addition to physical abilities or adaptations. To fully appreciate the concept of community "it is necessary to consider that it is not only based on relationships but also on partnerships and coalitions... this goes beyond the location of our (occupational therapy) practice. It suggests coming together with other people and feeling a sense of connection" (Fazio, 2008, p. 10). Communities can be a local place geographically or a social network of people with common culture, interests, and values, such as the Christian community, the business community, or, more broadly, the global community.

For therapists who wish to design goals and interventions for clients that promote participation in the community, it is important to combine client-centered and community-centered approaches. The client-centered part focuses on individual skills, motivation, and use of available supports, such as friends and family, while the community-centered perspective "emphasizes accessibility and acceptance within physical, social, and cultural environments" (Dudgeon, 2009, p. 182). In this context, disability must be associated with problems in participation in life situations (World Health Organization, 2001).

If disability causes loss of social roles, what is needed for an individual to re-establish them? A systems approach would focus not only on the individual's social abilities or disabilities but also on the groups in which the person chooses to participate. This may involve return to employment, with both skill building for the client and education and adaptation for others in the workplace. Taking part in service groups also involves the use of some degree of social competence depending on the level of the group. A good guideline is Mosey's (1986) five developmental group levels, all of which may be found in adult groups in the community. A therapist's role may be to explore social group options in the client's community and to evaluate the level of interpersonal skills necessary for effective participation in each of them. For many occupational therapy intervention plans or other health care discharge plans for clients with disability, this part of the process is overlooked. Yet, unless the client retains a high degree of social competence, without matching client social interaction ability with that required by the group, no amount of training on the part of a client will prepare him or her to participate successfully within the social contexts of community groups. In an unpublished study, Cole surveyed some of the social groups in a small town in Connecticut using occupational therapy graduate students to observe and evaluate different levels of social and activity groups in the community using Donohue's (1999, 2009) Social Profile Assessment. The preliminary findings are listed in Table 14-6. While not conclusive, these group levels can serve as a guideline for estimating the likelihood that clients at a particular interaction skill level will be able to participate effectively.

Client skills needed for participation at each group level are listed in Table 14-6. While no group fits neatly into any one category, the groups listed in column two represent an average of the observed interactions during a 30-minute time period. For example, during a bingo game, most people pay close attention to matching numbers called with those on their card, following the rules set out by the caller. This is an associative level interaction until the whole group takes a break for coffee or tea. At that point, informal conversations between players may occur, which requires basic cooperative level interaction skills. To prepare a client to participate in a bingo game, attention must be paid to how well he or she listens, focuses attention, and understands the rules or norms. Basic conversation skills should also be in place so that the client is prepared to participate in casual socialization.

Social Support Groups

The healing power of social support groups is well documented. In 1978, Bernie Siegel, renowned cancer surgeon and professor at Yale University, started Exceptional Cancer Patients, a specialized form of group therapy to facilitate personal change and healing through guided exploration of the links between body, mind, and spirit (Siegel, 1986). Support groups of all kinds fulfill the need for social connection and emotional validation during times of crisis and along the road to recovery. The basic premise of social support groups is peers helping peers through group meetings and interactions. Either temporary or ongoing support from one of these groups can empower individuals to overcome the sometimes overwhelming barriers to successful social participation. Recovered individuals may often be found leading and organizing self-help social support groups of all kinds, a social role that also serves as a part of their own "therapy."

Finding Peer Support for Self-Help

The concept of support groups is not new. For centuries, extended families and local villagers served as social supports for all their members, which was easier to do when people lived most of their lives in close proximity to one another. Support for the recovery from addiction dates back to 1935, when the infamous Bill W. and Dr. Bob cofounded Alcoholics Anonymous in Akron, Ohio. Their approach defined the well-known 12 steps of recovery from alcohol addiction using the concept of community—people with alcohol abuse habits helping one another to apply the spiritual values of the 12 steps in their everyday lives. Many other disability peer groups now use similar principles to what was dubbed in the 1980s *a self-help revolution* (Leerhsen, 1990). Four basic categories of support groups exist today:

Table 14-6

COMMUNITY GROUPS AT FIVE LEVELS OF INTERACTION

SOCIAL ACTIVITY GROUP LEVEL	COMMUNITY GROUPS FUNCTIONING AT THIS LEVEL	INDIVIDUAL INTERPERSONAL SKILLS NEEDED TO FUNCTION SUCCESSFULLY AT THIS LEVEL
Parallel	• Protestant church service • Catholic mass • Exercise group • Aerobics class • Adult education class	• Trust and follow leader direction • Trust others to follow rules • Show awareness of other members
Associative	• Social bingo game • Quilting class • Family christening service • Pet therapy visit to senior center • Board games—Monopoly, Scrabble	• Show cooperation, take turns • Focus on performance of task • Some competition as motivation • Seek help with the task • Willingly give assistance to others
Basic cooperative	• Support groups—information sharing • Weight watchers weekly meeting • Bat mitzvah service • Choir rehearsal • Beach volleyball—recreational	• Begin to express ideas • Respect rights of others • Begin meeting needs of others • Experiment with member roles • Can identify and meet group goals • Motivated to complete activity
Supportive cooperative	• Support groups—self-disclosure • Grandma's surprise birthday party • Family Thanksgiving dinner • Women's issues discussion group • Card party—social bridge game • Gourmet group dinner party	• Express positive and negative feelings • Show caring for other members • Enjoy equality and compatibility among members • Participate in mutual need satisfaction • Comfortable with self-disclosure • Able to trust other members • Give/receive social identity support
Mature	• Fundraiser committee meeting • Wedding reception • Baby shower • Sorority or fraternity meeting • Boy scout leaders training meeting • Writers critique group • Total quality management group—sales department	• High-level task performance • Assume variety of group roles without prompting • Members self-lead • Balance between performance and socialization

Adapted from Donohue, M. V. (1999). Theoretical bases of Mosey's group interactions skills. *Occupational Therapy International, 6,* 35-51.

1. Addictive behaviors—Alcohol, drugs, gambling, overeating, sex offenses, etc

2. Physical or mental illness—Parkinson's, multiple sclerosis, bipolar disorder, etc

3. Transitions and crises—Widows' bereavement, parents without partners, job search, etc

4. Friends and relatives of those with the problem—Alzheimer's caregivers, parents of children with disabilities, Al Anon, etc

The power of peer-to-peer support does not replace traditional medical treatment for these disorders, but often surpasses it as a reinforcement of a person's commitment to the recovery process, including abstinence from harmful substances, dietary and lifestyle changes, and therapeutic changes in attitude and behavior, as well as compliance with medical regimens. For example, a study of changing social network support for drinking found that drinkers' social networks (that encourage continued drinking) can be changed when support group involvement such as Alcoholics Anonymous specifically encourages such changes in social groups (Litt, Kadden, Kabela-Cormier, & Petry, 2007). People simply do better at facing challenges and overcoming obstacles when other people support and encourage them, especially others who have similar illness experiences or are facing similar challenges. Social support groups offer something the medical professionals cannot—the spiritual connection of friendship (Leerhsen, 1990).

What do peers offer each other? Some examples include the following:

× Exchanging information, such as evaluating Web sites, books, media, and methods

× Listening and accepting each other's experiences

× Suggesting solutions to common problems

× Providing sympathetic understanding

× Establishing social networks both in the community and online

How does one find a good support group? Most groups built around self-help are fully organized and run by volunteers. Most community health centers offer listings of local meetings, for example, bereavement support, divorced and separated support, families of those with mental illness support, irritable bowel syndrome support, mood disorders support, and well-spouse support groups (Connecticut Self-Help Network, 2004). These groups meet regularly on weekdays or evenings in local churches, temples, or other community centers, usually with peer organization and leadership. These face-to-face meetings

often serve refreshments and are informally structured to promote open discussion and interaction. Leaders have many resources for starting and running such groups. For example, the Connecticut Self-Help Network Consultation Center in New Haven publishes a free Starter Package Kit for peer leaders, covering topics such as how to locate a meeting place, techniques for recruiting group members, guidelines for group discussion, and dealing with problem behaviors such as inappropriate expression of anger. However well led, support groups led by peers do not replace traditional medical treatment or therapy. For people new to support group membership, those led by professionals such as psychologists, social workers, occupational therapists, or members of the clergy may be a safer place to start.

Clubhouse Centers for Mental Health

A good example of a successful self-help group center is Bridge House, a three-story Victorian that houses a wide array of social and activity groups for people with persistent mental health conditions (Figure 14-1). Funded by a state grant, Bridge House hires those in recovery to organize and lead groups; recruit and orient members; assist members with housing, budgeting, medical insurance, and job-seeking issues; as well as keep records for research purposes. Bridge House, based on a Fountain House model (Peck, 2000), provides a daily routine from 8 am to 4 pm, including low-cost meals, social meetings, and activities designed to train member volunteers in job-related skills by including them in the daily operation of the Clubhouse. Attending Bridge House is voluntary and offers a friendly alternative to the stigma that has traditionally been associated with mental illness within the workplace and in the community. Through their participation in the daily programs, members feel a sense of belonging and mutual respect that is shared by co-workers, neighbors, and friends. In this upbeat atmosphere pictured in Figure 14-2, a paid director works side by side with a volunteer member in giving an orientation and tour of Bridge House for new members.

Bridge House serves as an example of the many publicly funded consumer-operated programs that are effective for people with mental health conditions transitioning from hospital or day treatment programs to independent living in the community. Occupational therapists may be involved on a number of levels in using this type of transitional program, either by direct participation or by referral of selected clients who could benefit from the Clubhouse approach

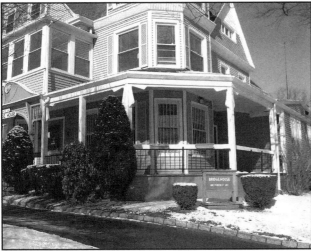

Figure 14-1. Bridge House, a "bridge" to the community for people with mental health conditions.

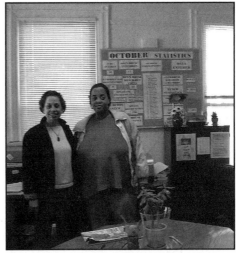

Figure 14-2. Phyllis and Utasha conduct an orientation and tour of Bridge House.

(Swarbrick & Pratt, 2006). Self-help groups, such as those at Bridge House, target adults of working age who need training and assistance in finding and maintaining employment so that they can be self-supporting citizens of their communities.

The mental health "Clubhouse" falls under the general category of consumer-operated self-help services (COS) described by Swarbrick and Pratt (2006). In 1998, a large-scale randomized controlled trial was initiated by the Substance Abuse and Mental Health Services Administration (SAMHSA). In the state of New Jersey, there are 22 COS. They offer after-hours and weekend services organized by peers, peer decision-making and government, work-readiness peer support sessions, a wellness newsletter, and an annual 2-day workshop for peers.

Online Support Groups and Networks

In addition to face-to-face meetings, online self-help groups have provided needed support to thousands, without the necessity of geographic proximity. In 2006, Yahoo listed more than 30,000 support groups focusing on a wide range of health-related topics within its hosted domains, and many others exist on health-related or other Web sites. For people with uncommon ailments, finding others who share their problems becomes easier online. The quality of online support groups varies widely and should be used with caution. In a good online support group, the same members continue to participate even after they have received needed help because of the sense of community that forms with high group cohesiveness (Grohol, 2004).

To find local groups on the internet, start with the national self-help clearinghouse Web site listing groups by problem or disability, region, and state. Each state has a listing also, such as the Connecticut Self-Help Network, which cross-references support groups by town and by topic and provides meeting sites and contact numbers that are updated frequently. Still, finding a good fit for one's own needs is not always easy. Therapists and educators may need to assist clients in searching and finding the right fit for their specific social support needs.

Self-help Web sites are also an invaluable resource for friends, family, and caregivers of people with various health conditions. For example, Obsessive-Compulsive Disorder (OCD) Resources Online (www.ocdonline.com) gives helpful tips for the mother of an adult daughter with OCD: (1) recognizing the symptoms such as excessive hoarding, checking, washing and cleaning, or re-arranging, (2) *not* getting tricked into participating in these rituals, as this only serves to reinforce maladaptive behaviors, and (3) monitoring the degree to which compulsive behaviors interfere with social participation and facilitating getting her daughter into treatment (Melville, 2008).

Work-Related Interventions

In recent years, public attention has focused on putting underserved populations back to work. People with persistent mental illness, estimated anywhere from 1% to 40% of the population depending on the type and definition used (Sadock & Sadock, 2003), fall into this category. Because the onset of mental illnesses, such as schizophrenia and bipolar disorder, usually begins in early adulthood and interferes with cognitive and social functioning despite medication, this population of adults of working age find themselves unable to maintain jobs, homes, or stable relationships. From a public health perspective, the cost of their care is high, and cost-cutting measures have only shifted the burden as unsupported people with persistent mental illness join the ranks of the homeless or fill beds in nursing homes or prisons. For this reason, public policy has given priority to programs that support their employment.

Traditional approaches focusing on client abilities, such as pre-vocational training and sheltered workshops, have not been supported by research. Despite participation in traditional programs that train and place people with persistent mental illness, less than 15% successfully maintain competitive employment, the lowest rate of any disability group (Strong & Rebeiro, 2003). From a systems perspective, this problem necessitates a shift to addressing environmental barriers, such as social stereotypes of mental illness; competitive, inflexible, and highly stressful work cultures; and disincentives built into the disability support payment systems (Strong & Rebeiro, 2003). Strong has called the plight of those with mental illness a "cycle of disempowerment and despair," (1998) described in Figure 14-3.

By the year 2000, supportive employment programs, such as job coaching, the practice of a professional coach accompanying the client with mental illness to the worksite and providing on-the-job support, had established some degree of success. Currently, several supported employment models using a community-based approach operate nationwide (and globally), including Transitional Employment Programs (TEPs), Programs of Assistive Community Treatment (PACT), and the Clubhouse model.

Transitional Employment Programs

TEPs have been adopted by state and local governments as a means of reducing costs by training and placing *hard-to-serve* populations, such as the homeless, people with persistent mental illness such as schizophrenia, people with alcohol and drug dependence, and others with poor employment histories. For example, Washington, DC, has a public- and grant-funded eight-step TEP for people older than 21 years of age:

1. Participant referral and enrollment—Such as people sleeping in public parks or those recurrently hospitalized for mental health conditions

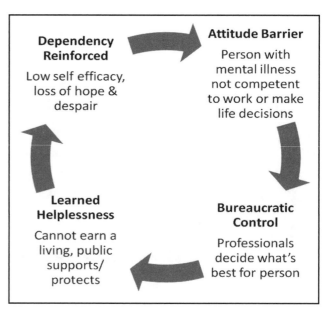

Figure 14-3. Strong's cycle of disempowerment and despair. (Adapted from Strong, S. (1998). Meaningful work in supportive environments: Experiences with the recovery process. *American Journal of Occupational Therapy, 52,* 31-38.)

2. Program orientation—Program explained in detail, responsibilities and benefits

3. Intake, assessment of life and work skills, and assignment to case manager

4. Supportive services such as counseling, medication, detoxification as determined by case manager

5. Job readiness and life skills training—3 weeks

6. Employability activities, such as subsidized employment, education including GED preparation, vocational training, or on-the-job training

7. Job club—Additional coaching and intensive job searching assistance/support

8. Job retention and follow-up—6 months of on-the-job support (Department of Employment Services, 2009)

TEPs vary greatly from location to location and are mostly grant- or state-funded programs. Common elements include consideration of personal skills and preferences, direct individualized assistance with finding and keeping a job, and a goal of sustained employment. One version of this type of program is the Bridge program in New York City in which occupational therapy students offer intense social and educational instruction in preparation for completing high school or college programs (Gutman, Kerner, Zombek, Dulek, & Ramsey, 2009).

Programs of Assistive Community Treatment

Programs of Assistive Community Treatment (PACT) or (ACT), founded in the 1970s, have a long record of success in working with people with persistent mental illness. These involve an interdisciplinary treatment team of professionals, including psychiatrists, psychologists, nurses, case managers, substance abuse specialists, and vocational specialists, who regularly meet with clients in their homes, workplaces, and community settings. Once used mainly in relocating formerly institutionalized people with persistent mental illness to the community, PACT or ACT programs have more recently shifted their emphasis to supported employment. These programs have a good record as measured by percentage of job placement for clients (Schonebaum, Boyd, & Dudek, 2006).

The Clubhouse Model

The Clubhouse model, such as Bridge House described earlier, is a widely replicated and well-defined model of psychiatric rehabilitation and community support. The International Center for Clubhouse Development defines parameters for certification to more than 100 Clubhouses in the United States and many more abroad. Clubhouses offer a range of employment initiatives, including the following:

- Transitional employment, in which client members work and get paid a prevailing wage directly by an employer. Support staff members cover absences, and positions are time limited (6 to 9 months) and are reserved for mental health clients.

- Supported employment, in which a case manager accompanies the client to work.

- Independent employment, which offers individual assistance in job seeking for competitive employment positions.

Clubhouses such as Bridge House use a professional self-help model in which client members and staff work together to help clients achieve their goals of getting a job and/or an education and establishing a home and friendships. Clubhouse environments provide a network of supportive relationships using voluntary work and education as mechanisms for recovery. Work of the Clubhouse includes cleaning, cooking, business management, keeping records, video production and marketing, and human relations training. Membership provides a positive work environment and a strong base for building human relationships and self-esteem (Schonebaum et al., 2006).

Evidence for Supported Employment

A longitudinal study comparing PACT and Clubhouse models found that both maintained 15% to 25% weekly employment rate, with no significant difference in placement rates, total jobs worked, or hours worked per week. However, when examining quality factors, Clubhouse programs achieved significantly higher numbers: 66% higher for job duration and 17% higher wages earned. Schonebaum and colleagues (2006) attributed Clubhouse successes to their work-ordered daily routines and their emphasis in sustained social support networks. A randomized controlled trial comparing these two programs looked at both work factors and continued engagement and retention over a 2-year period (Marcias et al., 2006). They found PACT programs superior in engagement and retention (clients continued to use professional services, such as medication and counseling), while Clubhouse members demonstrated better work performance and duration and earned higher wages. This difference may also reflect the populations served by these models, with many ACT clients needing extra support and many Clubhouse participants incapable of participation in peer government opportunities.

Therapists who wish to design interventions combining client and community approaches need to know what factors make a work environment supportive. Strong and Rebeiro (2003) found the following to be key features of the workplace culture:

- An accepting and inclusive atmosphere

- Support for diversity of all kinds

- Clearly communicated expectations from management

- Assistance in understanding workplace values and norms

- Assistance with necessary patterns of interaction with supervisors, coworkers, customers, and others in order to achieve work goals

Because therapists currently have little control outside the realm of health care, having an impact on work cultures relies on building partnerships with employers, using advocacy and diplomacy, opening lines of communication between employers and health care professionals, and emphasizing the strengths of peer group participation.

How does work affect recovery for people with persistent mental illness? In an ethnographic study, Strong (1998) identified the following themes for workers in ceramics and gifts shop, an affirmative business in Ontario, Canada:

- *Living with a label*—Constant internal battle to maintain control and dignity in a world that victimizes, blames, and labels them as *crazy*.

- *Becoming a capable person with a future*—People with mental illness are known to have diminished self-concept and a distorted sense of self-efficacy (Davidson & Strauss, 1992). Working helped them redefine themselves through concrete demonstration of accomplishment as well as a paycheck.

- *Getting on with life*—Workers used their worker status as a starting point for joining the mainstream of adult development in other ways, such as getting their own apartment and forming reciprocal relationships with friends and partners.

- *Finding a place in the world*—Feeling useful and experiencing a sense of belonging with others who have shared their illness experience. Workers reported receiving support, advice, and validation of their feelings from coworkers.

This study offers some insight for the role of the worker role in rebuilding or establishing a social identity for people with mental illness. The findings suggest that social support of peers may play the same role for people with mental illness that the adolescent peer group plays in initial development of identity. The research on the Clubhouse model in providing social support networks adds further evidence of the importance of occupation to social participation and life satisfaction for those with mental health conditions (Weiss, 2009).

Team Building in the Workplace

The notion of occupational justice as a basic human right to perform tasks, activities, and occupations necessary to thrive and to fully participate in life and in society (Wilcock, 2006) suggests that everyone (not only those with mental illness) could use a more supportive work environment. Most jobs require teamwork to some extent, and the basic requirements of teamwork look surprisingly similar to those of supportive work environments: cooperation, acceptance of diversity, mutual respect, open communication, and a shared burden of work toward a common goal. While members of a team may have different backgrounds, different roles, and different job descriptions, they all work better together when the group dynamics serve to support each person's efforts. Good teamwork requires social skills, competence, and communication. Small business expert Laura Harris (2008) has this advice for owners: (1) make your employees a real part of the team, (2) establish a clear vision of what success means for your company—and how the day-to-day work fits into the plan, (3) put each business process in writing—making goals and procedures clear to all

so that no one is indispensible to the success of the company, and (4) create a compensation system that rewards employees for team results—design your business so that the team works together to fulfill goals. Encourage healthy competition but ensure that individual goals align with corporate goals. That alignment makes an employee part of the team, creating a harmonious atmosphere (Harris, 2008).

If a team consists of members working together toward a common goal, what skills and abilities do members need to enable them to be a good team player? On sports teams, coaches encourage players to share the responsibility for winning the game. Do not hog the ball, and watch for opportunities to pass it to someone closer to the goal. Players take different positions on a team based upon their particular strengths and skills in kicking, throwing, running, endurance, blocking the opponent, or avoiding obstacles. Many parents encourage their children to play team sports, hoping that the teamwork and sportsmanship learned there will better prepare them for careers and other aspects of adult life.

The sports analogy generalizes to work, educational, recreational, and community settings. For example, when a supervisor tells an employee he or she is not a team player, there is little doubt about what that means. A committee whose leader is *not a team player* may try to do the whole task himself or herself instead of delegating tasks and sharing responsibility. But, the analogy goes beyond that of leadership style. In fact, between 40% and 50% of the U.S. workforce uses work teams to manage business, produce products, and provide services (Hirokawa, 2003). Corporations and businesses rely on teams based on the belief that these groups make better decisions and come up with more effective solutions to problems than one person alone. In reviewing the research, Hirokawa (2003) finds that high-quality group decisions rely on the following three characteristics influencing the final choice:

1. A proper understanding of the problem

2. Appropriate choice-making objectives

3. An accurate evaluation of the positive and negative qualities of available choices

The quality of the decision depends upon a significant degree of interaction and communication among the group members and the open exchange of information, reasoning, and opinions or judgments. When groups make poor decisions, three types of constraints were identified by Hirokawa (2003):

1. *Cognitive constraints*—Little is known about the problem, time is sharply limited, or the problem itself is exceedingly complex

2. *Affiliative constraints*—Friendships or adversarial relationships among members unduly influence team interactions by preventing members from addressing all of the functional requirements of the task

3. *Egocentric constraints*—At least one member has a highly pronounced need for control

To better understand how these constraints interfere with good group decision making, try applying them to the group processes used by the U.S. Congress when designing and voting on the national economic stimulus package.

Teams in Government—A Case for Intervention

Consider the task of the U.S. Congress in coming up with an acceptable Economic Stimulus Package during President Obama's first 3 weeks in office in January 2009. *While the disastrous state of the economy was evident, how much overall understanding did members of the House and Senate actually have of the underlying issues?* Yet, with severe time constraints, senators and congressmen could not adequately investigate or even debate the pros and cons of different actions to include in the plan. *What affiliative constraints influenced Democrats and Republicans when deciding which way to vote? Which members of these parties exerted the greatest influence in what would be included in the final bill sent to the President?* The wisdom of this multibillion dollar group decision remains to be seen. But, the constraints or barriers limiting the process are obvious. Political groups have much to gain from a reflective analysis of their interactions when solving problems and making decisions that have such far-reaching consequences for the nation, regions, states, towns, and neighborhood.

The traditional wisdom of group dynamics tells us that groups that communicate openly and interact effectively over time develop a certain closeness or group cohesiveness that allows them to work together without the interference of internal constraints. In cohesive groups, members may express both positive and negative emotions without fear of rejection, a highly desirable dynamic of support groups or therapeutic groups (Cole, 2005; Yalom, 2005). However, the business world has only recently studied the effects of emotion in self-directed corporate teams (Clark & Sline, 2003). Since the 1980s, U.S. corporations have incorporated Japan's model of self-directed teams as the most effective means for corporations to respond to global competition and high-speed information processing in today's global market. However, the

interdependency that results from lateral communication on multiple issues can raise anxiety, create information overload, and, under time constraints, lead to emotional outbreaks (Clark & Sline, 2003). These researchers studied emotion-triggering events reported by 186 members of work teams.

Volunteer Work Teams

Volunteering has many similarities to a paid worker role. Formal volunteering for community organizations often involves working with others on teams or committees, defined goals and responsibilities, and a weekly schedule or routine times during which the work must be done. Given today's high unemployment and competitive environment, volunteering might be a temporary alternative role for many working-age adults. Some employment agencies suggest that volunteering can provide job training and social networking that can lead to paid employment. But beyond the practical aspects, volunteering has benefits similar to work in building social identity and boosting self-efficacy through participating in a valued and meaningful work role in the community (Strong & Rebiero, 2003).

The most common tasks performed by volunteers are as follows:

- Fundraising/selling items to raise money (29.5%)
- Coaching, refereeing, tutoring, or teaching (27.8%)
- Collecting, preparing, distributing, or serving food (26.4%)
- Providing information, including ushering, greeting, ministry (22.7%)

The above volunteer statistics refer to work performed for charitable or service organizations. However, the definition of volunteering has expanded and changed to include many tasks informally performed for others, such as giving rides, meals, care, and support to friends and neighbors outside the household. Civic engagement does not exclude payment, which could come from public funds, research grants, or pro-rated fees for service. As a new idea in sociology, civic engagement includes public influence as well as public service. For example, people with mental or physical disability may seek to change how others, the media, and society view and define people with disabilities and to educate the public and thereby influence public policy affecting their health condition.

Therapists and counselors may seek to assist clients in exploring, locating, or establishing volunteer roles as a means of social participation. In the absence of a fulfilling or necessary work role, volunteer roles can help clients maintain skills, feel a sense of accomplishment, and remain connected to others in their community. Research overwhelmingly supports the connection between volunteering and maintenance of health and well-being. For many people who have faced personal loss or suffering, volunteering becomes a part of the healing process, as noted earlier in the section on social support groups. More on volunteering will be discussed in Chapter 15.

Friendships and Family Relationships

Parenting Issues

When a couple has a child, everything about their life changes. Taking care of an infant's basic needs only begins the journey. As the popular television show Supernanny has affirmed, many parents who do not establish reasonable social norms for their children find their home life to be uncontrolled and chaotic. Social interactions within families with young children parallel the development of any group—without clearly established norms, members (in this case children) create their own, often inappropriate norms that, once established, become difficult to change. Such families clearly illustrate the need for both directive and facilitative leadership in order to establish not only expectations for reasonable interpersonal behavior, but a daily schedule structured around the occupations of their everyday lives (Cole, 2005). Occupational therapy practitioners and others who have training in group leadership and dynamics are well equipped to assist parents in facilitating social participation within the shared activities of everyday family living. The script titled, "Family Crisis Intervention," at the end of Chapter 11 is a good example.

Very young children need clear direction from parents, mature adults who can guide their behavior according to the social norms of their own culture. Like directive group leadership, directive parenting takes the form of modeling appropriate expression of emotion, showing respect for others, and considering the needs of other members of the group, such as sharing, taking turns, listening, and giving as well as receiving support (Figure 14-4). When parents do not handle their own emotions well, children imitate this also. Staying in control, treating children with respect, and giving clear boundaries for what behaviors are acceptable prevents children from learning dysfunctional behaviors. Yet, life happens,

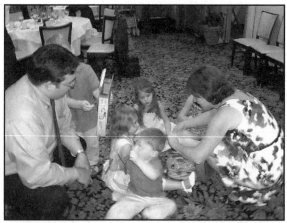

Figure 14-4. Mom and uncle help kids share toys and play fair, giving equal attention to each child during an extended family gathering.

and parents cannot always be perfect role models for their children. Children also need discipline, to experience some sort of negative consequence to let them know when they have crossed the line into unacceptable territory. That is when knowledge of positive discipline is needed.

Positive discipline, based on the philosophy of Alfred Adler (1958) and Rudolph Dreikurs (Dreikurs & Grey, 1968), emerged in the 1970s as a form of parental adult education in the community (Nelsen, 1981). Permissiveness abounded at that time, and parents raising multiple children began to feel the need for structure and guidance. This approach warned parents that punishing children produced only negative results: resentment, revenge, retreat, rebellion, and reduced self-esteem. The most recognized example of a negative parenting pattern is physical or verbal abuse, which tends to repeat unless intentionally changed. In a recent episode of the television show Supernanny, an abusive father learned to recognize the hurt he was inflicting on his children by doing a therapeutic activity: throwing darts at enlarged photos of his three young daughters, which were mounted on a dart board. This symbolic exercise provided this father with a visual reminder of how his verbal and physical abusive responses were harming his children psychologically. As advised by Jo Frost (Supernanny), Dad used the mental image of the dart exercise to stop himself from losing emotional control when faced with his children's misbehavior. Instead, he learned how to use positive discipline to shape his children's behavior by encouraging them to express their own emotions in more socially acceptable ways.

As proponents of positive discipline point out, children usually misbehave because they are unhappy with the way things are and need parental attention

Table 14-7

INEFFECTIVE PARENTAL RESPONSES

- Ordering, commanding
- Warning, threatening
- Moralizing, preaching
- Advising, giving solutions
- Questioning, interrogating
- Analyzing, diagnosing
- Persuading with logic, arguing
- Judging, criticizing, blaming
- Always praising and/or agreeing
- Name calling, ridiculing
- Reassuring, consoling
- Withdrawing, distracting, humoring

or intervention to set things right. Deep down, they really want to belong. Using positive discipline, Nelsen (1981) suggests "getting into your child's world" (p. 10) and regarding his or her mistakes as "wonderful opportunities to learn" (p. 67). The key to positive discipline is allowing children to experience the logical consequences of their misbehavior and to facilitate their social learning from that experience. This takes time on the part of parents, time that must be set aside for learning and practicing how to structure a consequence for children that directly relates to their misdeeds. The first step, as mentioned in Chapter 1, is to clearly communicate the important rules that children must follow. These are social norms and expectations for children who belong to this social group, the family. For example, refraining from hitting one another, treating every family member with respect, and complying with parents' requests might be on the list. In positive discipline parent classes, some of the common complaints of parents were as follows:

- Children fighting with each other
- Refusing to pick up toys, rooms
- Not getting to bed on time
- Not doing assigned chores
- Lateness with getting up and getting ready for school
- Refusing to do their homework
- Cannot enjoy family activities because of misbehavior
- Will not listen or comply with parental direction

Once rules are clear, consequences can be specifically enforced when a child breaks a rule (e.g., imposing a "time out" for a designated period of time or losing a privilege such as playing a computer game). Within the limits of keeping children safe, they can be allowed to experience natural consequences. For example, when they refuse to go to bed on time, they will be very tired and cranky in the morning. However, they will not learn this lesson without parental intervention. A discussion of the consequence and an insistence that the child get up and attend school the next morning regardless of being tired needs to be enforced for the child to learn the desired lesson. One mother actually took her child to school in his pajamas and marched him into his second grade class late, much to his embarrassment.

Another important element of positive discipline is active listening. Children need for their parents to understand how they are feeling and why they behave the way they do. Parents model respect by giving children an opportunity to explain their point of view before deciding on disciplinary action. In parent effectiveness classes, parents learn to avoid ineffective responses (Table 14-7) and to substitute more effective and positive responses that include acknowledging the child's feelings and defining the problem without bias and in simple, direct terms the child can understand (Gordon, 1992). Parents should always choose the response that facilitates the development of social and problem-solving skills.

Parent effectiveness includes a six-step problem-solving process for children and parents that incorporates active listening and empathy statements discussed in Chapter 3. The following are possible statements made by a child that call for an empathetic parental response:

- I'm not having any fun. There's nothing to do.
- I can't do this math problem by myself. It's too hard!
- All my friends went to the beach. I have no one to play with.
- Oh boy! A snow day!

For practice, use the formula described in Chapter 3 to identify how the child is feeling with the most accurate words you can think of and compose a statement recognizing the feeling while encouraging the child to come up with a solution. The following six steps recommended are by Gordon (1992):

1. Define the problem in an unbiased way, including situation and feelings

2. Gather possible solutions by brainstorming with the child, getting suggestions from the child without judgment

3. Evaluate or test the logical consequences of each proposed solution

4. Decide on the best solution—discuss and make a commitment

5. Implement the solution

6. After completion, evaluate the result with the child to facilitate social learning

Programs that support positive parenting may be found on the internet. Finding some of these can become an interesting learning activity.

Family Support for One Another

It is true that once people become parents, those roles continue throughout life. Adult children also need social support, and, as they marry and have children of their own, life circumstances can take unexpected turns. Many families who function well under normal circumstances can benefit from professional or community interventions from time to time. Examples of crises that can cause unusual stress are divorce, loss of one's job, serious illness, or moving to a new location. Even when individuals are coping fairly well, the love and support of family often sustains them through difficult times (Figure 14-5).

Family therapy is one form of intervention for families going through difficult situations that place unusually high levels of stress on family systems. While some professionals offer specialized training in family therapy, often, situations arise within which basic communication, group problem-solving, or conflict-resolution strategies can apply. Teachers, occupational therapists, or other community leaders may find themselves in a position to help families find ways to support one another by applying the basic skills described in Chapters 1 and 3. Examples of family therapy sessions may be found at the end of Chapters 2, 8, and 11.

Making New Friends and Repairing Relationships

For many reasons, such as illness or injury, change of employment status, moving to new locations, or

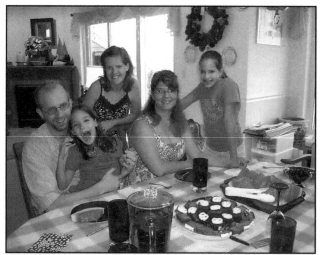

Figure 14-5. This family supports one another by welcoming Uncle Eric's fiancé into the family.

changes in economic status, adults may find themselves separated from former social groups and feeling lonely and isolated. The obvious remedy might be finding interesting groups in the community to join, as a way to reconnect. Karbo (2006) suggests five ways to find a new friend:

1. *Signing up for a group travel adventure*—People tend to bond more easily when away from their usual daily routine

2. *Taking a class*—Where you are likely to meet others with common interests

3. *Getting a dog*—Walking a dog gets you out of the house and invites others to approach a friendly pooch (and you)

4. *Tracking down old school friends*—It is a small world when it comes to finding former friends who may also have relocated or changed status

5. *Take a fresh look*—Consider befriending the people you see each day, at work, the grocery store, the gym, your condo clubhouse

Use some of the social skills discussed in this and earlier chapters to start conversations and begin building new relationships

Therapeutic Groups for Developing Social Interaction Skills

Group therapy, including group psychotherapy and occupational therapy activity groups, has a long history in health care, a predominantly American 20th century phenomenon (Cara, 2005). Beginning in the 1950s, diverse aspects of group therapy including therapeutic factors (hope, altruism, universality), interventions (feedback, role playing, reality testing), and leader traits (direction, warmth, passivity) became the subject of research. The conclusion at the century's end is that, for whatever reasons, group therapy does seem to work (Barlow, Burlingame, & Fuhriman (2000). Within both residential and outpatient health care institutions, group therapy has flourished, especially in the treatment of mental health conditions, with most if not all interventions occurring in groups. The benefits to group members include learning and practicing communication skills and leader-modeled skills, such as empathizing, active listening, clarifying issues, and giving and receiving feedback. Another advantage of groups is the opportunity for members to acquire personhood skills by observing and imitating each other (Corey & Corey, 2002). Personhood skills include courage, willingness, being present, belief in the group, ability to cope, nondefensiveness, self-awareness, sense of humor, and inventiveness.

Yalom's Therapeutic Factors Revisited

The well-recognized expert Irvin Yalom (2005) provides the latest updates on his well-researched therapeutic factors of group psychotherapy. These are the reasons why group therapy surpasses individual treatment for addressing interpersonal and social issues for participants. The following are the 12 general categories of therapeutic factors and brief definitions.

1. *Interpersonal input*—Group members learn how they are perceived by others. This factor was highly valued by participants.

2. *Catharsis*—Getting one's story told, often including intense emotional discharge. This is best accomplished within a cohesive group.

3. *Cohesiveness*—Belonging and being accepted by group members. This involves continued close contact with others, as well as trust that one is valued without judgment or condition and can share even embarrassing or negative experiences without being rejected.

4. *Self-understanding*—An intellectual comprehension of the relationship between past and present, such as understanding the causes of problems, also referred to as insight.

5. *Interpersonal output*—Improving skills in getting along with others, developing trust, and working out difficulties with relationships.

6. *Existential factors*—A shared recognition among members that life is not fair, one cannot avoid pain, and everyone is ultimately alone, no matter how close they feel to others.

7. *Universality*—Members feeling that they are not alone and that others in the group share equally distressing interpersonal and social problems.

8. *Instillation of hope*—A belief that the group can really help its members to overcome distressing emotional events.

9. *Altruism*—Helping others and having them value one's help increases one's feeling of self-worth. This feeling parallels the benefit of helping oneself by serving others that occurs in both caregiving and community volunteering.

10. *Family re-enactment*—The re-emergence of ancient memories and feelings originating with one's primary family group. This factor is more highly valued by therapists than members.

11. *Guidance*—Advice or suggestions from others for working out life's problems.

12. *Identification*—Involves imitative behavior or the ability to learn by watching other members or the leader/therapist.

While Yalom justifies all of these factors with theory and empirical data, the most valued by clients or participants is number 1, rank ordered to the least valued, number 12.

Client-Centered Activity Groups

Client-centered therapy, made popular by Canadian occupational therapists, follows the principles of Carl Rogers (1951), including (1) self-direction—the belief in each person's ability to make choices, (2) self-actualization—the person's capacity to attain personal completeness, and (3) unconditional positive regard—a cultivated attitude toward a client or patient that facilitates trust, respect, and self-disclosure. In activity groups, Cole (2005, 2008) provides guidelines for group leadership that support these client-centered values (see Chapter 1). These guidelines ensure that, whatever the activity, each member will have multiple opportunities for input, expression of emotion, discussion and interpretation of the meaning of the experience, and an invitation to personalize the experience with group input. For example, groups of people with depression might become engaged in a letter writing task to assist them with building their own social networks for support. In this activity, each person makes a choice about to whom their letter should be addressed, and the group is sequenced with ample time for discussion, sharing, and expression of emotions. A well-trained leader will also facilitate interpersonal interaction and ensure that each member feels empathy and support from other members, enacting several of the therapeutic factors discussed by Yalom.

Learning Activities

Support Groups Learning Activity

Choose a disability category from the following list: stroke, multiple sclerosis, bipolar disorder, obesity, attention deficit disorder, arthritis. Briefly describe the scope of the disability, focusing on potential barriers to social participation.

Internet search: Search the internet to identify three Web sites that offer online support in real-time or ongoing, reliable information about the disability and possible solutions to common problems, and information about local face-to-face meetings in a specific community, including contact information, phone numbers, and time and place of meetings.

Written narrative: If you had a client with this disability, how would you introduce the topic, guide the client to possible support groups, and outline the potential benefits and pitfalls? Write the exact words you would use to motivate the client to follow your guidelines.

Community Integration Learning Activity

To be able to meet basic needs while living independently in the community, clients need to be able to access needed services close to home. Let us assume your client has recently moved to a new community after a prolonged rehabilitation and is now able to drive short distances during the day. For this assignment, you will need a local street map, a pencil and protractor or string for drawing a circle, and a partner to work with who has access to a car. (Note: For urban dwellers, the scenario can be modified to services available within a reasonable walking distance from the client's apartment.)

Instructions: One partner role-plays the client, and the other the therapist. Together, compile a list of 10 essential services or resources, for example:

1. Grocery store
2. Bank/ATM
3. Library/computer café
4. Hair dresser/barber
5. Clothing or department store
6. Church, temple, religious group
7. Medical clinic/emergency walk-in clinic
8. Restaurant(s) within client's price range
9. Fitness center/gym/sports or recreational facility
10. Park or safe outdoor area for walking

Your list will be different for each client, depending on his or her age, interests, and priorities.

Windshield survey: Using a local street map, identify the client's home—this will be the center of your circle. Identify the scale in miles, and measure 5 miles—this will be the radius of your circle. With a string and pencil or a protractor, use the client's home as the center, and draw a circle encompassing a 5-mile radius. Everything within the circle will be within 5 miles of the client's home. With your partner, drive around the area within the circle, and identify as many resources on your list as you can. Write the names and addresses of these places, and look up the phone numbers in the telephone book or on the internet. Also, during your windshield survey, make notes about safety issues, ease of parking, accessibility, and price range or any other relevant information (adapted from Madison, 1982).

Written narrative: Make a complete list of resources within 5 miles, including addresses, telephone numbers, and brief descriptions, including potential facilitators or barriers for accessing these services. Note which services are missing from your survey, and suggest ways to overcome this barrier for the client. Discuss the social skills and social cognition that would be needed for the client to successfully participate in the process of procuring needed items or services from each of the places on your list, regardless of whether you found them within the 5-mile area you surveyed. *What interventions might be needed in order for the client to interact successfully in this community to meet basic needs?*

Script: Social Skills Training Group— Basic Conversations

Seating Chart

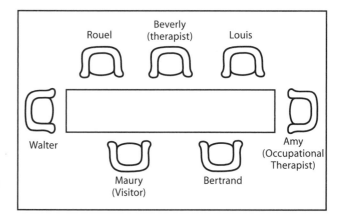

Characters and Scenario

The following is based on an actual group led by Amy, an occupational therapist, and Beverly, a speech-language therapist on a head injury unit at large state hospital. Their visitor, Maury, is also an occupational therapist. The four male members, all in their 20s, have good verbal skills and no difficulty speaking, but their head injuries are moderately severe, and they all have difficulty using good judgment in social situations. All of their names have been changed to protect their right to confidentiality.

Action Begins Here

Amy: Welcome, everyone. As you can see, we have a guest today. This is Maury. *(gestures toward guest)* He is here to see how we are learning social skills. He is writing a book for professional health care students. I'd like each of you to introduce yourselves to him, demonstrating some of the social skills you have learned. Let's start with you, Bertrand.

Bertrand: *(turns to look at Maury and makes eye contact)* I'm Bertrand. *(they shake hands)*

Maury: Nice to meet you, Bertrand.

(Bertrand turns back to Amy with an uncertain look)

Amy: Go on.

Bertrand: This weekend, I had two conversations with my family, and I used the social skills to start conversations.

Maury: What did you talk about?

Bertrand: The football game. *(nods from Louis and Beverly)*

Amy: Yes, that's right. It was Super Bowl Sunday, wasn't it?

Bertrand: Yeah. But I had to come back here before it ended…*(mumbles)*

Amy: Okay, Bertrand. Let's continue around the circle. Walter, your turn.

Walter: Hi, I'm Walter. *(turns to right, makes eye contact)* How far did you have to come today?

Maury: I drove up from Madison, about an hour.

Amy: That's a good question, especially with the weather outside. *(all turn to look out the window)* What's it doing out there?

Walter and Rouel: Snowing.

Rouel: *(without prompting)* Hi, I'm Rouel. What are you writing about, Maury?

Maury: Well, this week I'm writing about how social skills training, like you're doing right now, helps people to participate socially in their families and communities. Thanks for asking. But before we move on, would you repeat your name? I didn't quite hear it.

Rouel: *(louder)* Rouel. *(spells it out)* R-O-U-E-L.

Amy: That's better… just don't look upset when you have to repeat something. You do have a more unusual name.

(Rouel nods and smiles)

Beverly: Maury and I have already met. Louis, your turn.

Louis: *(looks straight ahead)* My name is Louis.

Amy: Who are you talking to?

Louis: Oh, sorry. *(stands up, moves chair backwards, reaches hand across the table to shake hands with Maury—they shake)*

Maury: *(laughs)* Nice to meet you, Louis.

Louis: *(sits, looks annoyed)* Why is everyone laughing?

Amy: *(to the group)* Does anyone think Louis overreacted? *(all raise their hands)* What could he have done instead?

Bertrand: Stay in his seat and just turn toward Maury.

Louis: That's hard to do in these chairs. They don't swivel.

Amy: The chairs don't, but your body does.

(Louis moves his chair with loud scraping noise to face group)

Amy: Okay, that's good. Now, let's review some lessons we've learned already. What three things do we need to have a friendly conversation?

Bertrand: People, place, and… *(pauses, thinking)*

Walter: …topic to talk about *(finishes Bertrand's sentence)*

Amy: Very good. Each of you, give an example of where you could meet someone to talk to *(looks at Bertrand)*

Bertrand: A restaurant.

Walter: The 7-11 store.

Rouel: The library.

Amy: Are you supposed to talk in the library?

Bertrand: No, unless you whisper.

Rouel: How about the gym?

Amy: Good idea. Louis where else can you find someone to talk with?

Louis: Gas station?

Amy: Well, maybe. Did you go anywhere over the weekend to practice your religion?

Louis: I went to church, but you aren't supposed to talk there.

Amy: That's true, during the service, but what about afterwards?

Louis: Oh, yeah. There's coffee sometimes, and you welcome new people. My parents do.

Amy: Not you?

Louis: *(looks down)* Not usually.

Amy: Moving on, what's a good topic to talk about? Bertrand.

Bertrand: Sports. I like to talk about sports.

Walter: *(spontaneously)* Movies.

Beverly: Good one. What movies have you seen lately?

Rouel: Slum Dog Millionaire. That was good, too.

Beverly: I meant you could ask someone as a topic to talk about.

Rouel: *(nodding and smiling)* Okay, I know, the weather.

Beverly: Good one. How about you, Louis?

Louis: Books.

Amy: What question could you ask someone about a book?

Louis: Have you read a good book lately?

Amy: If I said yes, then what?

Louis: *(grinning)* What was it?

Beverly: That was a great review. Now, let's begin today's activity. Each of you will pick a card and start a conversation with someone here using the topic on the card. *(holds out stack of cards)* Who wants to start?

Rouel: I will. *(picks a card and reads)* "Someone you admire and why." *(pauses, looks at Louis)* I admire my ex-wife, the mother of my children. She's a good mother... *(mumbles another sentence, looking down)*

Beverly: Who are you talking to?

Rouel: Louis. Oh, yeah. Who is someone you admire?

Louis: Derek Jeter, New York Yankees, cause he gets all the girls. *(group smiles and laughter)*

Amy: Okay, now pass it on. We're communicating with all the group members.

Louis: *(to Bertrand)* What about you?

Bertrand: I forgot the topic *(looks uninterested)*

Amy: Why don't you pick another card?

Bertrand: *(picks one and reads)* "Talk about a problem with keeping promises." I made lots of promises, and I feel bad when I don't keep them. Everyone should keep their promises. Don't you think so, Walter?

Walter: Yes. I break most all of them. Now, I try not to make promises to people any more. *(looks down sadly)*

Amy: Ready for a change of topic?

Walter: Yes. *(Beverly passes him a card, he reads)* "What do you do when you feel lonely?" I find a comfortable chair and watch a TV show. Do I pass to the right? *(Beverly nods)* Louis, what do you do when you're lonely?

Louis: Go to the library and find a good book.

Amy: That's a pretty good answer. But who are you talking to?

Louis: *(moves chair to face group from the corner of the table. Faces Bertrand.)* What do you do when you get lonely?

Bertrand: See if there's a game I can watch, or go to the gym and play racquetball. See if there's someone who wants to play...

Rouel: *(jumps in without prompting)* You'd find someone to be with... that's what I'd do, too. Or I'd call someone. *(face lights up)*

Walter: Who would you call? *(seems genuinely interested)*

Rouel: Maybe my mom, or my uncle. Who would you call, Walter? *(very sincere tone)*

Walter: Maybe I'd call Louis. He likes to watch sports. *(Louis looks up, pays attention)*

Amy: Time out. What did you notice about this last topic? How did you all do with keeping it moving?

Rouel: It was more interesting. We all got involved.

Beverly: I saw better eye contact and heard more emotion in your voices. Did anyone else notice that?

Bertrand: Yes. Rouel just talked, and I didn't have to ask him a question.

Amy: Great. You all did a good job today. For homework, I'd like each of you to start a conversation with someone using one of these topics or one of your own. We'll discuss how you did next time. Okay? *(nods)* Does anyone have any questions before we end?

Maury: I just wanted to say thank you for letting me come today. I understand much better now what you learn in the social skills group.

Beverly: See you all next time.

The End.

Discussion

1. What basic social skills are being taught by the leaders of this group?

2. To what extent do the leaders follow Cole's group leadership guidelines discussed in Chapter 1?

3. What basic communication skills from Chapter 3 can you identify in this scenario?

4. How are the leaders of this group facilitating interaction among the members?

5. Considering that these participants are hospitalized for significant behavioral and cognitive disabilities, how can they use the social skills they are learning to increase their social participation outside the hospital?

6. In considering the extent of disability, what health and community services would these clients need in order to be able to live independently?

7. If you were asked to lead this group, what might you do differently and why?

8. In what other adult populations might a group like this be useful? Give examples.

Acknowledgment

The author wishes to acknowledge the contributions of occupational therapists Amy Peloski and Anne Golensky for sharing their expertise in the area of social skills training with diverse populations.

References

Adler, A. (1958). *What life should mean to you.* New York, NY: Putnam & Sons.

Barlow, S. H., Burlingame, G., & Fuhriman, A. (2000). Therapeutic application of groups: From Pratt's thought control classes to modern group psychotherapy. *Group Dynamics Theory, Research, and Practice, 4* (1), 115-134.

Bellack, A., Mueser, K., Gingerich, S., & Agresta, J. (2004). *Social skills training for schizophrenia* (2nd ed.). New York, NY: Guilford Publications.

Cara, E. (2005). Groups. In E. Cara & A. MacRae (Eds.), *Psychosocial occupational therapy: A clinical practice* (2nd ed.). Clifton Park, NJ: Delmar Learning Thompson.

Clark, C., & Sline, R. (2003). Teaming with emotion: The impact of emotionality on work-team collaboration. In R. Hirokawa, R. Cathcart, L. Samovar, & L. Henman (Eds.), *Small group communication: Theory & practice.* Los Angeles, CA: Roxbury Publishing.

Cloud, J. (2009). The mystery of borderline personality disorder. *Time 2008, the year in medicine from A to Z.* Retrieved January 28, 2009 from www.time.com/time/printout/0,8816,1870491,00

Cole, M. (2005). *Group dynamics in occupational therapy* (3rd ed.). Thorofare, NJ: SLACK Incorporated.

Cole, M. (2008). Client centred groups. In J. Creek & L. Laugher (Eds.), *Occupational therapy and mental health* (4th ed.). London, England: Elsevier.

Connecticut Self-Help Network. (2004). *Starting a self-help group: Starter package kit.* New Haven, CT: The Consultation Center.

Corey, M., & Corey, G. (2002). *Groups: Process and practice* (6th ed.). Monterrey, CA: Brooks Cole, Thompson Learning.

Davidson, L., & Strauss, J. S. (1992). Sense of self in recovery from severe mental illness. *British Journal of Medical Psychology, 65,* 131 -145.

Department of Employment Services. (2009). *Transitional employment program: A way to work initiative.* Retrieved February 6, 2009 from www.does.dc.gov/does/cwp/vies,a,1232,q637871.asp

Dickerson, D., Bellack, A., & Gold, J. (2007). Social/communication skills, cognition, and vocational functioning in schizophrenia. *Schizophrenia Bulletin, 33,* 5, 1213-1220.

Dijkers, M. (1998). Community integration: Conceptual issues and measurement approaches in rehabilitation research. *Topics in Spinal Cord Injury Rehabilitation, 4,* 1-15.

Donohue, M. V. (1999). Theoretical bases of Mosey's group interactions skills. *Occupational Therapy International, 6,* 35-51.

Donohue, M. V. (2009). *The social profile.* Retrieved from www.Social-Profile.com

Dreikurs, R., & Grey, L. (1968). *A new approach to discipline: Logical consequences.* New York, NY: Hawthorne Books, Inc.

Dudgeon, B. (2009). Community integration. In E. Crepeau, E. Cohn, & B. Schell (Eds.), *Willard & Spackman's occupational therapy* (11th ed., pp. 181-191). Philadelphia, PA: Lippincott, Williams & Wilkins.

Encyclopedia of Mental Disorders. (2009). *Social skills training.* Retrieved January 28, 2009 from www.minddisorders.com/Py-Z/Social-skills-training

Fazio, L. (2008). *Developing occupation-centered programs for the community* (2nd ed.). Upper Saddle River, NJ: Pearson Prentice Hall.

Gordon, T. (1992). *Parent effectiveness training.* Pasadena, CA: Effectiveness Training Associates.

Grohol, J. (2004). *What to look for in quality online support groups.* Retrieved April 15, 2010 from www.psychcentral.com/archives/support_groups.html

Gutman, S., Kerner, R., Zombek, I., Dulek, J., & Ramsey, C. A. (2009). Supported education for adults with psychiatric disabilities: Effectiveness of an occupational therapy program. *American Journal of Occupational Therapy, 63,* 245-254.

Harris, L. (2008). *Surrender to win: Regain sanity by strategically relinquishing control.* Corpus Christi, TX: Greenleaf Publishing.

Hirokawa, R. Y. (2003). Communication and group decision-making efficiency. In R. Hirokawa, R. Cathcart, L. Samovar, & L. Henman (Eds.), *Small group communication: Theory & practice.* Los Angeles, CA: Roxbury Publishing.

Karbo, K. (2006). Friendship: The laws of attraction. *Psychology Today, Nov-Dec,* 91-95.

Leerhsen, C. (1990). Unite and conquer: America's crazy for support groups. Or maybe support groups keep America from going crazy. *Newsweek, February 5,* 50-55.

Liberman, R., Eckman, T., & Marder, S. (2001). Rehab rounds: Training in social problem solving among persons with schizophrenia. *Psychiatric Services, 52,* 31-33.

Liberman, R., & Fuller, T. (2000). Generalization of social skills training in schizophrenia. In J. Meder (Ed.), *Rehabilitation of patients with schizophrenia* (pp. 7-14). Krakow, Poland: Biblioteka Polish Psychiatry.

Liberman, R., Glynn, S., Blair, K., Ross, D., & Marder, S. (2002). In vivo amplified skills training: Promoting generalization of independent living skills for clients with schizophrenia. *Psychiatry Internal & Biological Processes, 65,* 137-155.

Liberman, R., Wallace, C. J., Blackwell, G. A., Eckman, T. A., Vacaro, J. V., & Kuchnel, T. G. (1993). Innovations in skills training for the seriously mentally ill: The UCLA Social and Independent Living Skills Modules. *Innovations & Research, 2,* 43-59.

Linehan, M. (1993a). *Cognitive-behavioral treatment of borderline personality disorder.* New York, NY: Guilford Press.

Madison, T. M. (1982) Windshield survey: A micro approach. In M. Stanhope & R. N. Knollmueller (Eds.), *Handbook of community and home health nursing: Tools for assessment, intervention and education.* St. Louis, MO: Mosby.

Marcias, C., Rodican, C., Hargreaves, W., Jones, D., Barreira, P., & Wang, Q. (2006). Supported employment outcomes of a randomized controlled trial of ACT and clubhouse models. *Psychiatric Services, 57,* 1406-1415.

Melville, S. (2008). *Helping someone with OCD: Tips for supporting people with obsessive-compulsive disorder.* Retrieved January 13, 2009 from www.obsessive-compulsive-disorder.suite101.com/article.cfm/helping_someone_with_ocd

Morrison, R. L. (1990). Interpersonal dysfunction. In A. S. Bellack, M. Hersen, & A. E. Kazen (Eds.), *International handbook of behavior modification and therapy* (3rd ed., pp. 503-522). New York, NY: Plenum Press.

Mosey, A. C. (1986). *Psychosocial components of occupational therapy.* New York, NY: Raven Press.

Nelsen, J. (1981). *Positive discipline.* Fair Oaks, CA: Sunrise Press.

Peck, W. (2000). Fountain House: Cutting edge services for the mentally ill. Retrieved April 16, 2010 from www.allbusiness.com/healthcare-social-assistance/582200-1.html

Rogers, C. (1951). *Client-centered therapy.* Boston, MA: Houghton-Mifflin.

Sadock, B. J., & Sadock, V. A. (2003). *Synopsis of psychiatry: Behavioral sciences/clinical psychiatry* (9th ed.). Philadelphia, PA: Lippincott, Williams & Wilkins.

Schonebaum, A. D., Boyd, J. K., & Dudek, K. J. (2006). A comparison of competitive employment outcomes for the clubhouse and PACT models. *Psychiatric Services, 57,* 1416-1420.

Siegel, B. S. (1986). *Love, medicine & miracles: Lessons learned about self-healing from a surgeon's experience with exceptional patients.* New York, NY: Harper & Row.

Strong, S. (1998). Meaningful work in supportive environments: Experiences with the recovery process. *American Journal of Occupational Therapy, 52,* 31-38.

Strong, S., & Rebeiro, K. (2003). Creating supportive work environments for people with mental illness. In L. Letts, P. Rigby, & D. Stewart (Eds.), *Using environments to enable occupational performance* (pp. 71-80). Thorofare, NJ: SLACK Incorporated.

Swarbrick, P., & Pratt, C. (2006). Consumer operated self-help services: Roles and opportunities for occupational therapists and occupational therapy assistants. *Occupational Therapy Practice, 11,* CE 1-8.

Tauber, R., Wallace, C., & Lecomte, T. (2000). Enlisting indigenous community supporters in skills training programs for persons with severe mental illness. *Psychiatric Services, 51,* 1428-1432. Retrieved January 13, 2009 from www.psychiatryonline.org/cgi/content/full/51/11/1428

Weiss, T. (2009). *Fountain house: Where it all began.* Retrieved February 28, 2009 from www.psychservices.psychiatryonline.org/cgi/content/full/50/11/1473

Wilcock, A. (2006). *An occupational perspective of health* (2nd ed.). Thorofare, NJ: SLACK Incorporated.

World Health Organization. (2001). *International classification of function, disability, and health.* Geneva, Switzerland: Author.

Yalom, I. (2005). *Theory and practice of group psychotherapy* (5th ed.). New York, NY: Basic Books.

Additional Resources

Harned, M. S., Chapman, A. L., Dexter-Mazza, E. T., Murray, A., Comtois, K. A., & Linehan, M. M. (2008). Treating co-occurring axis I disorders in chronically suicidal women with borderline personality disorder: A 2-year randomized trial of dialectical behavior therapy versus community treatment by experts. *Journal of Consulting and Clinical Psychology, 76,* 1068-1075.

Linehan, M. (1993b). *Skills training for treating borderline personality disorder.* New York, NY: Guilford Press.

Litt, M., Kadden, R., Kabela-Cormier, E., & Petry, N. (2007). Changing network support for drinking: Initial findings from the network support project. *Journal of Consulting and Clinical Psychology, 75,* 542-555.

chapter 15

Older Adult Interventions to Facilitate Social Participation

Marilyn B. Cole, MS, OTR/L, FAOTA

Changing demographics in the aging population necessitate a rethinking of the needs of the two different developmental stages of older adulthood: Laslett's Third and Fourth Ages (1989, 1997). As discussed in Chapter 9, these life stages reflect very different interests and goals regarding social participation. Research has validated this distinction, noting significant changes in social relationships, social priorities, and occupational interests (Adams, 2004; Baltes & Smith, 2001). Accordingly, this chapter will discuss two different sets of interventions. Facilitating current life roles by overcoming common barriers such as mobility, vision, and hearing impairments; restructuring one's life in retirement; and programs addressing wellness and prevention best meet the Third Ager's need to continue active social participation. Because the Fourth Age begins with the onset of disability, these older adults present more significant health challenges and require more traditional therapeutic approaches. However, while their physical needs require attention, their social interests and goals may vary significantly, and therapeutic activities need to be guided by individual social priorities. Interventions include issues of caregiving, reminiscence, sensorimotor approaches, adult day care and nursing home programs, and end-of-life issues.

Third Age Interventions

Older adults enter the Third Age at retirement, an event that sets in motion a whole spectrum of

life changes, including loss of worker role, loss of income, disrupted routines, and exclusion from work-related social networks. Spiritually, retirement initiates a reflective process about what to do with the rest of one's life: fulfilling one's dreams, enacting social changes, seeing the world, relaxing at home, or finally writing that novel. The outcome of this spiritual journey can take several years of exploration, experimentation, education, and self-analysis, often punctuated or interrupted by unrelated life events: a divorced son or daughter moving back home, a failed investment, an unanticipated health crisis, or the discovery that happiness and fulfillment do not always happen as expected. Even when well-planned, transitioning to retirement represents a time of increased vulnerability, greater stress, and higher risk for physical and mental health conditions. Staying socially connected remains paramount in providing the social and emotional support people need as they restructure their lives in retirement. For this reason, interventions for Third Agers should always facilitate social participation.

Transitioning to Retirement

The transtheoretical model of behavior change (TTM; DiClemente & Velasquez, 2002) is useful for understanding and facilitating the transition to retirement because it emphasizes the importance of the older adult's readiness for change and addresses the complexities of the change process itself (Miller & Cook, 2008). TTM includes five intentional stages of change:

Cole, M.B., & Donohue, M.V. *Social Participation in Occupational Contexts: In Schools, Clinics, and Communities* (pp 273-292).
© 2011 SLACK Incorporated

Table 15-1

PLANNING FOR CHANGES IN RETIREMENT (SIX GROUP SESSIONS)

1. **Pre-contemplation**
   - List five potential changes you will face following retirement
   - List five negative outcomes you would like to avoid
   - List five goals you may want to accomplish after retirement
   - Share and discuss with the group

2. **Contemplation**
   - Knowledge acquisition—Discuss normal Third Age life tasks
   - List five life roles you wish to acquire/continue after retirement
   - List five activities or occupations that give your life meaning
   - Share and discuss; choose two roles and two occupations as priorities

3A. **Preparation**
   - Decision-making process—List several options for change
   - List pros and cons for each
   - Choose best option—List steps or sequence of tasks to accomplish; example: exercise at home, join a gym, learn a new sport?

3B. **Building Social Supports (preparation continued)**
   - List five non-work-related social groups you currently belong to
   - List five relatives or friends you can always count on for support
   - What are gaps? How can you nurture your important relationships?
   - Research what additional community groups you could join

4. **Action**
   - Choose one goal to address for this session
   - List steps to take this week to begin implementation
   - Locate a specific local group to visit: make phone call, get directions
   - Discuss with members what support you need to carry out plans

5. **Maintenance**
   - Report experience and discuss barriers
   - Choose a partner to contact by phone, e-mail, or in person each week after group ends—set weekly goals and report back to each other

---

1. *Pre-contemplation*—Only a vague awareness of the need for change
2. *Contemplation*—Gaining awareness of the importance of change within 6 months
3. *Preparation*—Creating a plan to be executed within 1 month
4. *Action*—Implementing the plan, which is continued for next 6 months
5. *Maintenance*—Measures to continue new behavior and prevent relapse to old patterns

This evidence-based model may explain why some people, failing to plan and mentally prepare for retirement, become overwhelmed with the sudden lack of structure and feel marginalized by loss of meaningful occupational and social roles they once performed at work.

As pointed out by the popular media, no formula for a successful retirement currently exists for Third

Agers. During the next decade, retiring baby boomers will undoubtedly reinvent aging in many unanticipated ways (Johnson, 2002). Although many people plan financially for retirement, their readiness for the social and emotional changes often remains in the stage of pre-contemplation. A potential intervention for older adults anticipating retirement based on application of the TTM stages is outlined in Table 15-1. Such programming can be designed, marketed, and offered by health professionals through community agencies that support wellness and prevention for older adults. Pilot programs are needed to provide sufficient evidence to gain public or private funding.

The following 12-week occupational therapy group protocol was designed to help new retirees to contemplate, prepare, and try out some of the actions necessary for a successful transition to retirement. Groups of six to eight new retirees provide social support for each other throughout the 12 sessions, led by a trained facilitator. The leader or planner should design worksheets, handouts, and discussion questions for each topic. Refer to Cole (2005) for more about how to design group protocols (Table 15-2).

This program was developed to take place as a joint effort between a town senior center and a local library. The particulars for sessions were intended to come from the retirees themselves, who work as a team to create their own program and to make it relevant to their particular needs (M. Cole, unpublished grant application, 2008).

Prevention and Well-Being

Promotion of health and wellness represents one of six focus areas contained in the American Association of Occupational Therapy's (AOTA) centennial vision (Baum & Christiansen, 2005). For Third Agers, wellness factors take a high priority, including staying informed and taking actions that promote energy, longevity, and zest for life, therefore enabling the management of potentially disabling conditions and fulfillment of social participation goals. AOTA's focus on wellness reinforces *Healthy People 2010's* goals of facilitating older adult engagement in satisfying relationships with others, working and playing, and contributing to thriving communities and nation (Centers for Disease Control, 2010).

For community-dwelling older adults coping with disabling conditions, two of the greatest challenges for continued social and occupational participation are remaining in one's home and community mobility (Bettman, 2009). While occupational therapists are uniquely qualified to provide prevention programs that increase occupational performance, reduce health risks, and overcome barriers to community participation, health care legislators and third-party payers have been slow to recognize the cost-reduction benefits of wellness programs (AOTA, 2008; Bettman, 2009). What is prioritized within the United States health care system emphasizes personal independence and cost containment over social connectedness (Coppola, 2008). Advocates of wellness programs can cite ample evidence of the health-sustaining qualities of occupations for the well-elderly as well as its cost-effectiveness (Clark et al., 1997, 2001; Hay et al., 2002; Mandel, Jackson, Zemke, Nelson, & Clark, 1999). The U.S. Centers for Disease Control and Prevention predict that by 2030 the number of older adults will double, and 95% of these adults will likely live independently (CDC, 2008). Their publication, *Healthy People 2010*, lists as a primary goal, "to increase the quality as well as the number of years of healthy life…" including entering into satisfying

relationships with others, working, and contributing to society (Bettman, 2009; CDC, 2008, 2010). But keeping older adults healthy has benefits greater than saving health care dollars; it also increases the nation's social capital by making available the energy, skills, and life experiences of willing seniors to better serve the unmet needs of our society.

Lifestyle Redesign

The well-elderly study (Jackson, Carlson, Mandel, Zemke, & Clark 1998) gives a good example of an occupational therapy intervention program with Third Age older adults. The program emphasizes the power of occupations by educating participants about the health-relevant consequences of their occupations. Each of eight modules forms a structure for several small group (8 to 10) meetings, which include some form of didactic presentation, peer exchange, direct experience, and personal exploration. Each module begins by guiding small groups of community-living older adults through an "occupational self-analysis" (p. 330). The format allows members to learn, discuss, problem solve, and make choices according to their own interests and needs. Within the groups, members also have ample opportunity to provide one another social and emotional support. The module content areas are as follows:

- Introduction to the power of occupation—Discussion of how occupational choices affect well-being and create daily structure and meaning

- Aging, health, and occupation—Building healthy occupational habits and activities

- Transportation—Alternative ways to access and participate in the community

- Safety—In the home and neighborhood, crime prevention strategies, body mechanics

- Social relationships—Dealing with loss, maintaining friendships, and finding new friends

- Cultural awareness—Learning and sharing diverse aspects of group members and appreciating how culture shapes our daily occupations and social expectations

- Finances—Learning skills of budgeting, managing money, and engaging in affordable occupations

- Integrative summary—Lifestyle redesign journal. Reviewing the collected occupational knowledge and experience of the group using writing and photographs to construct individual roadmaps for the road ahead

Table 15-2

TRANSITION TO RETIREMENT GROUP PROTOCOL

1. Introduction and overview
   - Who are we? Introductory activity to get to know each other, sharing reasons for joining the group
   - Review outline for next 11 sessions
2. Perceptions of retirement
   - Visions worksheet: Best and worst scenario
     - ¤ What is the best retirement scenario you can imagine? Where are you living, with whom, what are you doing, what is a typical day like for you?
     - ¤ What is the worst scenario? What are your greatest fears?
   - Discussion of answers. What steps can be taken to avoid the worst, accomplish the best?
   - What are some goals we can set for ourselves?
3. Time management: Importance of routines
   - Role of routines when working
   - What is your ideal daily schedule?
   - What is a good occupational balance—work, leisure, self-care, social participation?
4. Redefining work in retirement
   - What are the benefits of a work role?
   - How can these be recreated in a meaningful way in retirement?
     - ¤ Maintaining one's home
     - ¤ Helping family members
     - ¤ Volunteering/civic engagement
     - ¤ Personal projects (writing, genealogy, scrapbooks)
5. What is the meaning of "leisure" time?
   - Worksheet of leisure interests
   - What are cultural differences in perceptions of leisure activities?
   - What is it about identified leisure interests that hold the most meaning for you?
6. What is appropriate self-care in retirement?
   - What is a healthy lifestyle?
     - ¤ Physical fitness
     - ¤ Mental fitness
     - ¤ Monitoring and maintaining health
     - ¤ Diet and nutrition
     - ¤ How can healthy habits be established and maintained?
7. Financial well-being—scaling back, setting priorities, making the most of income
   - Create a budget using monthly income and major living expenses
   - Keep a daily log of money spent for 1 week—keep receipts, categorize
   - What are some ways to save money on electricity, food, entertainment, other?
   - What are some potential ways to supplement income when needed?
8. Creating social support networks
9. Participation in the community—finding what's out there, good fit with skills
10. Managing belongings—deciding what you need, finding homes for what is no longer needed
11. Feeding the spirit—in what groups or activities do you find meaning/enrichment?
12. Continuing the learning curve—what new skills, experiences, roles await you?

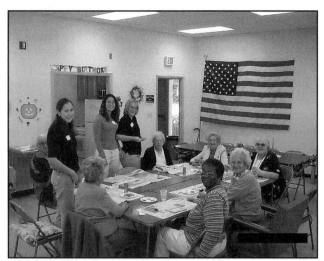

Figure 15-1. Elm Terrace Arts & Crafts Group.

The lifestyle redesign program, typically lasting about 9 months, has been adapted for older adults in many different phases of aging, including younger old (50 to 65), middle old (65 to 88), and oldest old (85+), and in many different settings, including family homes, senior apartment communities, and assisted-living facilities (Bettman, 2009). The successful adaptation and facilitation of this program requires a good understanding of the basic principles of occupational science, such as participation in occupation as a central route to health and psychosocial well-being and the experience of identity and meaning through occupation (Hay et al., 2002). Trained leaders viewed themselves as coaches or collaborators. Group facilitation skills also include the use of a client-centered and culturally sensitive approach, techniques to encourage group interaction, and modeling of social support behaviors, such as active listening and expressing empathy for one another (Cole, 2005). The group cohesiveness that develops within each group plays a significant role in providing support for promoting lifestyle changes.

One module that particularly promotes social participation is called "Relationships and Occupation" (Mandel et al., 1999). Because occupations can provide the context for starting and sustaining friendships and relationships, the group members are asked to reflect upon what activities they enjoy doing with their spouse, relatives, or friends. They discuss ways that occupations can help them connect with others and how occupations help them to avoid social isolation. Some associated activities are thinking of places to go with people you know, planning events or activities as a group, experiencing and discussing difficulties with communicating and planning all the steps of a group activity, bringing photos documenting some significant occupational events in their lives, such as sharing holiday traditions, or the celebration of life events. Sharing personal stories is encouraged among the group, as well as identifying ways to use occupation to repair broken relationships, to better understand or tolerate different cultural perspectives, or to help cope with lost relationships. What stories can you tell about the role of occupations in your relationships?

Wellness Interventions

Wellness groups for older adults have been initiated by occupational therapy fieldwork students at Quinnipiac University. Their fieldwork began with focus groups of older adults living independently in subsidized apartments. They used a client-centered approach to determine the occupational needs, interests, and priorities of these groups. Working in pairs, the students then designed a series of five group sessions addressing identified needs. Some of the topics were fall prevention, mental and physical fitness, patio gardening, scrapbooking, and structuring ways to learn from and about each other. For example, one group brought in photographs of the place where they were born, ranging from Poland, Japan, Germany, Italy, and Russia. This inspired a conversation between an American World War II veteran and a survivor of the Nagasaki atomic bombing that helped end the war, two very different sides of the same story. This group still meets weekly 2 years after the students began it, focusing on arts and crafts, scrapbook making, and sharing memoirs (Figure 15-1). Another group begun by students still meets to walk together for exercise each morning and has set up a call schedule to share information and to help keep one another safe. This illustrates the need for intervention with older adults to help them form and sustain social networks that keep them connected.

Community Mobility and Driver Safety

Transportation is clearly a conduit to community connectedness, whether for life maintenance or socialization (Womack, 2008). Social participation for most older Americans depends upon driving their own car to social gatherings. In fact, 89% of road trips taken by older adults involve either driving or riding in a private vehicle, while only 5% report use of public transportation (Houser, 2005). In 2001, 25% of all licensed drivers were over 65 (Center for Transportation Analysis, 2006). In an American Association of Retired Persons (AARP) survey of people older than 50, 91% were licensed drivers (2002). These facts highlight the importance of driver maintenance as a key factor in community-based social participation for older adults.

For most of the U.S. population, driving means independence. Losing this ability can leave older adults socially isolated and dependent on others, a growing source of stress for both older adults and their adult children (Burkhardt, Berger, Creedon, & McGavock, 1998). Yet, statistics show an increased accident fatality rate for drivers older than 65, a trend that is predicted to increase as the population of older adults grows (Center for Transportation Analysis, 2006).

Driver safety programs and screenings are one way to address the road safety issue (National Highway Traffic Safety Administration [NHTSA], 2005). Since 1970, the AARP has conducted driver safety refresher classes, available in many communities nationwide for those older than 50 years. This course, taught by trained volunteers in adult education settings, includes the following topics (among others):

×   Knowledge of traffic signs and rules of the road

×   Tests of reaction time, problem-solving while driving, and avoiding distractions

×   Review of what to do in a crash

×   Effects of alcohol and medication on driving alertness

×   Essential car maintenance

×   Driving in adverse road conditions (i.e., snow, ice, rain, heavy traffic)

The AARP driver manual advises looking for the following signs that driving is unsafe for an older adult:

×   Frightened or uncomfortable behind the wheel, fear they might hurt someone

×   Friends or family have expressed concern or felt unsafe as a passenger

×   Physical exhaustion while driving

×   Frequently getting lost or mind wandering

×   Having several "close calls" or minor scrapes

×   Physician or clergy has told them to stop driving

×   Cannot hear or see well enough, or cannot react fast enough

The program also recommends having a written emergency plan if stranded on the road, such as names and phone numbers of nearest relatives/friends and a sequence of actions to take. Carrying a cell phone and car charger might be an additional safeguard, as well as joining a roadside assistance program such as American Automobile Association or similar local on-call service. Routinely carrying credentials, cash and credit card, bottled water, and essential medications may also be a useful preparation for emergencies.

Occupational therapists can obtain an advanced certification in older driver safety through the AOTA, enabling them to evaluate sensory, cognitive, motor, and emotional functioning affecting driving ability, as well as on-the-road assessments. Occupational therapy's goal is to ensure that older drivers continue to be "transportation independent" in a way that is safe for them and the community (AOTA, 2007). In writing an evaluation for judicial use in decisions about driving cessation, the occupational therapy report would include a source of referral (whether state, family, or physician initiated); a summary of physical, cognitive, perceptual, and general functional abilities; evaluation findings; a summary of road test if performed; and recommendations regarding partial restrictions when appropriate (within 10 miles of home, only in daylight, etc.). If driving continuation cannot be recommended, alternate means of transportation can be suggested according to availability (AOTA, 2007).

In reality, there are many gaps in knowledge of older driver safety, including insufficient evidence of the validity and reliability of older driver assessments and screening tools; nonavailability of alternative public transportation in most areas; and a hesitancy on the part of medical professionals, families, and licensing agencies to require "giving up the keys" without having more options for "making a safe transition" from driver to passenger (NHTSA, 2005). This government agency is charged with conducting research and creating demonstration programs to improve traffic safety pertaining to older drivers (NHTSA, 2005). Yet, to date, no studies were found validating driver assessments for older adults with dementia or relating such assessments with safe driving or accident prevention (Martin, Marottoli, & O'Neill, 2009).

In the health and social sectors, the social norms of independence and emotional consequences of dependence and social isolation continue to influence driving continuation, according to a meta-analytic study (Classen, Winter, & Lopez, 2009). Driving cessation or reduction impacts the ability to meet day-to-day needs (Burkhardt et al., 1998), making driving continuation a priority due to problems accessing or affording alternative transportation and not driving limiting social participation (Kerschner & Aizenberg, 1999). Older adults in some studies believed that the consequences of driving cessation, such as loss of valued roles, social isolation, depression, and threats to their identity, posed a greater risk than safety issues (Johnson, 2002; Kostyniuk & Shope, 1998). Family and friends have the greatest influence on older adult driving decisions, sometimes easing concerns about sadness, anger, and loneliness (Johnson, 1998), and other times failing to communicate concerns about driving-at-risk as separate from family roles and relationships (Sterns, Sterns, Aizenberg, & Anapole, 1997). The authors of the meta-analytic study (Classen et al., 2009) conclude four themes or "Ds" from their synthesis:

1. *Destinations* captured the personal meaning of places important to them, and inability to reach them resulted in disruption of familiar routines and socialization.

2. The omission of effects of *drugs* on driving in the studies suggests more data are needed.

3. A *disconnect* emerged from older adults, families, and professionals when attempting to obtain help from service providers.

4. A need for more *diverse* mobility options was inferred as studies reported lack of alternatives and difficulties with scheduling, costs, and physical use of available alternatives. Volunteer drivers, door-to-door van services, and public bus routes are cited as needed alternative providers of community mobility for older adults.

In assessing risk of continued driving for older adults, studies cited mobility as the higher priority than safety. In the face of intervention by family and friends, some older adults willingly used self-regulation and greater caution when driving. However, given the high priority of independence and autonomy, it seems unlikely that older adults will be convinced to stop driving until viable alternatives for community mobility are developed. *How can professionals advocate for increased transportation services for older adults in their communities?*

Enabling Volunteering and Civic Engagement

Volunteering has many well-documented health benefits for older adults, including preventing depression, increasing both physical and mental health, and promoting a sense of well-being (Lum & Lightfoot, 2005; Mutchler, Burr, & Caro, 2003). From the perspective of society, some studies have suggested that older adults, with their skills, energy, continued good health, and rich life experience, represent "this country's only increasing natural resource—and the least used one" (Fried, Freedman, Endres, & Wasik, 1997, p. 216).

An evaluation of the client's skills and abilities, as well as limitations and barriers, is the first concern of the occupational therapist. In many ways, preparing to volunteer resembles preparing a resumé for employment, and in fact, some volunteer placement agencies require the potential volunteer to submit a resumé. Many community organizations depend on volunteers to supplement the work of paid employees. This requires a commitment of time and energy, and potential volunteers need to be willing to make such a commitment.

The next step in searching for volunteer opportunities requires a clarification of the client's reasons for volunteering. Some common reasons include:

- *Substitute work role*—Career exploration, learning new skills

- *Altruistic*—Furthering a cause the client believes in

- *Socialization*—Making new friends

- *Structure time*—Get out of the house and do something useful for others

- *Egoistic*—Using talents, be creative, mentor others

- *Leisure focus*—Doing something the client enjoys

Interventions that assist the client in clarifying his or her volunteer desires and specific interest areas will greatly facilitate the location of appropriate opportunities. One only needs to enter the word *volunteering* on any internet search engine to find thousands of volunteer opportunities (Table 15-3).

Most internet clearinghouses identify organizations within a few miles of one's local area and classify them according to specific areas of interest. However, many clients, especially those with a lower socioeconomic status, may not have internet access or the skills necessary to use these services. The occupational therapist should be prepared to search the internet and narrow down options that are appropriate for the client. To do the job right, the occupational therapist needs to investigate the job descriptions for volunteers and to analyze the specific tasks required. Follow-up phone calls or on-site visits may be required to assess the many task demands and contextual factors involved, especially for clients with a disability that must be accommodated.

Volunteer Roles

Once the client's skills and priorities have been identified, the client's reasons for volunteering need to be matched with the types of volunteer jobs available. One volunteer clearinghouse (www.nottinghamcvs.co.uk) categorizes the types of volunteer roles as follows:

- *Practical, immediate action*—Concrete tasks like feeding the homeless

- *Helping people solve their problems*—Advocacy, crisis intervention

- *Getting the organization's job done*—Managing, office tasks, fundraising

---

Table 15-3

EXAMPLES OF VOLUNTEER CLEARINGHOUSE WEB SITES

Retired Senior Volunteer Program (RSVP)	www.seniorcorps.org/joining/rsvp
Quintessential Careers (paid and unpaid)	www.quintcareers.com/volunteering.html
Service Corps of Retired Executives (SCORE)	www.score.org
Volunteers in Service to America (VISTA)	www.americorps.gov
AARP Community Service Web site	www.aarp.org/giving-back
End Childhood Hunger	www.strength.org
Serviceleader.org	www.utexas.edu/lbj/rgk/serviceleader/volunteers
National Retiree Volunteer Coalition (NRVC)	www.civicventures.org/public_service.cfm
Volunteer Abroad	www.volunteerabroad.com
Volunteer Match	www.volunteermatch.org/

× *Concern for people and relationships*—Providing caregiving, social support

× *Influencing and promoting change*—Political action, lobbying for social change

The Web site offers a questionnaire to help identify which type of role applies to the individual.

Clients need to feel that the volunteer role they perform has both a personal and an organizational meaning, and this requires a good match between meeting client needs, such as socialization or an outlet for skills and creativity, and meeting the needs of recipients of service. According to Merrill (2000), for people to view their volunteering positively and sustain their interest, there needs to be a balance between giving and receiving.

Common Barriers to Volunteer Participation

Many other factors contribute to this mutual satisfaction of needs. Some are adequate training and coordination of volunteers, clear expectations of the volunteer role, adequate supervision and positive reinforcement, flexibility in time constraints, and willingness to accommodate to physical and social contexts. When problems arise, the occupational therapist may facilitate mutual problem-solving in the volunteer workplace.

× *Lack of structure*—Volunteer roles vary widely in the amount of structure they provide. Some, such as the AARP Driver Safety Program, are highly structured with specific job descriptions and a training program for each role (AARP, 2002). Others, such as friendly visitor programs, depend on the volunteers to structure their own schedule and work. Studies of burnout and drop-out show that volunteers are more likely to leave a volunteer job because of too little structure

and role ambiguity (Ross, Greenfield, & Bennett, 1999). The occupational therapist can work with clients and volunteer supervisors to organize and structure the volunteer role according to the needs of both.

× *Inadequate supervision*—For direct service roles, such as adult literacy or soup kitchens, feedback in the form of appreciation or suggestions may come directly from the recipients. Volunteers in these types of settings report an increase in satisfaction with volunteering. However, there are many behind-the-scenes fundraising or administrative roles that do not provide much feedback or appreciation. Volunteers need guidance and feedback in order to serve more effectively and to reap the benefits of volunteering, such as daily meaning and a sense of well-being. Some organizations have performed their own studies of volunteer retention and have developed strategies for giving needed feedback, such as recognition events or awards. However, occupational therapists can advise volunteer organizations in providing the effective supervision to meet the needs of specific clients or client groups. For example, volunteers with mental health issues need a great deal of reassurance and direction with regard to appropriate social behaviors and boundaries. Knight (2004) identifies several keys to continued volunteer participation for those with mental health conditions, including peer support networks, use of home health aides, individual case management, and crisis intervention programs.

× *The stigma of disability*—Perhaps the most disturbing barrier to volunteer participation is social stigma. The social attitudes of volunteer recruiters play an important part in the successful placement of those with mental or physical disabilities. A study by Lauber, Nordt, Falcato, and Rossler (2002) found two categories of social attitude toward volunteers in psychiatry: 1) antipathetic, including a negative view of mental illness and a desire for social distance, and 2) socially responsible, including a positive attitude and an interest in social issues. Advocacy is needed to overcome the barrier of stigma for all types of disability, and this may become the focus of occupational therapy for specific clients who wish to participate in specific community services.

× *Unreasonable expectations*—Some areas of volunteering involve greater levels of stress and emotional burden than others. In studying volunteer burnout with people with AIDS, emotional overload was a common reason for dropout (Ross et al., 1999). Caregiving roles for many special populations have a similar risk, and this needs to be considered in the occupational therapy volunteer role analysis. Some volunteers have a greater capacity for emotional involvement than others. For example, those who volunteer in bereavement or hospice programs need a high tolerance for dealing with intense emotions of others. Physical limitations also place volunteers at risk for burnout, such as too many hours or not enough coverage for specific roles. Older adults may need to consider energy limitations and fatigue when scheduling volunteer hours.

× *Time constraints*—In assisting clients with volunteer roles, occupational therapists need to be aware of the balance of activities that make up a client's lifestyle. Linda Fried, director of the Center for Aging and Health at Johns Hopkins University, suggests that 15 hours a week of volunteering are needed for older adults to reap health benefits (Marek, 2005). However, the amount of time clients can devote to volunteer roles will vary widely, and occupational therapists need to consider each client's individual needs. Working with activity patterns, daily routines, and time management becomes the focus of occupational therapy in this area.

× *Physical and social contexts*—Volunteers with disabilities will need a variety of physical and social adaptations to the contexts of volunteer roles. Physical adaptations will be similar to those needed for adapting work settings and work task demands. Social support has perhaps the greatest influence of volunteer satisfaction and well-being (Sadler & Marty, 1998). Positive relationships with volunteer coworkers is a powerful motivator in volunteer retention and sustained interest. Many older adults depend on volunteering to meet their needs for social contact, while others need to feel needed, useful, and appreciated. Building social environments that support volunteer participation must include opportunities for social interaction and positive reinforcement (Cole, 2008).

Enabling Citizen Participation for Older Adults

Another aspect of civic engagement involves exercising one's rights as a citizen to participate in the democratic process of government. Letts (2003) describes a potential role for occupational therapists enabling older adults to participate in community-organizing initiatives. To do so, therapists need to clearly articulate how political and social infrastructures within communities influence occupational performance and social participation for older citizens (e.g., public policies regarding public transportation, housing, public health, accessibility, and safety). Grassroots organizations can pave the way for older adults to have a voice in policy decisions that directly affect their social and occupational participation at the community level. Letts (2003) believes that citizen participation is "as valid for occupational therapy to focus on as dressing, even more meaningful for some clients" (p. 72). Some of the skills that occupational therapists bring to such grassroots groups are small group facilitation, instrumental support, linking groups to funding sources, and evaluating progress based on initial goals or funding source requirements. Enabling citizen engagement often requires occupational therapists to modify the social and political contexts to accommodate the participation of older adults as monitors, advisors, and advocates through organized efforts.

Overcoming Vision and Hearing Impairments

Vision and hearing, both of which tend to diminish with aging, remain necessary components of communication, interaction, and social participation for most older adults. Unfortunately, many older adults and their caregivers assume that vision loss comes with normal aging and, therefore, do not seek professional assistance (Huefner, Kaldenberg, and Berger, 2008). Occupational therapists have the skills to enhance occupational performance and social participation for those with low vision through a variety of learned strategies, adaptive technologies, and environmental adaptation. Without adequate vision, community mobility and even room-to-room mobility within one's home may become severely limited. Visual rehabilitation and professional consultation can help older adults with low vision to maintain their independence and to continue social roles for as long as possible. Some of the strategies include the following:

- ✗ Increased lighting within the home, closely attending to specific task lighting, reducing glare, well-lit passageways to essential areas such as kitchen and bathroom, and lighting the faces of people with whom they are speaking

- ✗ Training people with specific retinal problems to use their preferred retinal focus to maximize remaining vision for important tasks and communication situations

- ✗ Increasing contrast between furniture and floor, steps and stairways, dishes and food, and background colors inside cabinets and drawers in order to better locate needed items for tasks

- ✗ Substitute other senses such as tactile indicators (tape, puff-paint) for reading dials on the stove, thermostats, telephone number pads, and television remotes

- ✗ Auditory alarm clocks, thermostats, and scales also assist older adults in staying organized and keeping schedules

- ✗ Keeping items in consistent locations avoids losing track of them, such as cell phone, flashlight, or magnifying glass kept in pockets for easy access when performing daily tasks

- ✗ Reducing clutter and eliminating barriers to mobility can reduce risk of falls. For example, furniture should be arranged so that tactile sense can assist when walking across a room, without low obstacles such as coffee tables interfering with easy passage to seating areas

Use of these strategies and others can enable older adults to continue their performance of social roles and should be communicated with other family members or caregivers who can help to maintain them.

Likewise, hearing impairments are often untreated because of lack of knowledge about technical auditory enhancements, such as hearing aids, amplified telephones, and headphones. One study of older adults' adaptation to use of hearing aids showed that group rehabilitation programs, which included participation of supportive spouses or peers, helped older adults to better adapt to using hearing aids and increased their social participation significantly (Taylor, 2003).

Fourth Age Interventions

The Fourth Age begins with dependency for at least one essential activity of daily living and indicates the need for change in life structure to access needed assistance. People with age-related disabilities represent the more traditional health care recipients whose disabilities present challenges to aging in place and continued social participation. For people who are 80 and older, evidence shows that perceived social support can more than double life expectancy, especially for women (Lyyra & Heikkinen, 2006).

Caregiver Issues

For older adults with disability, caregivers may provide a major source of social support, especially when aging in place. Health care provided in one's own home can enable even a frail elderly individual to remain living in the community. When family caregivers live in the home, social interaction centers around care in daily life, and the individual is less likely to depend upon community mobility in order to participate socially with others. Many caregivers of older adults are themselves older: of spousal caregivers of older adults with disabilities, 89% were older than 65 and 53% were older than 75 (Spillman & Black, 2005). Caregiving is an occupation as well as a life role, and its definition varies with culture.

The culture of caregiving for older relatives may stem from earlier experiences with parenting one's children. However, with older adults, there are issues regarding the older adult's emotional acceptance of care from people with whom they have differently defined relationships, such as from a son or daughter-in-law, younger sibling, or grandchild. Acceptance or denial of disability can have varying effects on the quality of caregiving and the emotions involved. When a caregiver underestimates or overestimates the amount of care necessary, this can easily create barriers to the social well-being of the recipient of care. For example, Sally's mother lived alone with mild dementia, and Sally, as the primary caregiver, did not realize the extent of her mother's disability until the electricity was shut off due to nonpayment. Upon closer investigation of her mother's apartment, Sally realized that unopened mail had been stashed under the bed, and trash had not been properly disposed of for several weeks. Neither had her mother done any laundry, but wore the same dirty clothes and underwear for weeks at a time. Sally lived nearby and checked on her mother

Table 15-4

SIGNS OF SENSORY DEPRIVATION IN OLDER ADULTHOOD

- Decline in autonomic postural responses
- Poor visual tracking and left/right discrimination
- Poor body awareness
- Poor hearing, one to two word responses
- Short attention span
- Poor problem-solving ability
- Flat affect, show little emotion
- Unable to carry on ordinary social conversations

often but was so preoccupied with her own growing family and job that she failed to realize the extent of her mother's disability. Some issues for review include caregiver education, use of professional consultants with regard to care, and the potential for various types of abuse.

Elder Abuse

Four types of abuse have been documented for elders: physical (including sexual), psychological, neglect, and exploitation. Physical abuse by those known to the disabled older adult may go unreported because of the dependent relationship. Most states have laws protecting seniors against such abuse when it is noted by health professionals. Psychological abuse, which involves use of disrespectful language and disparaging treatment, probably more commonly occurs because of the family caregiver feeling frustrated or overburdened or simply not understanding the nature of his or her relative's disability. Caregivers may also deny their own need for respite, support, and education, interventions that would reduce the risk of abusive or negative social interactions with the recipient of care.

Neglect of the older adult's care needs may easily be unintentional on the part of the caregiver, such as in the case of Sally mentioned earlier. Daughters, sons, spouses, and siblings may assume a level of physical, perceptual, or cognitive functioning in their aging relative that has, in fact, declined. Neglect exists when a caregiver fails to perform for older adults those self-care and life management tasks that they cannot do for themselves. While a form of neglect, withholding such care may reasonably occur because

the older adults deny or minimize the extent of their disability, a phenomenon especially common in people with dementia. Neglect may also occur when emotions create barriers to communication. Sam needs a prescription refilled but he is embarrassed to admit that he spent all his money on a gift for his grandson. Jeanne is afraid that if she complains about her recent fall, her daughter will insist that she give up her apartment and move to a retirement home. Self-neglect can also occur for similar reasons, when the value of autonomy surpasses the admission of the need to ask for help.

Older adults who live alone are most in need of social contacts, and this makes them especially vulnerable to certain types of financial exploitation. The media frequently reports the latest scams. Unscrupulous individuals may attempt to win the trust and friendship of older adults in order to sell them something they do not need or get them to donate money to a phony cause. The AARP bulletin recently reported teams of burglars ringing doorbells to offer handyman services to unsuspecting seniors. While one would-be worker lured the older adult outside to inspect peeling paint on the garage, the other team member entered and went through the house, stealing jewelry, cash, and the like. An insurance salesman threw an ice cream party for members of a senior housing project in order to sell them bogus insurance products. Some of the ladies told the occupational therapy fieldwork students they thought he was so generous to offer them all free ice cream and failed to recognize the obligation they took on by signing up.

Sensory Deprivation

For more severely disabled or homebound older adults, caregivers need to provide an appropriate amount of sensory stimulation in order to avoid the onset of sensory deprivation. In such circumstances, caregivers should be educated to recognize the signs of sensory deprivation, which include a loss of the ability to socialize (Table 15-4). Sensory deprivation can mask the symptoms of other illnesses or sensory impairments and can also be reversed with increased social and sensory stimulating activities. In nursing homes, residents who do not have sufficient opportunity to participate socially may also be at risk for sensory deprivation.

Social Expectations of Caregiving

In addition to cultural values for family caregiving, the assumptions of the U.S. health care system leave family members little choice when picking up the slack of early discharge from hospitals and outpatient aftercare (Bookwalter & Siskowski, 2009).

Families either uninsured or unable to pay the high cost of long-term care spend an average of $5,531 annually per family for caregiving-related expenses. In addition, the calculated value of unpaid labor of adult family caregiving is currently $350 billion annually (Gibson & Houser, 2007). More than half of family caregivers are employed (59%), including both men and women. Intense caregiving, a function of level of burden and personal choice, may feel equivalent to having two full-time jobs, extended over an average of 4.3 years (AARP, 2004). While employers are required to offer 12 weeks of unpaid family leave, restricted definitions of family and other legal exceptions allow employers in some states to deny workers this option.

Adult Day Care Social Programs

The move to a skilled nursing facility drastically diminishes a person's opportunities for social participation. Leaving behind the long-established routines of interaction with family, neighbors, and friends, a new nursing home resident's daily contact with caregivers and other unfamiliar residents can seem unnerving. Add to that the disabilities that caused an older adult to need assistance with self-care in the first place, and the experience can easily be overwhelming. While nursing home staff make an effort to ease the transition by allowing familiar objects, family photos, and even furniture to be placed in their bedrooms, residents still need assistance to establish social relationships within their new environment.

Some of the social programs offered for residents at most nursing homes are church services, exercise groups, group games, field trips, and social dining programs. In recent years, residents themselves have organized activities through community meetings and other forms of self-government (Haight, 2005). Other groups within the skilled nursing facility include in-service training for staff, programs and support groups for volunteers, educational groups for families, and memorial services for residents and families when one of them dies (Haight, 2005). While these groups do not directly represent interventions, their subject matter often involves educating those people who have the most opportunity to meet social needs of residents or to facilitate their social participation.

Pet Therapy

Pets have a health-sustaining effect on many health conditions, including heart disease, chronic pain, and stress-induced illness. For nursing home residents, studies have shown that interacting with pets, dogs in particular, reduces loneliness (Banks & Banks, 2002), decreases agitated behaviors, increases

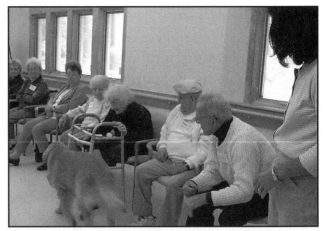

Figure 15-2. Mary plays ball with therapy dog Griffin during a pet therapy session.

mental function (Kawamura, Niyama, & Niyama, 2007), and increases social interactions (Richeson, 2003). The therapeutic use of pets has been linked with sensory modulation—petting a dog or cat reduces stress, heart rate, and anxiety and produces pleasurable tactile sensations. The unconditional acceptance of animals has been associated with psychological well-being and connectedness, thereby supporting attachment theory (Colombo, Buono, Smania, Raviola, & DeLeo, 2009; Kleinman, 2009) (Figure 15-2).

Therapy dogs undergo a certification that ensures an even temper and level of obedience with their handlers. A visit from a therapy dog and owner team may occur as follows:

- Group of older adults gather in a central location, with an introduction to the process by staff members, assuring that the dog is friendly and obedient and will not harm anyone.

- Dog and handler enter the room with dog wearing muzzle and leash or harness. The handler leads the dog around the circle, giving each resident an opportunity to pat the dog on the head, and allowing the dog to sniff his or her hand.

- Handler then removes the muzzle and harness or leash and obedience exercises are demonstrated.

- The dog demonstrates retrieving a ball or toy with handler.

- Each resident has the opportunity to throw the ball and play with the dog. Free play and giving of dog treats may be incorporated. This may take 15 to 20 minutes. Then, the dog leaves.

- Discussion of the experience with the dog is facilitated, giving residents an opportunity to share stories of their own pets and other experiences with animals.

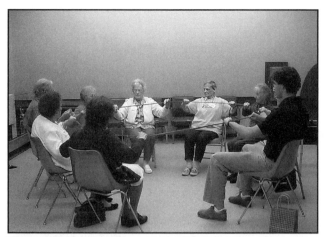

Figure 15-3. Ross Five Stage Group Stage II: Movement.

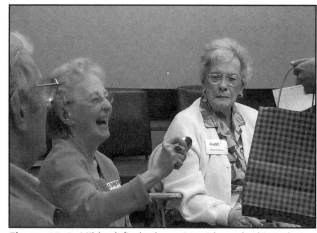

Figure 15-4. Mildred finds the coin without looking during a stereognosis activity.

Ross' Five Stage Groups

Although cognitive deficits make socialization particularly difficult, older people with dementia still need to be able to communicate their thoughts and feelings and to feel connected and supported by other people. Mildred Ross (1997, 2004) developed the five stage groups to assist residents with social participation through a controlled, theory-based sequence of sensory input. Occupational therapists use knowledge of sensory integration in planning and adapting activities for small groups of individuals with moderate to severe disabilities. The titles of the five stages represent the goal of each stage, and therapists vary the activities according to the interests and preferences of members.

1. Stage I: *Orientation.* The goal is to recognize each member by name, capture their attention, and direct their focus to the group as a whole. Passing an object with unusual sensory qualities, such as a strong smell (lotion, herbs), sound (squeak, rattle, gong), or texture (soft, rough, heavy), will accomplish this. The act of passing an object to another person alerts members to each other, and watching each member's reaction to the object begins the process of social awareness. This stage takes about 1 minute and should not involve lengthy discussions or unrelated emotional expressions—these come later in Stages III and IV.

2. Stage II: *Movement.* A physical activity that requires movement, muscle tone, and changes in body and head position continues to increase member alertness and cognitive and physical readiness for participation with others. The sensory input should match but not exceed member ability. The leader may introduce objects such as a ball, a parachute, or an elastic theraband

(Figure 15-3) to facilitate group interaction during the movement phase. Reactions of members often show corrected postural alignment, changes in facial expression, mood elevation, and renewed energy. Members can imitate the leader or take turns imitating each other's movements. The focus on interaction distinguishes this phase from just fitness or exercise groups, which are parallel groups. Leaders should facilitate social engagement within the context of the movement activity, bringing the interaction to an associate group level.

3. Stage III: *Visual-Motor-Perceptual Activities.* This stage combines motor and perceptual features in an activity that enhances awareness of self and environment. Throwing bean bags at a basket in the center of the circle, for example, requires eye-hand coordination, depth perception, grasp and release, trunk stability, and controlled arm movement. The activity encourages more precise sensory processing and a more organized and planned response. Adding a game quality, such as cheering one another, or dividing into teams and keeping score, further encourages the social nature of the interactions. Other appropriate activity suggestions are identifying tools or objects in a bag; identifying sounds, smells, shapes, or weights; tying knots; braiding or winding yarn/string/rope; sequencing a story from pictures; or putting together a floor puzzle. These also combine movement and perception (Figure 15-4).

4. Stage IV: *Cognition.* Previous stages have prepared members for the thinking that this social activity requires. Group discussions, problem-solving, organizing and planning, and other group efforts requiring verbal and nonverbal

communication among members characterize Stage IV activities. Cognitive activities can take the form of storytelling; verbal expression of emotions in relation to paintings, photographs, music, or poetry; creating artwork or writing poems, letters, or memoirs to be shared with the group. This activity may last up to 30 minutes depending on the activity demand and the attention span of members. The outcome may meet or exceed the cooperative group level of interaction. When possible, leaders should model and encourage members to give each other feedback and emotional support. The goal is to facilitate the highest level of social participation possible among the members.

5. Stage V: *Closure.* The therapist gauges the timing of closure by watching member responses to the previous activity. Signs of fatigue or irritation, wandering attention, or distractibility signal the need to wind down the level of stimulation and cognitive demand and to bring the session to a positive ending point. Only short, familiar activities should be introduced during closure. A brief summary of the happenings in the group and an affirmation of each member's contributions reinforces the experience of positive social connection for members to carry with them throughout the rest of their day (Cole, 2005; Ross, 2004).

Ross' five stage groups can also guide programming for older adults in other settings. Leaders of a local adult day care social program used Ross' principles in creating a daily schedule of activities (pictured in Figure 15-5). Daily activities follow the sequence of morning refreshment and greeting one another, group fitness movement activities, group games involving perception and cognition, and creative craft activities after lunch. A mid-afternoon snack amid casual conversations promoted closure and preparation for departure at the end of the day.

Reminiscence and Life Review

Since the 1960s, reminiscence has developed as a popular psychosocial intervention that is used by many health professionals, family caregivers, and volunteers (Gibson & Burnside, 2005). Although suitable for any age group, older adults are the most frequent participants in reminiscence and life review groups. Reminiscence may be defined as the act or process of recalling the past (Butler, 2002). Butler stresses that, because older adults need to reminisce as part of their preparation for death, health professionals need not only to attend to physical needs but also become good listeners, facilitating the opportunity for the older client to "achieve resolution and celebration,

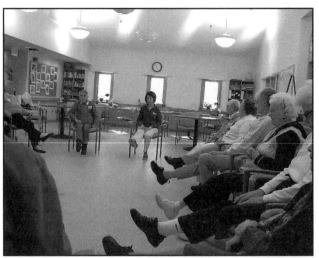

Figure 15-5. Baldwin Adult Day Care Social Program uses Ross' five stages to sequence daily activities.

affirmation and hope, reconciliation and personal growth in the final years" (Butler, 2001, p. 9).

Reminiscence has four interdependent parts, according to Gibson (2004):

1. *Remembering*—Awareness of a memory

2. *Recall*—Sharing the memory with others, verbally or in written or artistic form

3. *Review*—Evaluating the memory, alone or with others

4. *Reconstruction*—Modifying judgment or emotional tone of the memory through reflection, reasoning, and integrating alternate viewpoints

This process can be facilitated individually, but groups have some distinct advantages. Elders tend to reminisce as a natural part of group interaction. For example, consider that almost every family gathering endures the re-telling of stories of the "good old days" by one or more aging relatives. Groups of similar age in community centers or nursing homes also tell each other these stories. The more each life is shared, the greater trust and confidence develops among members. The resulting cohesiveness facilitates greater self-disclosure and greater courage to explore significant but more painful memories (Birren & Deutchman, 2005). Integration of both positive and negative issues requires individuals to rethink, reflect, and consider some alternative viewpoints from supportive others, which are necessary steps toward the resolution of unfinished issues and unsatisfying past relationships. Group leaders encourage the development of group cohesiveness by asking reflective open questions that encourage discussion and expression of understanding and empathy of members toward one another. Modeling of self-disclosure and sharing of nonjudgmental responses may help group members to learn how to provide one another encouragement and needed support.

End-of-Life Occupations

Occupations near the end of life can be experienced more intensely than at other times, often with a "mixture of sadness and satisfaction for being able to use occupations to put closure on a life well lived" (Coppola, 2008, p. 49). Finishing important personal projects, such as written memoirs, family photo albums, needlework, quilts, artwork, or gardens, can symbolize leaving things of this world behind, while continuing connections with important others. Enabling occupations such as these for people in nursing homes or otherwise nearing the end of their Fourth Age can promote feelings of well-being and acceptance for both elders and their families.

Summary

This chapter has reviewed a variety of interventions that promote social participation across the continuum of the Third and Fourth Ages of older adulthood. Some of these represent traditional therapeutic programs, while others move into areas of health promotion, wellness, civic engagement, and advocacy, potentially new areas for health care professionals.

Script: Nursing Home Team Meeting

Seating Chart

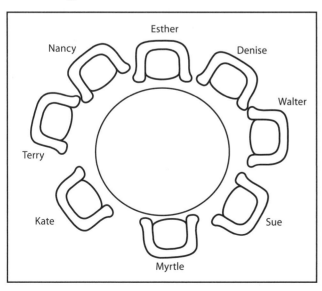

Characters and Background

The client is Margaret, who is in Stage 6 dementia.

Nancy: Head nurse and team leader for the dementia unit at a skilled nursing facility. She organizes the periodic reviews of clients and sets goals collaboratively with other professionals. She is friendly and makes a point of including family members in the review meetings.

Esther: Licensed practical nurse, responsible for hands-on activities of daily living, dressing, bathing, toileting, transporting, etc.

Walter: A social worker whose job it is to facilitate family involvement with the residents (clients) and to understand the cultural background. Also monitors social needs of clients.

Terry: Pastoral care. Because this is a Catholic facility, her role is to serve the spiritual needs of residents, providing access to religious services, private prayer meetings, Bible or daily devotional reading, and communion. She supervises volunteers who will meet with residents as often as needed.

Sue: Certified occupational therapist assistant who provides consultation and occupational therapy services as needed and leads daily groups using Ross' five stage group format.

Myrtle: Recreation therapist who provides daily exercise groups and several socialization groups, such as sing alongs, group games, movie nights, and holiday events.

Denise: Dietitian who provides individualized diets for residents with special needs.

Kate: Daughter of Margaret, the resident being discussed.

Dr. Ash: Not present at the meeting but makes a brief visit to group via the telephone. He gives the last word on medical issues.

Action Begins Here

Nancy: Come in Kate, we're ready to discuss Margaret now. How are you these days?

Kate: Busy as always. *(enters room, sits, and places box of chocolates on the table)*

Nancy: Are those for us?

Kate: Yes. A token of my appreciation for taking good care of my mother. *(chorus of thank you)*

Walter: As you know, we're doing our quarterly review of each resident. *(passes Kate a clipboard)* Would you please sign our attendance sheet?

Kate: *(signs)* I just saw Mom sitting in the day room. She's tapping her feet to the music playing in there, but she has her eyes closed.

Myrtle: Yes, she usually participates in the exercise program each morning, especially when we do it to music. She seems to enjoy it.

Kate: That's nice to hear.

Nancy: *(looking at a chart)* I'm going to read each goal we set last quarter, and we'll discuss her progress as a group. The first goal is *(reads)* "Resident will safely walk around public areas of the unit and refrain from entering private or exit areas."

Esther: She's getting used to the alarm bracelet, but she has attempted to walk out the stairwell exit and has been found in other residents' private rooms. We'll have to continue to watch her more closely.

Kate: Excuse me. Are you referring to the metal band around her left wrist? Just now, she was trying to get it off, and her wrist is kind of red.

Esther: That's because she keeps rubbing the metal against her wrist. She'll get used to it eventually. Most residents do.

Nancy: Actually, the bracelet is on for her safety. It sets off an alarm if she should open an exit door or try to enter the elevators.

Kate: I can see why it bothers her, though. It's awfully tight. And she's left-handed. Maybe it should be on her other wrist.

Nancy: We could have the doctor look at her wrist. *(makes note)* Okay? The next goal is *(reads)* "Resident will feed herself 50% of each meal and maintain current weight."

Denise: She's doing pretty well with meals. Actually, she's gained weight. She's up to 110.

Kate: Excuse me. *(waves hand, but no one notices)*

Nancy: *(continues reading)* The note here says she has Ensure shakes each afternoon. Does that apply to the next goal, fluid intake?

Denise: Yes, she isn't inclined to drink during her meals. And she seems to enjoy the shakes, so that's the best way to get fluids into her.

Kate: Excuse me. Could we go back? I'm still concerned about the weight gain. My mother is a small woman, only 4'11". She's never weighed over 100 pounds her entire life. I'm sure none of her clothes fit her properly at that weight.

Esther: I've been meaning to call you about that. *(Esther stands and retrieves a large plastic bag full of clothes)* These are the things that no longer fit Margaret. We're going to need you to bring her some larger ones.

Kate: But she shouldn't weigh this much. Why is she drinking Ensure? Isn't that full of fat calories?

Denise: It's also full of nutrition, and she needs the fluid.

Kate: You said she feeds herself at meals.

Denise: At least 50%, yes.

Kate: What happens after she stops eating?

Esther: When residents don't feed themselves, we have volunteers who feed them.

Kate: So someone is feeding her the rest of her meals, AND she's having Ensure, too?

Nancy: With dementia, sometimes it's a good idea to have a little extra weight. When they move to a lower functioning level, it's harder to get them to eat. We're just planning ahead. *(smiles)* The next goal is, "Resident will participate in exercise groups three times a week and will spend 6 hours a day in the day room in the company of other residents."

Walter: Yes, she has been participating more than three times a week. However, she does tend to lose interest and wander off. We often find her in her room, rocking in her rocking chair and leafing through magazines. She reads aloud, even when no one is there.

Kate: My father was blind in his later years. She's used to reading aloud to him. By the way, I noticed Mom's not wearing her glasses. She had her eyes closed when I came into the day room.

Esther: Her glasses are broken. She took them off and was biting on them, so I put them in her drawer.

Kate: You should have called me. I could get them fixed.

Nancy: We think it's safer if she doesn't wear them. The lenses could fall and someone could step on them. We can't have broken lenses lying around.

Kate: But she can't see. How will she know where she's going when she walks? And I brought her some new magazines. How can she read them without glasses?

Terry: I do remember hearing her read the prayer book I gave her aloud. We can have a volunteer read the Bible to her if you like.

Walter: That's a good idea, Terry. But I think it's been a long time since she actually understood what she's reading. They're just meaningless sounds.

Myrtle: That's probably true. She doesn't answer when I ask her questions during activities. I don't even think she understands spoken words.

Kate: What's going on with her glaucoma? Is she getting her daily eye drops?

Nancy: *(flips through chart)* Actually, we had to stop those. She wouldn't do it herself, and she fights with Esther when she tried to do it.

Esther: She got combative and tried to hit me. I couldn't get her to open her eyes.

Kate: I know how she gets. I used to do it every day for her until 3 months ago when she was admitted. If you put the drops in her hand and let her think she's doing it herself, she'll cooperate.

Nancy: We can't have the nursing staff fighting with her and risk getting hit. We really had no choice.

Kate: But she has glaucoma. The disease will damage her optic nerve if she doesn't get those drops. Doesn't that concern you?

Nancy: With dementia, sometimes you have to let some things go.

Kate: Not this. I want to speak with her doctor.

Nancy: We'll try to get him on the phone for you. *(calls and speaks briefly on the phone)* I left a message with his service. Hopefully, he'll call back in a few minutes. Shall I go on to the next goal? *(nods)* "Resident will participate in sensory groups and will respond with eye contact and a smile when spoken to by others."

Sue: Margaret does respond nonverbally to a friendly voice, but seldom speaks. She will imitate and follow simple instructions in our sensory groups. She likes soft textures and interesting objects. She helped us do a floor puzzle last week.

Kate: Do you notice any difficulties with her vision?

Sue: It's hard to say. Most of our activities use movement and touch in addition to vision. It would be preferable for her to wear glasses if she needs them.

Kate: Could I ask for the occupational therapist to evaluate her visual perception?

Nancy: We could ask the doctor to refer her. Occupational therapy evaluations require his approval. *(the telephone rings, and Nancy answers, she speaks for a few sentences, and then announces)* It's Dr. Ash. Kate, would you like to talk to him?

Kate: Thank you. *(to the telephone)* Hello, Dr. Ash. Thank you for calling back. My mother has glaucoma, as you probably know. She's sitting with her eyes closed, and maybe that's because there's increased pressure due to the glaucoma. What do you think?

(pause)

Kate: No, she's not complaining of pain. But I don't know that she knows how.

(pause)

Kate: I was wondering if you could ask the nursing staff to reinstate my mother's eye drops.

(pause)

Kate: But couldn't I show them how I used to do it? *(pause)* I see. Also, her glasses are broken, and I'm wondering if I get them fixed whether she would be able to wear them to the activity groups.

(pause)

Kate: I see. So I'll just take them home, then. *(pause)* Yes, Nancy told me about the wrist band. I'll put her back on the line. *(hands phone to Nancy, who speaks briefly, then hangs up)*

Nancy: *(to Kate)* We'll put the alarm bracelet on her right wrist. Dr. Ash will check her wrist when he comes in day after tomorrow. He explained about the visual issues, didn't he?

Kate: Yes. I'll take the glasses and the clothes with me. *(stands to leave, taking bag of clothes)*

Walter and Nancy: Thank you for coming in. We'll see you next time.

The End.

Discussion

1. Describe the role of the person you played on the team. How did it feel to play this role?

2. What type of team organization did this meeting represent?

3. Who was the designated leader? What leadership roles did this person play?

4. What was the goal of this team meeting? Did the team achieve this goal?

5. List three conflicts that occurred during the meeting. How did the conflicts get resolved?

6. If you were leading this team, what would you have done differently and why?

7. Choose one character and describe how you would have changed his or her role if you had the opportunity.

8. What facilitators and barriers for social participation can you identify in this script?

9. What ethical issues does this script suggest, and how were they addressed?

10. How well were Margaret's health and well-being issues served?

References

Adams, K. B. (2004). Changing investment in activities and interests in elders' lives: theory and measurement. *International Journal of Aging and Human Development, 58,* 67-108.

American Association of Retired Persons. (2002). *AARP driver safety program* (5th ed.). Washington, DC: Author.

American Association of Retired Persons. (2004). *Caregiving in the US. National Alliance for Caregiving and AARP.* Retrieved February 19, 2009 from www.thefamilycaregiver.org/who_are_family_caregivers/care_giving_statistics.cfm

American Occupational Therapy Association. (2007). *Occupational therapy's role in judicial decisions about older drivers: A guide for occupational therapists.* Bethesda, MD: Author.

American Occupational Therapy Association. (2008). Occupational therapy practice framework: Domain and process (2nd ed.). *American Journal of Occupational Therapy, 62,* 625-683.

Baltes, P., & Smith, J. (2001). *New frontiers in the future of aging: From successful aging of the young old to the dilemmas of the Fourth Age.* Retrieved April 22, 2005 from www.valenciaforum.com/Keynotes/pb.html

Banks, M. R., & Banks, W. A. (2002). The effects of animal-assisted therapy on loneliness in an elderly population in long term care facilities. *The Journals of Gerontology Series A: Biological Sciences and Medical Sciences, 57,* 428-432.

Baum, C., & Christiansen, C. (2005). Person-environment-occupation-performance: An occupation based framework for practice. In C. Christiansen, C. Baum, & J. Haugen (Eds.), *Occupational therapy: Performance, participation, and well-being* (pp. 242-267). Thorofare, NJ: SLACK Incorporated.

Bettman, C. (2009). Wellness interventions in community living for older adults. *Occupational Therapy Practice, 14,* CE-1-7.

Birren, J. E., & Deutchman, D. E. (2005). Guided autobiography groups. In B. Haight & F. Gibson (Eds.), *Burnside's working with older adults* (4th ed., pp. 191-204). Sudbury, MA: Jones & Bartlett Publishers.

Bookwalter, R. & Siskowski, C. (2009). Family caregiver: Doing double duty. *Today in OT, May 16.* Retrieved May 20, 2010 from freeceus.angtherapist.com/?p=87

Burkhardt, J., Berger, A., Creedon, M., & McGavock, A. (1998). *Mobility and independence: Changes and challenges.* Bethesda, MD: Ecosometrics Inc.

Butler, R. N. (2001). The life review. *Journal of Geriatric Psychiatry, 35,* 7-10.

Butler, R. N. (2002). Age, death, and life review. In K. Doka (Ed.), *Living with grief: Loss in later life.* Washington, DC: Hospice Foundation of America.

Centers for Disease Control. (2008). *Statistics older adults.* Retrieved May 16, 2010 from www.cdc.gov/aging

Centers for Disease Control. (2010). *Healthy People 2010/2020.* Retrieved April 16, 2010 from www.healthypeople.gov/about/goals.htm

Center for Transportation Analysis. (2006). *National highway transportation safety admin.* Retrieved April 16, 2010 from www.dot.gov/statistics

Clark, F., Azen, S. P., Zemke, R., Jackson, J., Carlson, M., Hay, J., ... & Mandel, D. (1997). Occupational therapy for independent-living older adults: A randomized controlled trial. *JAMA, 278,* 1321-1326.

Clark, F., Azen, S.P., Carlson, M., Mandel, D., LaBree, L., Hay, J., ... & Lipson, L. (2001). Embedding health-promoting changes into the daily lives of independent-living older adults: Long-term follow-up of occupational therapy intervention. *Journal of Gerontology: Psychological Sciences and Social Sciences, 56(B),* pp. 60-63.

Classen, S., Winter, S., & Lopez, E. (2009). Meta-synthesis of qualitative studies on older driver safety and mobility. *Occupational Therapy Journal of Research, 29,* 24-31.

Cole, M. (2005). *Group dynamics in occupational therapy.* Thorofare, NJ: SLACK Incorporated.

Cole, M. (2008). Volunteering for older adults: Roles for occupational therapy. *Gerontology Special Interest Section Quarterly (AOTA), 30,* 1, 1-3.

Colombo, G., Buono, M., Smania, K, Raviola, R, & DeLeo, D. (2009). Pet therapy and institutionalized elderly: A study on 144 cognitively impaired subjects. *Archives of Gerontology & Geriatrics, 42,* 207-216.

Coppola, S. (2008). A transactional approach to understanding meanings and benefits of occupation in older adulthood. In S. Coppola, S. Elliott, & P. Toto (Eds.), *Strategies to advance gerontology excellence: Promoting best practice in occupational therapy.* Bethesda, MD: American Occupational Therapy Association.

DiClemente, C. C., & Velasquez, M. (2002). Motivational interviewing and the stages of change. In W. R. Miller & S. Rollnick (Eds.), *Motivational interviewing: Preparing people for change* (2nd ed., pp. 201-215). New York, NY: Guilford.

Fried, L., Freedman, M., Endres, T., & Wasik, B. (1997). Building communities that promote successful aging. *Western Journal of Medicine, 167,* 216-219.

Gibson, F. (2004). *The past in the present: Using reminiscence in health and social care.* Baltimore, MD: Health Professions Press.

Gibson, F., & Burnside, I. (2005). Reminiscence group work. In B. Haight & F. Gibson (Eds.), *Burnside's working with older adults* (4th ed., pp. 175-190). Sudbury, MA: Jones & Bartlett Publishers.

Gibson, M. J. & Houser, A. N. (2007). *Valuing the invaluable: A new look at the economic value of family caregiving.* Washington, DC: AARP Public Policy Institute. Retrieved May 20, 2010 from www.assets.aarp.org/rgcenter/il/ib82_caregivingcare-giving.pdf

Haight, B. (2005). Special groups. In B. Haight & F. Gibson (Eds.), *Burnside's working with older adults* (4th ed., pp. 115-130). Sudbury, MA: Jones & Bartlett Publishers.

Hay, J., Luo, R., Azen, S. P., Carlson, M., Mandel, D., LaBree, L., & Clark, F. (2002). Cost-effectiveness of preventive occupational therapy for independent-living older adults. *Journal of the American Geriatric Society, 50,* 1381-1388.

Houser, A. (2005). *Community mobility options: The older person's interest.* (Publication ID-FS44R). Washington, DC: AARP Public Policy Institute.

Huefner, K., Kaldenberg, J., & Berger, S. (2008). Vision-related issues facing older adults: Occupational therapy's role. *Gerontology Special Interest Section Quarterly, 31,* 2, 1-4.

Jackson, J., Carlson, M., Mandel, D., Zemke, R., & Clark, F. (1998). Occupation in lifestyle redesign: The well-elderly study occupational therapy program. *American Journal of Occupational Therapy, 52,* 326-336.

Johnson, J. (1998). Older rural adults and the decision to stop driving: The influence of family and friends. *Journal of Community Health Nursing, 15,* 205-216.

Johnson, J. (2002). Why rural elders drive against advice. *Journal of Community Health Nursing, 19,* 237-244.

Kawamura, N., Niyama, M., & Niyama, H. (2007). Long term evaluation of animal-assisted therapy for institutionalized elderly people: A preliminary result. *Psychogeriatrics, 7,* 8-13.

Kerschner, H., & Aizenberg, R. (1999). *Transportation in an aging society (focus group teport).* Pasadena, CA: The Beverly Hills Foundation. Retrieved April 15, 2009 from http://www.seniordrivers.org/researchers/researchers.cfm?selection=0

Kleinman, C. (2009). *Pet therapy part III: Therapeutic value.* Retrieved April 17, 2009 from www.community.advance-web.com/blogs/ltc_3/archive/2009/02/27/pet-therapy-part-iii-therapeutic-value.aspx

Knight, E. L. (2004). Exemplary rural mental health services delivery. *Behavioral Health care Tomorrow, 13,* 20-24.

Kostyniuk, L., & Shope, J. (1998). *Reduction and cessation of driving among older adults: Focus group.* (Report No. UMTRI-98-26). Ann Arbor, MI: University of Michigan Transportation Research Institute.

Laslett, P. (1989). *A fresh map of life: The emergence of the Third Age.* Cambridge, MA: Harvard University Press.

Laslett, P. (1997). Interpreting the demographic changes. *Philosophical transactions of the Royal Society of London. Series B, Biological Sciences, 352(1363),* 1805-1809.

Lauber, C., Nordt, C., Falcato, L., & Rossler, W. (2002). Determinants of attitude to volunteering in psychiatry: Results of a public opinion survey in Switzerland. *International Journal of Social Psychiatry, 48,* 209-219.

Letts, L. (2003). Enabling citizen participation of older adults through social and political environments. In L. Letts, P. Rigby, & D. Stewart (Eds.), *Using environments to enable occupational performance.* Thorofare, NJ: SLACK Incorporated.

Lum, T. Y., & Lightfoot, E. (2005). The effects of volunteering on the physical and mental health of older people. *Research on Aging, 27,* 31-55.

Lyyra, T. M., & Heikkinen, R. L. (2006). Perceived social support and mortality in older people. *Journals of Gerontology. Series B, Psychological Sciences and Social Sciences, 61,* S147-S152.

Mandel, D., Jackson, J., Zemke, R., Nelson, L., & Clark, F. (1999). *Lifestyle redesign: Implementing the well elderly program.* Bethesda, MD: American Occupational Therapy Association.

Marek, A. C. (2005). Fifty ways to fix your life. *US News & World Report, Dec. 27, 2004 – Jan. 3, 2005,* (p. 84).

Martin, A., Marottoli, R., & O'Neill, D. (2009). Driving assessment for maintaining mobility and safety in drivers with dementia. *Cochrane Database of Systematic Reviews,* January 21, 2009. Retrieved February 18, 2009 from www.cochrane.org/reviews/en/ab006222.html

Merrill, M. (2000). Exploring the value of volunteering. Retrieved April 16, 2010 from www.merrillassociates.com/topic/2003/08/exploring-value-volunteering-part-i/

Miller, P. A., & Cook, A. (2008). Interventions along the care continuum. In S. Coppola, S. Elliott, & P. Toto (Eds.), *Strategies to advance gerontology excellence: Promoting best practice in occupational therapy.* Bethesda, MD: American Occupational Therapy Association.

Mutchler, J. E., Burr, J. A., & Caro, F. G. (2003). From paid worker to volunteer: Leaving the paid workforce and volunteering in later life. *Social Forces, 81,* 1267–93.

National Highway Traffic Safety Administration. (2005). *Older driver traffic safety plan.* Washington, DC: US Department of Transportation. Retrieved April 15, 2009 from www.nhtsa.dot.gov/people/injury/olddrive and www.nhtsa.dot.gov/people/injury/olddrive/OlderDriverPlan/images/OlderDriverSafetyPlan.pdf

Richeson, N. E. (2003). Effects of animal-assisted therapy on agitated behaviors and social interactions of older adults with dementia. *American Journal of Alzheimer's Disease and Other Dementias, 18,* 353-358.

Ross, M. (1997). *Integrative group therapy: Mobilizing coping abilities with the five stage group.* Bethesda, MD: American Occupational Therapy Association.

Ross, M. (2004). A five-stage model for adults with developmental disabilities. In M. Ross & S. Bachner (Eds.), *Adults with developmental disabilities: Current approaches in occupational therapy.* Bethesda, MD: American Occupational Therapy Association.

Ross, M. W., Greenfield, S. A., & Bennett, L. (1999). Predictors of dropout and burnout in AIDS volunteers: A longitudinal study. *AIDS Care, 11,* 723-731.

Sadler, C., & Marty, F. (1998). Socialization of hospice volunteers: Members of the family. *Hospital Journal, 13,* 49-68.

Spillman B. C., & Black, K. J. (2005). Analyses of informal caregiving: Evidence from the informal caregiving supplement to the 1999 national long-term care survey. Results from the technical expert panel and recommendations. Washington, DC: U.S. Department of Health and Human Services (Contract No. HHS-100-03-0011).

Sterns, H., Sterns, R., Aizenberg, R., & Anapole, J. (1997). *Family and friends concerned about an older driver. (focus group report).* Washington, DC: National Highway Traffic Safety Administration.

Taylor, K. (2003). *Effects of group composition in audiologic rehabilitation programs for hearing impaired elderly.* Retrieved April 17, 2009 from www.audiologyonline.com/articles/pf_article_detail.asp?article_id=498

Womack, J. L. (2008). Occupations of older adults. In S. Coppola, S. Elliott, & P. Toto (Eds.), *Strategies to advance gerontology excellence: Promoting best practice in occupational therapy.* Bethesda, MD: American Occupational Therapy Association.

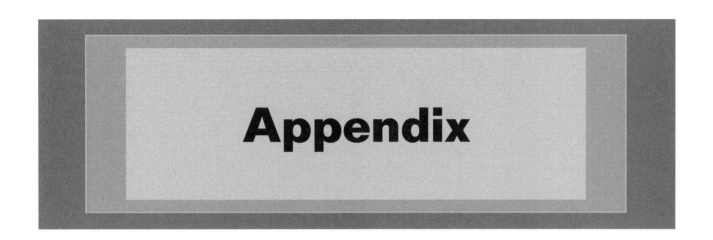

Appendix

Outline of *International Classification of Functioning, Disability and Health* (WHO, 2001)

Section on Activities and Participation

Chapter 7: Interpersonal interactions and relationships

d710   General interpersonal interactions
Basic interpersonal interactions
Complex interpersonal interactions

d730   Particular interpersonal relationships
Relating with strangers
Formal relationships
Informal social relationships
Family relationships
Intimate relationships

Chapter 9: Community, social, and civic life

d910   Community life
Recreation and leisure
Religion and spirituality
Human rights
Political life and citizenship

Reference:
World Health Organization. (2001). *International classification of function, disability, and health* (pp. 150-152, 158-160). Geneva, Switzerland: Author.

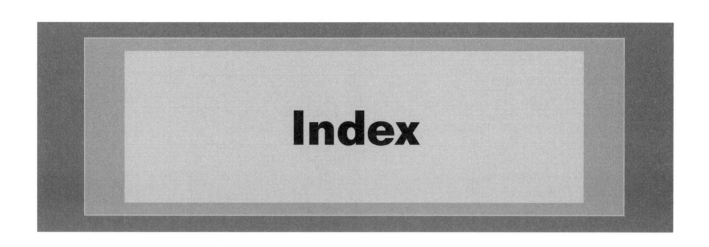

Index

active listening, 49–50
Adolescent Role Assessment, 189
adolescents, 109–125, 229–250
adult cognitive development, 131–132
adult psychosocial development, 127–128
advisory boards, 161
advocacy, 161
    roles, 142–143
after-school social skills, 217
aggression, 179
    in children, 178
aggressive boys, programs for, 211–212
aggressive tendencies, 58
alcohol abuse, 120, 232–233
alternative thinking, 206–207
anger management, 211
assertiveness training, 56–58
    aggressive tendencies, 58
    assertion, 56–57
    direct request, 57–58
    discretion, 58
    "I" statement, 57
assessment of social competence protocol, 191–193
associative group levels, 50–51
Atchley, R.C., 132–133
attachment theory, 100
attachments, 58–59
    supportive cooperative groups, 58–59
attending, as nonverbal behavior, 44–46
authenticity, 179
autism spectrum disorder, 217–219

Baltes, P., 133, 152–153
Bandura, A., 36–38
barriers to social development, 103–104
barriers to social participation, 20
Berkman, L.F., 187–188
bibliography, 238
board meeting script analysis, 22–27
bomb threats, 231
Bordieu, P., 68
Bowlby, J., 100
bullies, 209–211
    interventions for, 211
    victims of, 209–211
bullying, 120
    adolescents, 120
business groups, 92–93

cancer, 174–175
capital, social, 67–80
    Centers for Disease Control and Prevention, 75
    construct of, 38
    development of, 78
    features of, 70–71
    financial support group script, 77
    health, relationship, 74
    health care without borders, 74
    International Monetary Fund, 75
    measurement, Putman's indicators, 72–73
    national elections, 78
    peace, 78
    political capital, 78
    political capital network, 78

Cole, M.B., & Donohue, M.V. *Social Participation in Occupational Contexts: In Schools, Clinics, and Communities* (pp 295-306).
© 2011 SLACK Incorporated

Wait...There's More!

SLACK Incorporated's Health Care Books and Journals offers a wide selection of books in the field of Occupational Therapy. We are dedicated to providing important works that educate, inform and improve the knowledge of our customers. Don't miss out on our other informative titles that will enhance your collection.

Applied Theories in Occupational Therapy: A Practical Approach

Marilyn B. Cole MS, OTR/L, FAOTA; Roseanna Tufano LMFT, OTR/L

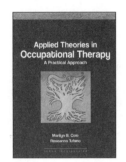

312 pp., Soft Cover, 2008, ISBN 13 978-1-55642-573-8, Order# 35732, **$42.95**

This text provides a comprehensive overview of theories and frames of reference in occupational therapy. Unlike other texts, there are no distinctions between specialty areas, as current and developing theories are applied to a continuum of health and wellness for all populations across the lifespan. Practical guidelines are included to assist with evaluation and intervention strategies.

Marilyn B. Cole and Roseanna Tufano examine the different levels of theory, the definition of each, and the various ways in which these levels guide occupational therapy practice. This timely text is divided into three sections: foundational theories that underlie occupational therapy practice, occupation-based models, and frames of reference. Students and practitioners are provided with specific guidelines as well as case examples and learning exercises to enhance their understanding of applied theory.

Group Dynamics in Occupational Therapy: The Theoretical Basis and Practice Application of Group Intervention, Third Edition

Marilyn B. Cole MS, OTR/L, FAOTA

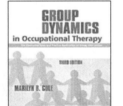

432 pp., Soft Cover, 2005, ISBN 13 978-1-55642-687-2, Order# 36879, **$52.95**

To lead effective groups, occupational therapists must develop the skills of group facilitation, design group experiences using different frames of reference, and adapt group interventions to a broad range of client populations. A core text for over 15 years, this third edition provides an updated perspective on the design and use of groups in emerging practice areas.

Marilyn B. Cole explains how group activities can serve the needs of clients with similar physical disabilities and mental health issues by working on shared goals and providing a context of cultural and social support for engagement in occupation.

Please visit **www.slackbooks.com** to order any of the above titles!

24 Hours a Day...7 Days a Week!

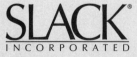